Stochastic Modeling for Medical Image Analysis

Stochastic Modeling
for Medical Image
Analysis

Ayman El-Baz
Georgy Gimel'farb
Jasjit S. Suri

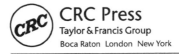

CRC Press
Taylor & Francis Group
Boca Raton London New York

CRC Press is an imprint of the
Taylor & Francis Group, an **informa** business

CRC Press
Taylor & Francis Group
6000 Broken Sound Parkway NW, Suite 300
Boca Raton, FL 33487-2742

First issued in paperback 2021
First issued in hardback 2019

© 2016 by Taylor & Francis Group, LLC
CRC Press is an imprint of Taylor & Francis Group, an Informa business

ISBN 13: 978-1-03-223754-1 (pbk)
ISBN 13: 978-1-4665-9907-9 (hbk)

Library of Congress Cataloging-in-Publication Data

El-Baz, Ayman S., author.
  Stochastic modeling for medical image analysis / Ayman El-Baz, Georgy Gimel'farb, and Jasjit S. Suri.
    p. ; cm.
  Includes bibliographical references and index.
  ISBN 978-1-4665-9907-9 (hardcover : alk. paper)
  I. Gimel'farb, Georgii L'vovich, author. II. Suri, Jasjit S, author. III. Title.
  [DNLM: 1. Image Interpretation, Computer-Assisted--methods. 2. Imaging, Three -Dimensional--methods. 3. Models, Statistical. 4. Stochastic Processes. WB 141]

RC78.7.D53
616.07'54--dc23   2015031035

Visit the Taylor & Francis Web site at
http://www.taylorandfrancis.com

and the CRC Press Web site at
http://www.crcpress.com

Contents

Notations

$\mathbb{A}$	Set of arcs, or edges in an interaction graph
$\mathbf{A}$	Set of clique families
$a_1, \ldots, a_{12}$	Coefficients of an affine transformation
a	Index of a clique family
$\mathcal{B}$	Deformable boundary
$\mathbf{b}$	Boundary point
$\mathbb{C}$	Set of all maximal cliques
$\mathbb{C}_a$	Clique family (a set of the cliques of type a)
$\mathbf{C}$	Covariance matrix
$C(\ldots, \ldots)$	Cost function
$\mathbf{c}$	Individual clique
D	Distance function
d	Distance
E	Energy
e	Error
$\mathbf{e}$	Eigen-vector
$F, \mathbf{F}$	Empirical probability; cumulative probability
$f(\ldots)$	Factor of a probability function; empirical probability
$\mathbb{G}$	Set or parent population of images
$\mathbf{g}$	Image vector
$g : \mathbb{R} \to \mathbb{Q}$	Image as a mapping of lattice sites to signals
$g(\mathbf{r})$	Image signal on a lattice site $\mathbf{r}$
$\mathbf{H}$	Hessian matrix of second partial derivatives
$H(\ldots)$	Entropy
$\mathbf{h}$	Histogram (nonnormalized empirical marginal)
h	Histogram component
J	Number of training samples
K	Number of regions; MGRF order
$\mathcal{K}(\ldots)$	Kernel
$\mathbb{L}$	Set of region labels
$\mathcal{L}$	Lagrangian
$L(\ldots)$	Likelihood function
$\ell(\ldots)$	Log-likelihood function
l	Region label
$\mathbb{M}$	Set or parent population of region maps
M	Signal mapping function
$m : \mathbb{R} \to \mathbb{L}$	Region or classification map
$\mathbf{m}$	Region map or classification map in vectorial form
$m(\mathbf{r})$	Region label on a lattice site $\mathbf{r}$

$\mathbb{N}$	Neighborhood (a set of neighbors)
$P(\ldots), p(\ldots)$	Probability density of continuous variables or a probability of discrete variables
$\mathbf{P}$	Probability distribution
$\mathbb{Q}$	Set of scalar or vectorial pixel/voxel-wise image signals
Q	Number of discrete signal values
q	Pixel/voxel-wise signal, e.g., intensity of color
$\mathbf{q}$	Signal vector
$\mathbb{R}$	Continuous or discrete set of pixels or voxels
$\mathbf{r}$	Site (pixel or voxel) in $\mathbb{R}$
$\mathbf{S}$	Vector of scalar sufficient statistics
s_x, s_y	Scaling coefficients
T	Size of (number of frames in) a digital video sequence
$\mathbf{T}$	Transformation matrix; image transformation
t	Temporal coordinate of a frame in an image sequence
$\mathbb{U}$	Set of scalar signals u or signal vectors $\mathbf{u}$
U	Random variable
u	Value of a random or deterministic variable; filter output
$V(\ldots)$	Gibbs potential function
$\mathbf{V}$	Vector of scalar values of a Gibbs potential
$\mathbb{V}$	Finite set of potential values
$\mathbf{w}$	Coordinate offsets defining a moving window
w	Weight, or coefficient
x, y, z	Spatial pixel/voxel coordinates
Z	Normalizing factor
α	Contrast factors
α	Parameter of a deformable model; factor
β	Control speed factor
$\beta(\ldots)$	Weights for signal interpolation
$\boldsymbol{\beta}$	Signal offsets
Γ	Interaction graph
γ	Coefficient; potential value
$\gamma(\ldots)$	Potential field
Δ	Increment
$\delta, \boldsymbol{\delta}$	Region indicators
ε	Error; small distance
ε_u	Fractional part of a real number u
ζ	z-coordinate offset; force evolving a parametric deformable boundary
η	y-coordinate offset
$\theta, \theta \equiv (\mu, \sigma^2)$	Shorthand notation for the mean, μ, and variance, σ^2
Θ	Set or vector of parameters
κ	Threshold
λ	Coefficient; region label; eigen-value, scale factor

μ	Mathematical expectation, or mean of a random variable
ν	Coordinate offset
Ξ	Speed function
ξ	x-coordinate offset
π	Prior; the number π
ϱ	Relative size, scale factor
σ	Standard deviation of a random variable
τ	Threshold
Φ	Gaussian cumulative probability function
$\varphi(q \mid \theta)$	Gaussian probability density with parameters θ
Ψ	Core distribution of a generic exponential family
$\psi(q \mid \theta)$	Discrete Gaussian with parameters θ
ω	Rotation angle
$\lvert \mathbf{A} \rvert$	Cardinality (the number of elements) of a finite set, vector, or matrix $\mathbf{A}$
$\nabla f(\mathbf{v})$; $\nabla_{f:\mathbf{v}}$	Gradient vector of a scalar multivariate function $f(\mathbf{v})$
$\mathcal{E}\{\mathbf{u} \mid P(\mathbf{u})\}$	Expectation of a random variable, $\mathbf{u}$, with distribution $P(\mathbf{u})$
$\equiv$	Is equivalent to
$\propto$	Is proportional to
$\lfloor u \rfloor$	Integer part of a real number u ($u \leq \lfloor u \rfloor < u + 1$)
$\lim_{n \to \infty} F(n)$	Limit of a function $F(n)$ if n tends to the infinity
T	Matrix-vector transposition
$\delta(s)$	Kronecker's delta-function: $\delta(0) = 1$ and $\delta(s) = 0$ for $s \neq 0$

Preface

Today's medical computer-assisted diagnostics (CAD) rely in a great part on fast and noninvasive anatomical (static) and functional (dynamic) imaging that visualizes inner organs of the human body and helps to monitor their state and condition. Earlier imaging modalities produced conventional photography, e.g., an x-ray film; however, at present a majority of CAD-related images are digital. Each static digital image is a collection of numerical values, measured for cells, or sites of a finite two-dimensional (2D) or three-dimensional (3D) lattice. The lattice is typically arithmetic, i.e., its sites are equidistant along the spatial coordinate axes. A 2D image is a slice through the body, i.e., it presents an intersection of an organ or a body part of interest with the lattice. Its 2D cells (typically, squares or rectangles) are traditionally called pixels, standing for picture cells, or elements. A 3D lattice embeds a whole organ or a body part, and its usually cubic 3D cells are called voxels, i.e., volume cells. Dynamic digital images, e.g., digital video streams, add a temporal (time) axis to resulting 3D and 4D spatiotemporal lattices.

The pixel/voxel-wise signal, usually called an *intensity* or gray level, measures physical properties of a small body area in the corresponding 2D/3D lattice site (cell). In particular, the signal is a quantized absorbed electromagnetic radiation in x-ray and computed tomography (CT) imaging or an acoustic pressure in ultrasound imaging (USI) or a magnitude of an emitted radio-frequency wave encoding spatial hydrogen distribution in magnetic resonance imaging (MRI), exemplified in Figure 0.1. The signals are mostly scalar, although in some cases they can be vectorial too, i.e., if several scalar signals are acquired per lattice site in a multichannel or multiband image, such as, e.g., a dual-echo MRI.

Solutions of almost every CAD task require the use of one or more modalities to collect images of certain medical objects and analyze these images. Individual objects or areas of interest occupy separate continuous or disjoint collections or configurations of the lattice sites and differ in visual appearances and shapes, which should be quantified in terms of signal patterns and the geometric properties of these configurations. Basic image analysis in CAD, surgical simulation, and other real-world medical applications includes linear or nonlinear filtering to suppress noise or the background of individual images, co-registration (alignment) of multiple interrelated images, segmentation (detection and separation) of goal objects or their meaningful parts from their background, and comparisons of the segmented area with the same object in other images acquired for the same subject at different times and/or places or with like objects for other subjects. These

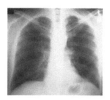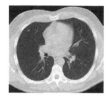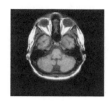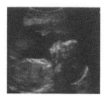

FIGURE 0.1
Popular digital medical images (from left to right): x-ray, CT, MRI, and USI.

operations are instrumental, in particular, for appearance and shape monitoring, object recognition, tracing appearance and shape changes, and shape
analysis on anatomical and functional medical images.

Image-guided CAD faces two basic challenging problems: (1) accurate
and computationally feasible mathematical modeling of images from different modalities to obtain clinically useful information about the goal objects
and (2) accurate and fast inferring of meaningful and clinically valid CAD
decisions and/or predictions on the basis of model-guided image analysis. Trade-offs between the high complexity of the medical objects and tight
clinical requirements to CAD accuracy and speed call for simple yet sufficiently powerful image/object models and basically unsupervised, i.e., fully
automated image processing and analysis.

Stochastic or *probabilistic modeling* considers static or dynamic images of
objects of interest, such as, e.g., lungs, kidneys, or brains in CAD applications, as samples from a certain spatial or spatiotemporal random field that
accounts for varying shapes and the visual appearances of goal objects. An
image set of combinatorial cardinality is modeled with joint and/or conditional probability distributions of signals, making signal configurations,
typical for the goal objects, considerably more probable than all other configurations. Long-standing experience with developing CAD systems has
shown that stochastic modeling–based medical image analysis outperforms
its heuristic *ad hoc* alternatives in most practical applications.

This book details original stochastic appearance and shape models with
computationally feasible and efficient learning techniques that hold much
promise for improving the performance of object detection, segmentation,
alignment, and analysis in a number of practically important CAD applications, such as, e.g., early lung cancer, autism, dyslexia, or cardiological
diagnostics. The models (Figure 0.2) focus on the first-order marginals
(i.e., marginal probability distributions) of pixel/voxel-wise signals and
second- or higher-order Markov-Gibbs random fields (MGRF) of these signals and/or labels of regions supporting the goal objects in the lattice. The
obtained accurate descriptions of visual appearances and shapes of the goal
objects and their background in terms of the signal marginals and spatial conditional dependencies between the signals in the MGRFs help to

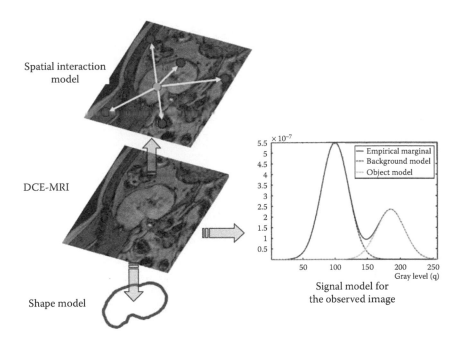

FIGURE 0.2
Modeling object/background appearance and object shape.

solve efficiently a number of important and challenging CAD problems, exemplified in part in this book.

The goals of a brief introduction to medical imaging, stochastic modeling, and model-guided image analysis, provided in this book, are twofold: (1) a textbook for graduate and postgraduate students in biomedical engineering and computer science to study the basics of medical image analysis and (2) a handbook providing engineers and researchers with useful means of and solutions in developing CAD systems. Figure 0.3 outlines an overall structure of the book and basic dependencies between and topics of the chapters (abbreviations indicate the contributing authors).

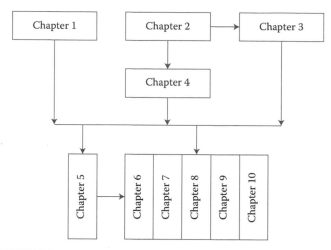

Ch.	Topic	Contributors
1	Medical Imaging Modalities	AEB + JS
2	From Images to Graphical Models	GG + AEB
3	IRF Models: Estimating Marginals	AEB + GG
4	MGRF Models: Estimating Signal Interactions	AEB + GG
5	Applications: Image Alignment	AEB + JS
6	Segmenting Multimodal Images	AEB + GG + JS
7	Segmenting with Deformable Models	AEB + GG + JS
8	Segmenting with Shape and Appearance Priors	AEB + GG + JS
9	Cine Cardiac MRI Analysis	AEB + GG + JS
10	Sizing Cardiac Pathologies	AEB + GG + JS

FIGURE 0.3
Basic dependencies between the book chapters.

Abbreviations

1/2/3/4D	one-/two-/three-/four-dimensional
AAM	Active appearance model
AD	Absolute difference
AIC	Akaike information criterion
a.k.a.	also known as
ARMA	SAR model with moving average
ASM	Active shape model
AUC	Area under the ROC curve
CAD	Computer-aided (-assisted) diagnostics
CE-CT	Contrast-enhanced CT
CE-CMRI	Contrast-enhanced CMRI
CMRI	Cardiac MRI
CN	Chang-Noble model
CRF	Conditional random field
CSA	Controllable SA
CSF	Cerebrospinal fluid
CT	Computed tomography
CTA	CT angiography
CWD	Continuous wave Doppler
DCE-CT	Dynamic contract enhanced CT
DCE-MRI	Dynamic contract enhanced MRI
DG	Discrete Gaussian
DM	Deformable model (active boundary)
DMG	Gradient-guided DM
DOG	Difference of Gaussians
DOOG	Difference of offset Gaussians
DSC	Dice similarity coefficient
DSI	Diffusion spectrum MRI
DTI	Diffusion tensor MRI
DWI	Diffusion-weighted MRI
EDV	End-diastolic volume
EF	Ejection fraction
EM	Expectation–maximization
ESV	End-systolic volume
fMRI	Functional MRI
FN	False negative
FoE	Field of experts
FP	False positive

FPR	FP rate
FRAME	Filters, random fields, and maximum entropy
GAC	Geodesic active contour (DM)
GAR	Geodesic active region
GEM	Generalized EM
GGMRF	Generalized GMRF
GI	Gastrointestinal
GLCH	Gray level co-occurrence histogram
GLDH	Gray level difference histogram
GLS	Geometric level-set-based shape-prior-guided DM
GMRF	Gauss-Markov random field
GPD	Gibbs probability distribution
GVF	Gradient vector flow guided DM
HD	Hausdorff distance
HL	Half-life
HVL	Half-value layer
ICA	Independent component analysis
ICM	Iterated conditional modes
IRF	Independent random field
IT	Iterative thresholding
LCDG	Linear combination of DGs
LCG	Linear combination of Gaussians
LDCT	Low dose CT
LS	Least square
LV	Left ventricle
MAP	Maximum *a posteriori* decision
MCMC	Markov chain Monte Carlo
MGRF	Markov-Gibbs random field
MHD	Modified HD
MI	Mutual information
ML	Maximum likelihood
MLE	ML estimate
MPM	Maximum posterior marginals decision
MPP	Markov point process
MR	Magnetic resonance
MRA	MR angiography
MRF	Markov random field
MRI	MR imaging
MRS	MR spectroscopy; multiple resolution segmentation
NMI	Normalized MI
NN	Nearest neighbor
PCA	Principal component analysis

PC-MRA	Phase-contrast MRA
PD	Proton density
PDE	Partial differential equation
PET	Positron emission tomography
PMD	Pulse-mode Doppler
PWI	Perfusion-weighted MRI
RBC	Red blood cell
RF	Radio frequency
RGB	Red-green-blue
ROC	Receiver operating characteristic
SA	Simulated annealing
SAR	Simultaneous auto-regressive
SIFT	Scale invariant feature transform
SPECT	Single photon emission CT
SPIO	Super-paramagnetic iron oxide
st.d., std	Standard deviation
TN	True negative
TOF-MRA	Time-of-flight MRA
TP	True positive
TPR	TP rate
US	Ultrasound
USI	US imaging
USPIO	Ultra-small SPIO
WN	Wilson-Noble model
w.r.t.	with respect to

1

Medical Imaging Modalities

As one of the basic monitoring tools, today's medical imaging effectively assists clinicians and radiologists in diagnosing diseases, taking therapeutic or surgical decisions, and guiding surgery operations. Recent advances in medical imaging modalities provide images with a menagerie of sizes, structures, resolution, and degrees of contrast. A two-dimensional (2D) image is a rectangular array of pixels containing measured scalar or vectorial visual signals (e.g., intensities or colors) that quantify properties of related spatial locations in a whole body or its part. The 2D image of a thin planar cross section of a 3D object is usually called a *slice*. A collection of the successive slices forms a 3D image, being an array of voxels.

Each imaging modality has advantages and limitations in providing structural and/or functional physiological information about every organ of interest. Figure 1.1 exemplifies most important and popular modalities, namely, magnetic resonance imaging (MRI); CT; ultrasound imaging (US, or USI); positron emission tomography (PET); and single photon emission computed tomography (SPECT). The MRI and CT provide both the functional and structural information, whereas the USI, PET, and SPECT give the functional information. The structural MRI falls into three basic categories: the $T1$-, $T2$-, and PD (proton density)-weighted MRI. The functional MRI is classed into the fMRI; dynamic contrast enhanced MRI (DCE-MRI); tagged MRI; perfusion-weighted MRI (PWI), and diffusion MRI. The latter includes the diffusion-weighted imaging (DWI), diffusion tensor imaging (DTI), and diffusion spectrum imaging (DSI). The functional CT is separated into the contrast-enhanced CT (CE-CT) and the CT angiography (CTA).

Pros and cons, selected applications, and anatomical and/or functional information of the basic preoperative modalities, such as the MRI, CT, USI, and nuclear medical imaging (NMI), are briefly discussed below. However, their instrumental design, as well as the intraoperative imaging modalities are out of our scope.

1.1 Magnetic Resonance Imaging

The MRI has become the most powerful and central noninvasive tool for clinical diagnostics. The human body to be imaged is entirely or partially

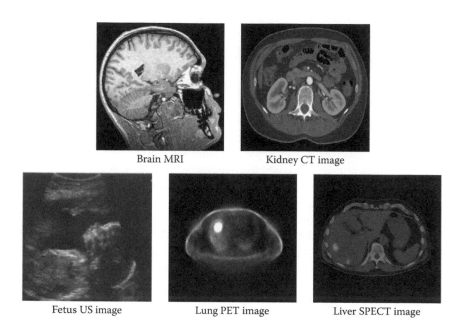

Brain MRI   Kidney CT image

Fetus US image   Lung PET image   Liver SPECT image

FIGURE 1.1
Most popular types of medical images.

placed into a strong external static magnetic field to aligns parallel all hydrogen (single-proton) nuclear magnetic spins in water molecules containing in different tissues, such as muscles, fat, and cerebral spinal fluid. Applied to the field radio frequency pulses form tissue-specific electromagnetic signals that encode spatial hydrogen distribution in the tissues and are measured to form an MR image.

The MRI contrast strongly depends on how the image is acquired, because a preselected gradient of the external field and strengths, shapes, and timing of sequences of the pulses highlight different components of the scanned areas. Generally, the MRI produces planar 2D slices, 3D volumes (spatial sequences of the slices), or 4D spatiotemporal images (temporal sequences of the 3D volumes) exemplified in Figures 1.2 and 1.3.

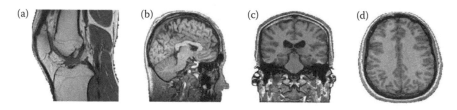

(a)   (b)   (c)   (d)

FIGURE 1.2
Typical 2D MR slices of a knee (a) and a brain in sagittal (b), coronal (c), and axial (d) 3D planes.

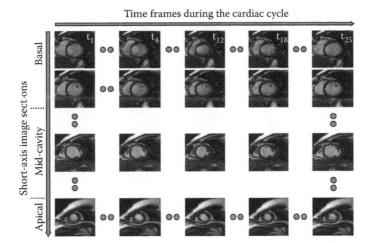

FIGURE 1.3
Typical 4D (3D + time) cardiac MR images acquired at different heart sections (from basal to apical) over the cardiac cycle. Each section is represented with a time series of 25 images.

1.1.1 Structural MRI

Signal strengths measured by the MRI depend primarily on nuclear magnetic relaxation properties in tissues. Time taken by nuclei to return to their baseline states after applying the radio frequency pulse is called the *longitudinal relaxation time* (T1) or the *transverse relaxation time* (T2), according to the component's orientation with respect to the magnetic field. Every tissue in the human body has its own T1 and T2 values, which depend on the proton concentration in the tissue in the form of water and macromolecules.

Main MRI contrast between the tissues is due to their different T1 values, so that the T1-weighted MRI is the most common clinical MRI scan, which is the best for demonstrating anatomical details. The T2-weighted scan amplifying the T2-contrast is used usually to discriminate between the fluid, abnormalities (like tumors, inflammation, or trauma), and surrounding tissues and is the best for revealing pathological details. In practice, the T1- and T2-weighted MR images provide the complementary information, so both are important for characterizing the abnormalities.

The proton (spin) density weighted scans tend to neither T1-, nor T2-contrast and demonstrate only signal changes due to different amounts of available hydrogen nuclei in water. The main advantage of the PD-weighted MRI is the increased contrast between fluid and nonfluid tissues. However, the contrast resolution is usually lesser, than for the T1- and T2-weighted MRI, because differences in the hydrogen concentration (i.e., proton density) of soft tissues are relatively small.

The best soft tissue contrast among all the medical imaging modalities is the main advantage of the MRI. Moreover, this imaging technology is

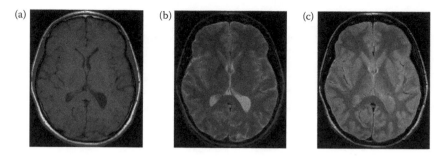

FIGURE 1.4

T1- (a), T2- (b), and PD-weighted (c) MRI brain scans. Note how their very different contrast reveals specific information about various brain structures.

dynamic and can be optimized to capture any anatomical part or disease process under investigation. In particular, imaging planes can be adjusted to anatomical areas studied, like axial, coronal, and sagittal ones in Figure 1.2, and multiple oblique planes can be captured with equal ease and signal intensities for tissues can be controlled by selecting the T1-, T2-, or PD-weighted scan, illustrated in Figure 1.4. Moreover, for each scan type, a special pulse sequence can be designed and other imaging parameters can be optimized in order to produce the desired image contrast.

1.1.2 Dynamic Contrast-Enhanced MRI

While the structural MRI provides excellent soft tissue contrast, but lacks functional information, the DCE-MRI is able to obtain superior information about the anatomy, function, and metabolism of target tissues. Unlike the structural MRI where the contrast depends mainly on the intrinsic magnetic relaxation times, T1 and T2, the DCE-MRI requires oral, rectal, intravesical, or intravenous administration of special contrast agents prior to the medical scan. An image series is acquired with high temporal resolution before, during, and several times after administering the contrast agent, so that the signal intensity in each pixel or voxel of the target tissue is changing from image to image in proportion to the contrast agent concentration.

The DCE-MRI is commonly used to enhance the contrast between different tissues, in particular, the normal and pathological ones. Typical DCE-MRI time series for the kidney, heart, and prostate are exemplified in Figure 1.5. The DCE-MRI has gained considerable attention due to the lack of ionizing radiation, increased spatial resolution, ability to inform about the hemodynamic (perfusion) properties of tissues, microvascular permeability, and extracellular leakage space.

The contrast agents make visible those anatomical structures, e.g., blood vessels, which cannot be easily visualized by altering magnetic properties of the water molecules in their vicinity. This in turn improves the visualization

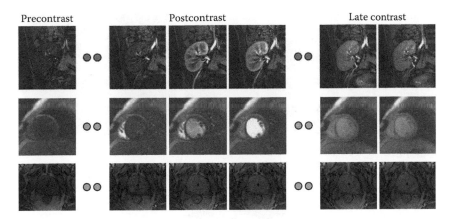

FIGURE 1.5
Dynamic MR images of kidney (top row), heart (middle row), and prostate (bottom row) at different times after administering the contrast agent. Note how the contrast is changing while the agent is perfusing into the tissue beds.

of tissues, organs, and physiological processes. Depending on the imaging modality, various contrast agents are in clinical use, in particular, paramagnetic, superparamagnetic, extracellular fluid space (ECF), and tissue-, or organ-specific agents for the DCE-MRI.

The most successful and widely investigated paramagnetic gadolinium-based agents include pure gadolinium (a rare nontoxic metal); gadopenthetic, gadoteric, gadobenic, or gadoxetic acids; gadodiamide; gadoteridol; gadoversetamide, and gadobutrol. Gadolinium decreases the T1-relaxation times in the vicinity of water protons in living tissues and thus enhances the detected signals to perform the high-contrast MRI of soft tissues. Such contrast agents are widely used for cardiovascular, oncological, and neurological MRI, because of no radioactive materials, or high frequency or x-ray radiation.

1.1.3 Diffusion MRI

The gadolinium-based and similar contrast agents still may be harmful to some patients, having, e.g., kidney problems. The functional diffusion MRI avoids any intravenous contrast agent or specialized hardware due to measuring random Brownian micro-movements of extracellular water molecules that indirectly characterize anatomical structures surrounding the molecules inside the body. Main types of the diffusion MRI are DWI, DTI, and DSI.

DWI relates image contrast to differences in the water molecule mobility by adding magnetic field gradients during data acquisition. An integral b-factor (in s/mm^2) expressing the degree of diffusion weighting of the sequence depends on the gradient values and time intervals of their application. A typical DWI is shown in Figure 1.6.

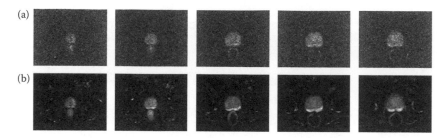

FIGURE 1.6
Typical prostate DWI with the b-value of 0 (a) and 800 (b) s/mm^2.

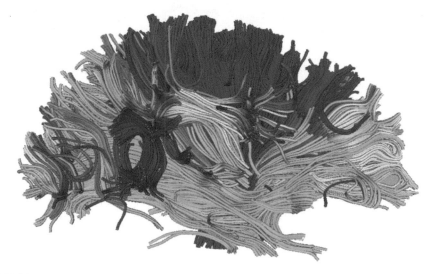

FIGURE 1.7
Color streamlines show likely nerve fiber bundles extracted from a DTI set.

DTI also measures the Brownian motion of water molecules to study the tissue microstructure *in vivo*, e.g., to study connectivity between different brain areas because the DTI can demonstrate the network of nerve fibers. A bundle of the connected brain nerves, obtained from a 3D DTI data set, is exemplified in Figure 1.7.

DSI generalizes the DTI and overcomes limitations of the latter in visualizing complex structures, such as, e.g., fibers that cross within a single voxel and thus cannot be directly captured with the DTI. The goal fibers follow directions of the maximal diffusion.

1.1.4 Functional MRI

The fMRI allows for observing specific brain functions and structures, which participate in these functions, by revealing brain areas, activated after certain

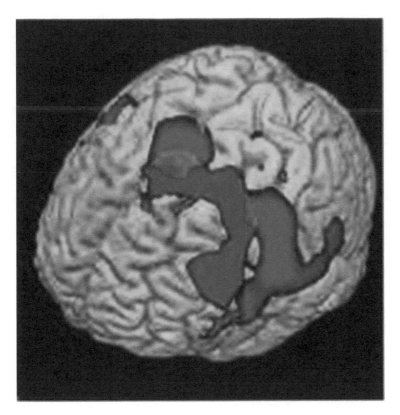

FIGURE 1.8
Brain fMRI with indicated activated areas of a normal reading person.

stimuli, and mapping changes of brain hemodynamics that correspond to mental operations. The fMRI acquires pairs of the brain images in a rest state and after some stimulation to define brain activation areas as any regions that differ in these two successive scans. Contrary to the electroencephalography (EEG), measuring integral surface information (brain waves) through electrodes mounted on the patients' scalp, the fMRI details the inner brain activities and allows for better understanding of how the brain is organized and assessing its neurological status and risk.

Figure 1.8 shows that the fMRI is capable to determine changes in a brain response after applying a certain stimulus (here, a text for reading).

1.1.5 Magnetic Resonance Angiography

Unlike the traditional angiography, placing a catheter into the body, the MRA examines the vascular anatomy noninvasively and thus is a valuable tool in preoperative evaluation of suspected intracranial vascular diseases. The phase contrast MRA (PC-MRA) suppresses background signals and

(a)   (b)

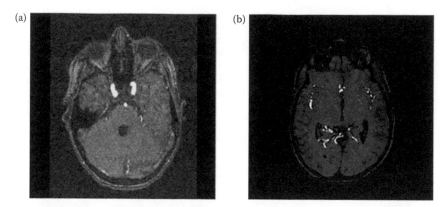

FIGURE 1.9
TOF-MRA (a) and PC-MRA (b) brain slices.

quantifies blood flow velocity vectors for each voxel. The time-of-flight MRA (TOF-MRA) is less informative, but it is faster and produces the higher-contrast images. Figure 1.9 presents typical 2D TOF- and PC-MRA slices of the brain.

1.1.6 Tagged MRI, MRS, and PWI

The *tagged MRI* visualizes cardiac motions in detail and helps in localizing heart diseases, such as coronary atherosclerosis, and evaluating global conditions, like heart failure and diabetes, that result in the heart wall dysfunction. A prespecified pattern of temporary markers, called tags, is placed inside soft-body tissues in order to measure motion in the tagged tissue by analyzing a sequence of images. This technique complements traditional anatomical images, and the tag lines allow for capturing detailed temporal information about the heart, including displacement, velocity, rotation, elongation, strain, and twist. Figure 1.10 shows a typical tagged MRI time series of the heart.

The MR spectroscopy (MRS) provides important information about the intracell chemical activity and also can be used to identify the size and stage of a tumor. As distinct from the conventional MRI, the MRS measures spectra of chemical compounds other than water and therefore it is often combined

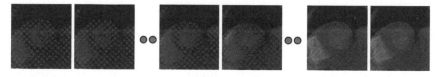

FIGURE 1.10
Tagged MRI: Time frames during the cardiac cycle.

with the MRI to help radiologists in making more well-grounded diagnostic decisions.

The perfusion-weighted imaging (PWI) visualizes the blood flow into brain vasculature and allows neuroradiologists to better understand brain perfusion by providing its important characteristics, such as blood volume and perfusion enhancement time.

1.1.7 MRI: Pros and Cons

The MRI as a whole has many advantages: because the patients are not exposed to any harmful radiation, the imaging can be repeated sequentially many times, and arbitrary 2D cross sectional images of a 3D body, including oblique planes, can be easily obtained. Due to superior resolution and far better contrast than other medical image modalities, the MRI helps in finding useful for diagnostics differences between similar, but not identical tissues.

At the same time, this data acquisition process is relatively long and complex because it is necessary to fix imaging parameters and pulse sequence for each scan. The MR images suffer from noise and artifacts, and the MRI signals depend on the imaging parameters and the pulse sequences used. These dependencies can become nonlinear beyond certain concentrations, leading to errors in the extracted physiology. Also, the MRI is unsuitable for patients with metallic implants due to strong magnetic fields and may be uncomfortable for some claustrophobic ones. Recent improvements of the MRI designs, making more open spaces and shorter exam times, aim to help the claustrophobic patients. However, there is often a trade-off between the open space and image quality.

1.2 Computed Tomography

One of the most popular and useful medical imaging modalities, the CT reconstructs internal object structures from multiple projections obtained by measuring transmission of x-ray radiation through the object. The x-ray source and the set of detectors are mounted on the rotating gantry of the CT device, so that both the source and the detectors remain opposite to one another when revolving around, or scanning the patient's body. While passing through the patient's body, each individual x-ray beam is absorbed (attenuated) by muscles, fat, bones, and other tissues. The detector, being opposite to the x-ray source, measures the beam magnitude integrating all the attenuations due to absorption along the way from the source. The multiple projections, i.e., the integral absorptions by the patient's body for multiple directions of the beams, allow for reconstructing point-wise x-ray attenuation coefficients for each location within the object. The coefficients are measured in integer Hounsfeld units (called CT numbers), which vary from −1000 (air) to +1000 (cortical bone), 0 corresponding to water. The reconstructed CT images are 2D/3D maps of these coefficients.

1.2.1 Structural CT

Historically, the CT images were acquired in an axial or transverse plane, being orthogonal to the long axis of the body. Recent developments in spiral and multislice CT enabled acquiring the volumetric (3D) images in a single patient breath-hold. For exploring anatomical structures, the volumetric data is easily represented by various planar cross sections. Figure 1.11 shows typical axial 2D CT images.

Today's multidetector CT scanners with 64 or more detectors obtain images with much finer details and in a shorter time. Continuous improvements in the scanning times and image resolution have dramatically increased the diagnostic accuracy. The structural CT allows radiologists to understand more in depth organs under examination and gain valuable information for diagnosis and treatment.

1.2.2 Contrast–Enhanced CT

Although the CT readily acquires structural (anatomical) information, its abilities to provide functional (physiological) information are limited. Administering contrast agents before a CT scan helps in acquiring finer image details. The resulting CE-CT has benefits in both disease diagnosis and preoperative guidance and planning, due to better contrast of anatomical structures, increased sensitivity of detecting pathologic lesions, and higher accuracy of lesion characterization. These benefits assist physicians in their clinical management.

Functional CT, called also *dynamic contrast enhanced CT* (DCE-CT), takes a sequence of CT scans at the same location to study changes of the contrast agent distributions in time (Figure 1.12). Like the DCE-MRI, the administration of contrast agents prior to the CT scan increases the image contrast and, therefore, helps to visualize finer details of tissues, organs, and physiological processes. Several types of noniodinated (barium sulfate) and iodinated

(a) 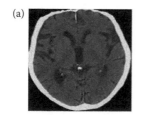 (b) 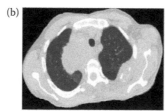 (c)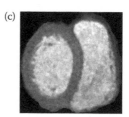

FIGURE 1.11
Axial brain (a), lung (b), and heart (c) CT scans.

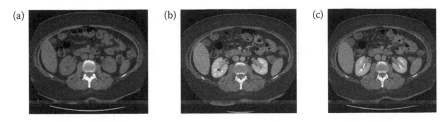

FIGURE 1.12
Abdominal DCE-CT scans before (a); 90 s after (b), and 180 s after (c) administering the contrast agent.

contrast agents are routinely used for both the traditional x-ray imaging (where these agents are often called *radiocontrast* ones) and the CT scans.

Generally, signal intensities in the x-ray imaging are proportional to electron densities. Since the early years of the x-ray radiography, a number of substances containing heavy elements with large atomic numbers, i.e., large numbers of electrons, were employed to achieve the better contrast. Depending on application, barium and iodine are the most common radiocontrast agents. The iodinated agents are either ionic (high-osmolar) or nonionic (low-osmolar organic) compounds, the former having more side effects, than the latter.

The medical DCE-CT scanning generally uses an insoluble barium sulfate powder to block the x-rays passage, so that organs filled with it become white on an x-ray image. This universal contrast agent helps in the x-ray diagnosis of problems in the upper gastrointestinal areas, e.g., the esophagus, stomach, and/or small intestine. Clear soluble iodine agents are generally harmless and usually injected as liquids into the body parts to be imaged. Most of the intravenous contrast dyes are iodine based, so that the iodine-containing agents are used for imaging the gallbladder, urinary tract, blood vessels, spleen, liver, bile duct, and other soft tissues.

1.2.3 CT Angiography

The noninvasive CTA visualizes the blood vessels throughout the body, e.g., in the brain, neck, lungs, and abdomen, after an intravenous contrast agent was injected (Figure 1.13).

Comparing with other imaging techniques, the CTA has reduced scan time and lower cost, but its main advantage is in detecting aneurysms (enlarged blood vessels) and narrowing or damages of vessels early in time for determining appropriate therapies.

1.2.4 Microtomography

The micro-CT (µCT) is a high-resolution CT for imaging small-scale internal structures. While spatial resolution of a typical medical CT scanner is about

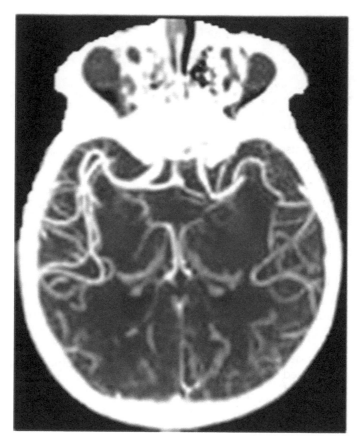

FIGURE 1.13
Brain CTA image.

1 mm, the micro-CT systems can acquire 3D images with voxel spacing of less than 0.1 mm and perform 3D microscopy of internal structures by getting about 2600 2D cross sections in a single scan. These technical advances have made the micro-CT practical for both *in vivo* and *in vitro* studies that need high-resolution images, e.g., for biomedical research.

1.2.5 CT Imaging: Pros and Cons

At present, the CT is faster and more widely available than other imaging modalities. Also, it is less likely to require sedating or anaesthetizing the patient, and it provides good spatial resolution, compared with the MRI, i.e., the CT allows for separating two inner structures at smaller distances from each other.

The main concern of the CT is the use of ionizing x-ray radiation, which may be harmful to patients and may induce cancer. Recent CT technologies use low radiation doses in order to reduce the radiation effects. However, the lower the dose, the lesser the image quality.

1.3 Ultrasound Imaging

The USI has been used in medical diagnostics for many decades, in particular, for studying body regions or structures and measuring the blood velocity. While generally all high-frequency sound waves, exceeding the upper limit of human hearing, are called "ultrasound," the typical USI operates in the range from one to ten MHz, the lower (1–3 MHz) and higher (5–10 MHz) frequencies being used for deep-lying, such as the liver, and closer to the surface organs, respectively. Due to the absence of ionizing radiation and cheapness, comparing to the MRI and CT scans, the USI is the modality of choice in many clinical applications, such as gynecology and obstetrics, requiring safe investigations. Moreover, the images are acquired in real time with rates above 30 frames/s. Recent advanced USI devices have become smaller and more portable, that only increased their popularity and usability. However, the USI produces low-quality images with no fine structural details and is hindered by the air (lungs, bowel loops) or bones. Its penetration depth is limited by the sound wave frequency even if obstructions are absent. The images highly depend on personal skills of operators performing the examination, and are affected by the patient body constitution (e.g., the image quality decreases if the sound wave is absorbed in a subcutaneous fat layer).

The anatomical USI uses 1D "amplitude" (A), motion (M), 2D "brightness" (B), compound, and 3D scanning modes.

The *1D A-mode*, or amplitude-mode scan, is acquired by transmitting short pulses along an US probe and plotting the amplitude of the backscattered echo pulses against the time of arrival, as shown in Figure 1.14. This mode exploits reflected echoes to determine a target depth or relative distances

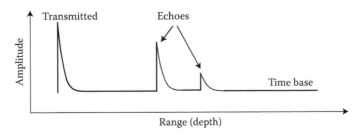

FIGURE 1.14
A-mode USI scan.

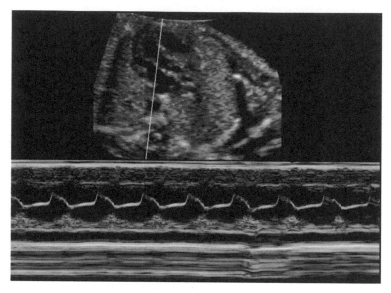

FIGURE 1.15
Typical screen shot of an actual M-mode scan for clinical obstetrical studies.

between different scanned regions, because the amplitude of the A-mode echoes is proportional to the target range for a given speed of sound.

The *M-mode*, or motion-mode scan, is primarily a continuous sequence of the A-mode scans to provide degrees of movement of different scanned tissues within the body. An example of a typical M-mode scan is shown in Figure 1.15.

The *B-mode*, or "brightness" mode, forms 2D images by scanning tissue cross sections. Each image scan-line consists of an A-mode scan, the brightness of each A-mode signal being proportional to the amplitude of the backscattered echo. The B-mode scans are typically used to visualize both stationary and moving anatomical structures.

The *compound USI*, or *sonoCT*, extends the B-mode for enhancing the image quality. A phase transducer acquires multiple coplanar B-mode images at different angles, and the echoes from these different directions are averaged (compounded together) into a single composite image in order to reduce noise, speckles, and clutter. Comparing to the conventional B-mode scans, the compound imaging needs more time for acquiring the data from multiple angles, and thus it has a reduced frame rate.

The *contrast-enhanced USI* helps to further investigate the physiological states and diseases. To enhance the image quality, a contrast agent is administered intravenously before the USI, the typical agents consisting of rigid or flexible tiny spheric microshells with albumin (human protein), or phospholipids, or polymers with microparticles of galactose, or perfluorocarbon, or microbubbles of nitrogen, perflenapent (flurocarbon), or sulfur hexafluoride.

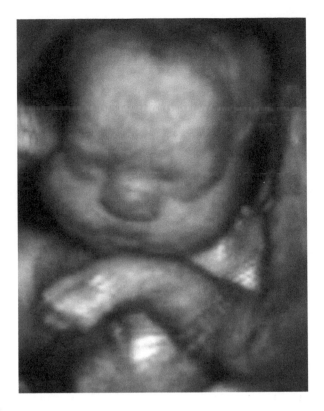

FIGURE 1.16
3D fetus USI.

The chosen bubble microshell and gas strongly influence reflection properties of an agent, which should differ from those of body tissues (e.g., the US reflected by the bubbles back to the transducer produces higher-energy signals).

The *3D USI* stitches together multiple 2D shots from different angles to produce a 3D image, such as, e.g., in Figure 1.16. A region of interest is scanned typically with a single sweep of a volumetric transducer, being able to acquire multiple cross sections.

Measuring the blood velocity with the USI is very important in clinical applications that require understanding flow patterns in the heart or evaluating the risk for various diseases and cardiovascular pathologies. In particular, the lower or higher blood rates can indicate the risk of a cardiac arrest or a stroke, respectively. The color blood velocity images are built by measuring either the continuous wave, pulse-mode, or B-mode duplex Doppler shift, or the time-domain signal correlation.

The *Doppler shift* (Figure 1.17) is the difference between the frequencies of the transmitted US and received backscattered echo wave. The latter frequency varies in line with the blood flow direction, i.e., whether the flow

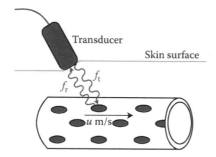

FIGURE 1.17
Measuring the Doppler shift: f_t and f_r—the transmitted and received frequencies; u—the velocity.

is moving from or toward the transducer. The blood velocity is a function of the Doppler shift estimated by either the continuous wave Doppler (CWD), or pulse-mode Doppler (PMD), or color Doppler method.

The *CWD* exploits continuous US waves, generated by a transmitting transducer coupled with a special receiving transducer. Because the transducers cover a relatively large area, which may include more than one blood vessel, the CWD has low sensitivity and depth discriminability and is recording the average blood velocity for all vessels in the whole covered area. On the other hand, the CWD can measure high blood velocities at any depth, e.g., it can record the highest velocities in any valvular structures.

The *PMD* is more selective and thus is typical for local velocity measurements over a small area. The same transducer alternates between transmitting the US pulses and receiving their echoes, and the operator can control the location of the sample volume. The highest measurable by the PMD frequency is limited due to so-called "aliasing." Therefore, the velocities above 1.5–2 m/s of the sample volumes located at the standard ranges in the heart cannot be recorded and high blood flow velocities for certain types of valvular and congenital heart diseases cannot be accurately measured.

The *color Doppler*, or B-mode duplex imaging interlaces the Doppler flow measurement with the B-mode USI in order to combine the blood flow map with the high-resolution image and thus localize the blood flow measurements. To superpose the flow map onto the image, the Doppler shifts are measured in a few thousand sample volumes over an image plane. As shown in Figure 1.18, the color codes, associated with each velocity, are displayed on the locations of these volumes on top of the B-mode image (this is why the method was called "the color Doppler").

The *time-domain signal correlation* measures the blood velocity by accounting for a specific "signature" of each red blood cell in the backscattered signal. Two US pulses are transmitted, and the time shift between the two instances of the same backscattered and recorded "signature" of a certain

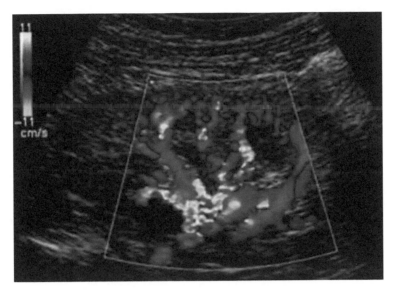

FIGURE 1.18
Color Doppler USI of blood movements toward the transducer (reddish points) and in the reverse direction (bluish points).

cell is estimated by correlation. The blood velocity is easily estimated then from the calculated time shift.

The time-domain correlation method does not limit the maximum blood flow speed to be recorded and performs significantly better than the Doppler-shift-based ones if the signal-to-noise ratio is relatively low, e.g., less than 10. Like the color Doppler method, the time-domain correlation can be extended to 2D signals and integrated with the B-mode USI (the integrated method is usually called the *color velocity imaging*).

1.4 Nuclear Medical Imaging (Nuclide Imaging)

This modality visualizes spatial distribution of a radioactive decaying isotope (radionuclide), which has been administered into the body. Emitted gamma rays or positrons are acquired by an appropriate radiation detector, e.g., a gamma camera (Figure 1.19). The resulting functional images are of low-resolution, noisy, and without anatomic or structural details, but demonstrate metabolic or biochemical activities in the body, specific disease processes, or damaged areas. However, this imaging, like the CT, may be harmful to patients due to ionizing radiation.

The emitted isotope radiation is quantified by measuring its half-life (the time required for radioactivity to drop to half of its starting value), half-value

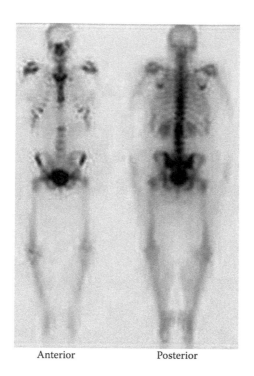

Anterior   Posterior

FIGURE 1.19
Nuclear medical imaging.

layer, and energy. For imaging, the half-life time should be short enough to reduce the patient radiation dose, but still sufficiently large to produce the image with radiation, which was not totally absorbed within the body. The half-value layer is the tissue thickness that absorbs half of the radioactivity produced. The layer of several centimeters indicates that most of the radiation is absorbed within the body, so that the required patient's radiation dose has to be too high. The radiation energy is usually measured in KeV, the typical gamma-radiation energies in the nuclear medical imaging being between 100 and 200 KeV. Gamma rays of the lower energies cannot leave the body to produce images, while the higher energies cause image distortions due to scattered and unwanted radiation penetrating the gamma camera. Table 1.1 shows the half-lives and energies of radionuclides, being commonly used in the nuclear medical imaging. In particular, Thallium-20 emitting x-rays with energies between 69 and 82 KeV and photons of 135 and 167 KeV is widely used for nuclear cardiac stress tests due to good imaging characteristics and reasonably small patient radiation doses. Iodine-123 and indium-111 isotopes have similar characteristics.

Typical nuclear medical images are produced by either a gamma-ray (rarely, x-ray) emission: a planar scintigraphy and single-photon emission CT (SPECT)—or a positron emission tomography (PET), which can

TABLE 1.1

Typical Radionuclides for Nuclear Medical Imaging

			Emission Type	
Radionuclide	Symbol	Half-Life	Gamma (KeV)	Positron (KeV)
Krypton 81m	^{81m}Kr	13.1 s	190	–
Rubidium-82	^{82}Rb	1.3 min	511	3.4
Nitrogen-13	^{13}N	10.0 min	511	1190
Fluorine-18	^{18}F	1.8 h	511	250
Technetium 99m	$^{99m}T_c$	6.0 h	140	–
Iodine-123	^{123}I	13.0 h	159	–
Indium-111	^{111}In	2.8 days	171, 245	–
Thallium-201	^{201}Tl	3.0 days	69–82 (x-ray)	–
Gallium-67	^{67}Ga	3.2 days	93, 185, 300, 394	–
Xenon-133	^{133}Xe	5.3 days	81	0.36
Iodine-131	^{131}I	8.0 days	364	0.81

also be combined with the CT or MRI, e.g., the PET/CT, SPECT/CT, and SPECT/MRI. A positron is an electron's antiparticle with opposite charge. Other types of radioactivity, such as, e.g., alpha-, beta-, or gamma rays, are used only for therapeutic applications, where a radionuclide is targeting tumor locations in order to destroy diseased tissues. The gamma- and beta-rays are not used for imaging due to their too high energies and too small half-value layers. For positron emission, a radiopharmaceutical is synthesized in a cyclotron. Typical examples: carbon-11, oxygen-15, fluorine-18, and nitrogen-13—are introduced into the body with biologically active molecules, in which one or more atoms have been replaced by their radioactive counterparts. The most common radiopharmaceutical in the clinical PET scanning is a sugar fluorodeoxyglucose, containing fluorine-18 and carbon-11 palmitate. A positron emitted by a radioisotope travels in the tissue for a short distance (typically, less than 1 mm depending on the isotope). Then it annihilates with an electron in the tissue, forming two gamma rays that produce better image quality, than other radioactive decay mechanisms.

The *planar scintigraphy* visualizes a 2D distribution of a radioactive (radiopharmaceutical) material within the human body. Typically, the material is taken internally, and its emitted radiation is captured by a gamma camera. Clinically, these scintigraphic images are beneficial for obtaining information and making diagnostic conclusions about the size and normal/abnormal behavior of inner organs. Also, certain abnormalities, e.g., lesions or tumors, which are difficult to find with other imaging modalities, can be visually detected in these images as brighter or darker than normal areas of higher or lower concentration of radiation, respectively.

The planar scintigraphy is widely used for detecting bone fractures as areas of the increased radiation; thyroid metastases and functionality (using

Iodine-131 or Technetium-99m) or parathyroid adenomas; and a heart stress (usually, using Thallium-201) due to a coronary steal and ischemic coronary artery disease. It can also diagnose pulmonary embolism with a two-phase ventilation/perfusion scan; obstruction of the bile ducts by a gallstone or a tumor, and gallbladder diseases, e.g., bile leaks of biliary fistulas. In the brain imaging, the planar scintigraphy helps usually to detect tumors, indicated by higher radiation uptakes, since the blood flow is often higher in the tumor than other tissues, or confirm the brain death (dead brain functionally) if the visualized carotid arteries are cut off at the base of the skull.

The *SPECT* imaging exploits the same principles as the planar scintigraphy and a similar imaging procedure, but reconstructs, like the conventional CT, a 3D tomographic image from a set of 2D nuclear medical images taken from different views. A radiopharmaceutical is injected into the patient, e.g., through blood; multiple scintigraphic images are acquired from the different angles, and a 3D distribution of the radiation energy is reconstructed from these 2D images considered the tomographic projections.

The SPECT images are clinically beneficial for measuring blood perfusion in the brain to indicate strokes or the Alzheimer's disease, and myocardial perfusion and blood flow patterns in the heart to detect the coronary artery disease and myocardial infarct. Like the planar scintigraphy, these images can also be used for bone scanning and detecting tumors. Other applications include detecting liver diseases, e.g., cirrhosis; assessing the kidneys functionality, e.g., to reveal renal artery stenosis or renal infarction, and studying the lung perfusion to indicate bronchitis, asthma, or pulmonary edema.

The *PET* produces a 3D image that provides functional information about specific processes in the body. Contrary to the SPECT, the PET's gamma camera detects pairs of gamma rays, following the annihilation of an emitted positron. Detecting the pairs, rather than single gamma rays, as in the planar scintigraphy and SPECT, allows the PET to produce images of better quality and resolution. However, the cost of the PET imaging is higher, and a cyclotron to provide the positron-emitting radionuclides, having typically very short half-life times, must be available just on-site.

The PET has been used in many medical applications. In particular, the PET with the fluorodeoxyglucose radiopharmaceutical (FDG-PET) was widely used in exploring possibilities of cancer metastases to spread to other sites. Other positron-emitting radionuclides are often used in the PET, too. For instance, the regional blood flow in the brain is measured with the radioactive oxygen-15, because its concentration is proportional to the brain perfusion and allows for detecting brain diseases associated with local areas of the increased or decreased uptake. In neurology, the PET is used in brain tumor evaluation and early identification of recurring degenerative disorders such as the Alzheimer's disease in order to plan assessment and surgical treatment of seizure disorders. The cardiac PET helps in measuring the blood flow and metabolism inside the heart; assessing myocardial fatty acid metabolism and infarction, and determining the need for a heart transplant or a bypass surgery.

The combined, or *hybrid PET/CT, SPECT/CT,* and *PET/MRI* add precise anatomic localizations and/or soft tissue images to functional nuclear imaging data. Both types of the images are captured sequentially, in the same session, and fused into a single superposed (co-registered) image. The PET/CT is typically used in lung cancer applications for diagnosing pulmonary nodules, surgical planning, radiation therapy, and cancer staging. The combined PET and CT images improve delineating lung nodule contours and estimating their volumes. The SPECT/CT helps in locating ectopic parathyroid adenomas, which may not be in their usual locations in the thyroid gland.

1.5 Bibliographic and Historical Notes

The MRI is based on fundamental principles of nuclear MRS [201]. An external radio-frequency pulse interacts with and changes directions of aligned unpaired spins [127,156,206], causing periodic energy absorption and emission. While relaxing back to their lower, or equilibrium energy state, the protons release energy in a form of spatially encoded electromagnetic signals, which are measured to build an image. Due to abilities to differentiate between similar, but not identical tissues [201] and other advantages (no exposure to harmful radiation, high resolution, both structural and functional information, etc.), the MRI plays an important role in assessing locations and extent of tumors, directing biopsies, planning proper therapy, and evaluating therapeutic results [207]. At present it is used extensively in many clinical applications, including detection of brain disorders such as autism and dyslexia [43–46,72,73,78,79,82,98–100,102,221,222,258,266,304], and diagnostics of myocardial diseases [96,97,165,166,275,276].

The DCE-MRI [61,208] helps in detection of pathological tissues, e.g., brain tumors [191], analysis of myocardial perfusion [18], detection of prostate cancer [106], and early detection of acute renal rejection [85,163,164,196,215,257, 313]. The super-paramagnetic contrast agents such as ferumoxsil or ferristene, are based on water insoluble iron oxide crystals, usually, magnetite (Fe_3O_4) or maghemite (Fe_2O_3; γ-Fe_2O_3), classified into super-paramagnetic iron oxide particles (SPIO) and ultra-small SPIO (USPIO) [274]. These agents are suitable for imaging the gastrointestinal tract, such as the stomach, liver, spleen, esophagus, etc. A few other types of agents, like perflubron, are used for the DCE-MRI, too.

Clinical applications of the fMRI [40] include epilepsy surgery [41], diagnosis of schizophrenia [42], and cerebral injury [280].

The functional diffusion MRI is detailed in References 128 and 172. At present, the DWI is a well-established MRI technique, which is successfully used for tumor localization and diagnosis [202,261], investigation of brain disorders, such as epilepsy, multiple sclerosis, brain abscesses, brain tumors, and hypertensive encephalopathy [11], and *in vivo* study of tissue microstructure [284]. The DTI [301], which is widely used to investigate neurological disorders, including addiction, epilepsy, traumatic brain injury, and various neurodegenerative diseases, is capable to reveal subtle abnormalities in a variety of diseases, such as stroke, multiple sclerosis, dyslexia, and schizophrenia [11,27,284]. The DSI is mapping axonal trajectories more accurately than other diffusion imaging techniques [301], but comparing with the DTI and DWI it requires many hundreds of images and long acquisition times [128].

The MRA is widely used to characterize vascular pathology, such as stenosis, dissection, fistula, and aneurysms [81]. Two its major categories: the TOF-MRA and PC-MRA,—rely on different physical effects and provide complementary information about the vasculature [148]. The tagged MRI [8,312] uses specific tags, e.g., lines of magnetic spin patterns inside soft body tissues to be examined for measuring the motion in the tagged tissue from the images [8,187,223]. While the more traditional MRI reveals only information about the motion at the boundaries of an object, the tag lines facilitate close examining of the strain and displacement of the tissue interior [8].

The MRS has been investigated for diagnosing patients with cancerous conditions in the brain [144], prostate [56,286], breast [149,150], cervix [197, 198], pancreas [57], and esophagus [74]. Unlike the conventional MRI visualizing the spatial water (hydrogen) density in tissues, the MRS generally detects the distribution of chemical compounds other than water [268]. The PWI has been shown to be superior to conventional MRI because its image contrast provides information about the location and extent of dead cells within a few hours of a stroke [13]. The dynamic susceptibility contrast (DSC) imaging is the most common PWI that has been thoroughly studied to measure the cerebral blood flow of the brain for patients with vascular stenosis [189], stroke [186], and brain tumors [237].

Basics of the CT, including the attenuation corrections, CT numbers, windowing, back projection, and reconstruction are detailed in References 139, 140 and 300. This imaging modality has been extensively used in clinical determination of a trauma's extent [182], tumor localization [87], detection of lung diseases [1,2,77,80,83,86,88–94], heart disease diagnosis [229], diagnosis of kidney diseases [272], study of dental problems [151], etc.

The DCE-CT has gained considerable attention for capturing parameters of physiological functioning and disease in the human body and has many clinical applications in brain and neck tumor diagnosis [28], lung nodule evaluation [285], prostate cancer examination [174], and therapy monitoring [209]. The CTA is widely used in clinical applications, in particular, for diagnosing the coronary artery disease of the heart [281], evaluating patients with acute ischemic stroke [293], diagnosing renal artery stenosis [108], and detecting acute pulmonary embolism [70].

Practical applications of the micro-CT, include investigation of small specimens and animals [142,292], evaluations of mineralized tissues, such as insect exoskeletons [218] and skeletal tissues [225], quantification of pulmonary fibrosis and investigation of airway microstructures of animals lungs [152], assessment of bone and soft tissue disease and therapeutic response of small animals [162], and assessment of induced cardiac stress [10].

The USI and nuclear medical imaging are described in detail in Reference 300. The A-mode [302] of the USI is often used in ophthalmology to measure eye dimensions prior to corneal thinning or lens replacement [300] and localize solid masses in the eye orbit or globe [302]. The M-mode scans are widely used in echocardiography and fetal cardiac imaging, e.g., for detecting heart valves and heart wall motion [300]; valvulopathies (like calcification), and cardiomyopathies (dyskinesis, aneurysm etc.), as well as measuring abdominal muscle thickness [39]. The B-mode applications include characterizing carotid artery plaques [161] and cardiac imaging [300]. Due to its higher resolution, the contrast-enhanced USI is used to examine the blood perfusion in organs, measure the blood flow rate in the heart and other organs, and detect hepatocellular carcinoma in the liver [306].

This 3D USI scanning mode is still under investigation, and further research is required to identify benefits of and indications for 3D USI [300]. Nonetheless, it has already shown promising results in studying the abdomen and pelvis and imaging fetal and uterine malformation [300]. Other specific applications of the 3D USI include the volume estimation of liver or breast masses, gallbladder, or gallstones; identification of the bladder cancer; measurement of the kidney long axis, and estimation of the cardiac valves dimensions [300]. Recently, 4D US scans were built to track movements of the organ-of-interest by acquiring multiple 3D image frames in a short period of time. However, one needs higher frame rates to obtain a real-time 4D USI scan.

2

From Images to Graphical Models

Rigorous clinical requirements to accuracy, limited time between acquiring data and making decisions, and very large data volumes make medical image analysis for computer-assisted diagnostics (CAD) a challenging task. Stochastic modeling that forms the basis for image analysis has to deal with intricate visual appearances and shapes of target static or dynamic objects (human body organs and processes), being difficult to quantify and formally describe. Typically, a menagerie of visual appearances and shapes of objects and processes of interest in 2D, 3D, and 4D medical images are modeled with probability distributions of spatial or spatiotemporal configurations of pixel- or voxel-wise signals (intensities) or probability distributions of particular features, defined as particular functions of these configurations.

To be accurate, a model has to account for considerable geometric and perceptive (contrast/offset) deviations between the images depicting objects of the same type or the same object, acquired at different times and/or places. The shapes and appearances of objects of the same class may vary considerably for different subjects and under changing external and internal body conditions, while objects from different classes may appear similar. Image acquisition at different times and places and with various modalities and protocols adds more shape and appearance variations, including notable geometric and perceptive (contrast/offset) deviations between the images of similar objects or even the same object. *Global deviations* affect the entire image, whereas *local deviations* change appearances and/or shapes of individual objects or their parts only. Frequent similar appearances and shapes of different static or dynamic objects make their detection, recognition, and other the statistical inference problems ill-posed. Large image sizes, i.e., numbers of variables (intensities) to be taken into account, and contradictory requirements of both fast and accurate model-based image analysis in a limited time between acquiring the images and making diagnostic decisions, which might be useful in clinical practice, also present a considerable challenge.

Realistic images, encountered in each diagnostic problem, form an extremely tiny subset of an entire set, or *parent population* of all possible images, which is of combinatorial cardinality. Complexity of models to focus on and describe each such subset reflects an attainable trade-off between feasibility, accuracy, and speed of inferring optimal or suboptimal diagnostic decisions with due account of the most typical shape and appearance deviations. This chapter gives a brief introduction to probabilistic graphical models, which are popular in the computer-aided medical diagnostics and consider each image as a sample of a particular multidimensional random process, e.g., a random field with a certain unconditional or conditional joint probability distribution or density of components. A majority of the widely used models, such as e.g., Markov random fields (MRF) with joint Gibbs probability distributions (GPD), called often Markov-Gibbs random fields (MGRF), belong to exponential families of p.d. with attractive modeling properties, including feasible learning and inference.

2.1 Basics of Image Modeling

Medical images visualize and allow to qualitatively and/or quantitatively analyze various parts (organs) of human body. The prime objective of stochastic modeling is to relate probabilities of individual images to objects-of-interest and their background by describing visual appearance and shapes of the objects in terms of signal configurations (co-occurrences) in and geometric properties of the associated image regions. Many medical objects are modeled as homogeneous spatial or spatiotemporal textures with repetitive local probabilistic characteristics. Such a homogeneity manifests itself in hard or soft constraints on signal configurations in subsets of adjacent and/or distant pixels or voxels.

Filtering in spatial and spectral domains helps to capture and quantify appearances of different objects. In particular, notable intensity changes found by linear filtering or nonlinear edge detectors allow for separating fine and coarse textures; e.g., the nonlinear DOOG (difference of offset Gaussians) edge detector facilitates the discrimination between textures with the same first- and second-order signal statistics (mean values, variances, and covariances).

To be jointly analyzed, multiple images of the same object or similar objects taken at different times, from different sensors, and/or from different viewpoints have to be co-registered, or co-aligned. Virtually all the computer vision applications, including medical image analysis, e.g., detecting and recognizing objects in various still images and video sequences, change detection in MRI and CT images of the same patient collected at different time, and combining images from different medical modalities for a computer-aided medical diagnostics, to mention just a few, require image registration at early and/or intermediate steps.

2.1.1 Digital Images, Videos, and Region Maps

Definition 2.1

An image, $\mathbf{g} = \{g(\mathbf{r}) : \mathbf{r} \in \mathbb{R}; \; g(\mathbf{r}) \in \mathbb{Q}\}$, is a collection of signal values obtained by mapping, $g : \mathbb{R} \to \mathbb{Q}$, a supporting set $\mathbb{R}$ of spatial or

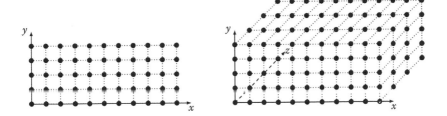

FIGURE 2.1
2D lattice of square pixels and 3D lattice of cubic voxels.

spatiotemporal locations, or sites, **r**, to a set Q of scalar or vectorial site-wise signals.

For a continuous static image, the set $\mathbb{R}$ is a bounded 2D plane or 3D volume with spatial (x, y)- or (x, y, z)-coordinates of the sites respectively: $x_{min} \leq x \leq x_{max}$; $y_{min} \leq y \leq y_{max}$, and $z_{min} \leq z \leq z_{max}$. Spatiotemporal 3D, (x, y, t), and 4D, (x, y, z, t), sites of a continuous dynamic video sequence have also the time coordinate, t; $t_{min} \leq t \leq t_{max}$. Continuous images and videos are typically quantified (digitized) by converting $\mathbb{R}$ into a rectangular arithmetic lattice (grid) with integer coordinates, $x, y, z, t \in \{0, 1, 2, \ldots, \}$. Discrete 2D and 3D spatial or 3D and 4D spatiotemporal sites, **r**, are called *pixels*, i.e., picture elements, and *voxels*, i.e., volume elements, respectively (Figure 2.1).

The signal set, Q, for a continuous image is a bounded scalar (1D) interval $[0, q_{max}]$ or a bounded volume of vectorial values, such as, e.g., $[0, q_{max}]^3$ in the 3D RGB color space. The quantification produces a finite set $Q = \{0, 1, \ldots, Q-1\}$ of scalar gray levels (intensities) for the most widespread digital grayscale CT, MR, and US images exemplified in Chapter 1. Site-wise vectors of discrete intensities characterize digital multimodality and multiband images, e.g., $Q = \{0, 1, \ldots, Q-1\}^3$ for the three-band RGB color images.

Medical image analysis produces and uses also special symbolic images, often called *region*, or *segmentation maps* $m : \mathbb{R} \rightarrow \mathbb{L}$, with a set $\mathbb{L}$ of symbolic labels of objects. Image segmentation partitions the lattice, $\mathbb{R}$, supporting an individual image, $g : \mathbb{R} \rightarrow Q$, or a stack of mutually aligned images into a collection of nonoverlapping and connected regions, i.e., connected subsets of pixels or voxels. Each region has specific visual appearance and possibly shape. If the regions may be disconnected, the segmentation, regions, and region maps are called frequently the *classification*, classes (objects), and classification (object) maps, respectively. The main goal of medical image analysis is mostly classification, rather than conventional segmentation, because image regions occupied by the same tissue or anatomical organ are not necessarily connected.

After ordering (scanning) the sites **r** along a fixed route without repetition, an entire digital image or its part can be considered a vector-column, e.g., $\mathbf{g} = [g(\mathbf{r}) : \mathbf{r} \in \mathbb{R}]^{\mathsf{T}}$ where T denotes the vector–matrix transposition. The sites $\mathbf{r} \in \mathbb{R}$ in this case are ordered by scanning the lattice $\mathbb{R}$ along a fixed and possibly disjoint route, such that each site appears in it only once. In other words, an entire digital image or its part can be considered either as a 2D, 3D, or 4D array, or an 1D vector-column of the site-wise signal values.

Let $|\mathbb{A}|$ denote the cardinality, or the number of elements of a finite set $\mathbb{A}$. Sets $\mathbb{G} = \mathbb{Q}^{|\mathbb{R}|}$ and $\mathbb{M} = \mathbb{L}^{|\mathbb{R}|}$ are called *parent populations* of the images $g : \mathbb{R} \to \mathbb{Q}$ and region maps $m : \mathbb{R} \to \mathbb{L}$, respectively, on a fixed finite lattice $\mathbb{R}$. The populations are typically of the combinatorial cardinality, $|\mathbb{G}| = |\mathbb{Q}|^{|\mathbb{R}|}$ and $|\mathbb{M}| = |\mathbb{L}|^{|\mathbb{R}|}$, respectively, although any practical image analysis problem deals with relatively small data sets, containing from few dozens to hundreds, and only in very rare cases thousands or more individual images. The cardinalities of the parent populations are combinatorial even for very simple images and maps.

2.1.2 Image Homogeneity

Stochastic modeling considers each particular digital image or region map as a sample of a multivariate random variable, or a random field specified with a joint probability distribution over the parent population. To define the model, visual appearances and shapes of objects to be analyzed in the images are most often considered statistically or structurally homogeneous. An acceptable and constructive universal formal definition of image homogeneity or closely related notions of self-similarity or repetitiveness of depicted objects is difficult (if possible) to give, although these properties are more or less obvious for human vision. Spatial, temporal, or spatiotemporal *statistical homogeneity* implies repetitive in space and/or time conditional probabilistic dependences between signals in neighboring lattice sites, i.e., hard or soft constraints on signal configurations, or co-occurrences in these sites.

Definition 2.2

A lattice site $\mathbf{r} \in \mathbb{R}$ is the neighbor of a site, $\mathbf{r}' \in \mathbb{R}$, if conditional probabilities of signals on $\mathbf{r}$ depend on the signals on $\mathbf{r}'$: $P_{\mathbf{r},\mathbf{r}'}(g(\mathbf{r}) \mid g(\mathbf{r}')) \neq P_{\mathbf{r}}(g(\mathbf{r}))$.

The set of all neighbors of $\mathbf{r}$ is called a *neighborhood*, and the union of the neighborhoods for all sites $\mathbf{r} \in \mathbb{R}$ forms a *neighborhood system* on the lattice $\mathbb{R}$. This system is typically described with a *neighborhood graph*, which nodes are the sites $\mathbf{r} \in \mathbb{R}$ and edges connect all pairs of the neighbors. To avoid impractical generalizations, statistical homogeneity is usually limited to exact or nearly exact translation or, less often, translation–rotation invariant local statistical properties, such as, e.g., shapes of pixel/voxel neighborhoods and conditional probabilities that govern signal co-occurrences or functions of these signals on the neighborhoods.

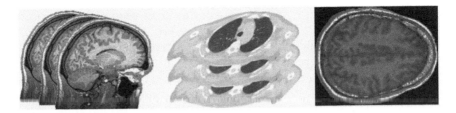

FIGURE 2.2
Textured 2D and 3D MRI.

Structural or *syntactic homogeneity* involves a library of basic texture elements called traditionally *textons* or *texels*, and a system of deterministic or probabilistic rules guiding their locations, poses, scales, and contrast with respect to each other and image background with due account of admissible adjacency and overlaps. Translational repetitiveness, or invariance of local signal patterns (configurations) is the simplest kind of homogeneity, which can be met in many artificial (human-made) textures, such as fabrics, nettings, or other regular mosaics. Such entirely or almost identical signal patterns can be considered as template texels that differ by spatial arrangement. But most of the medical images, such as in Figure 2.2 or Chapter 1, contain more intricate objects, which shapes and appearances only rarely can be modeled with the repetitive texels. Thus, the today's medical image analysis relies most typically on the statistical homogeneity.

Stochastic modeling for practical image enhancement, segmentation, object detection, and other applications seeks an reasonable trade-off between computational feasibility and accuracy of the model-based image analysis. Ultimately, both shapes and appearances of all objects-of-interest should have been characterized with a single model, being invariant to or at least accounting for unessential local and global geometric and perceptual (contrast/offset) image deviations that preserve the lattice continuity and do not affect visual object perception and classification. Because it is difficult to make such a model computationally feasible, less universal separate stochastic models of object appearances and shapes are typically used in the today's medical image analysis. The simplest models describe only marginal probability distributions of pixel/voxel-wise signals related to each object of interest, while more sophisticated models account also for selected characteristic spatial or spatiotemporal dependences between adjacent and/or distant lattice sites.

2.1.3 Probability Models of Images and Region Maps

Probabilistic or *stochastic models* are $|\mathbb{R}|$-variate functions of pixel/voxel-wise signals on a lattice $\mathbb{R}$ that specify unconditional (prior), conditional, or joint probabilities of an image, $\mathbf{g} \in \mathbb{G}$, and/or its region map, $\mathbf{m} \in \mathbb{M}$. *Descriptive models* allow for evaluating and comparing (at least, partially) these probabilities in order to solve individual image analysis or processing problems. In particular, such models facilitate co-alignment of a particular object or objects of the same type in different images, detection of certain objects, image retrieval from a database, image segmentation to outline regions occupied by certain objects and background, de-noising or restoration of a corrupted image, etc. More complete *generative models* add to descriptive abilities sampling of images from a probability distribution, i.e., simulation (generation) of images with realistic object appearances and/or shapes.

An *unconditional* model, $P_u : \mathbb{Q}^{|\mathbb{R}|} \to [0,1]$ or $P_u : \mathbb{L}^{|\mathbb{R}|} \to [0,1]$, called usually a *prior*, specifies a probability distribution or density of each unobserved (*hidden*) image, $P_u(\mathbf{g}) = (P_u(g(\mathbf{r}) : \mathbf{r} \in \mathbb{R})$, or map, $P_u(\mathbf{m}) = (P_u(m(\mathbf{r}) : \mathbf{r} \in \mathbb{R})$, in their parent populations*:

$$\mathbf{P}_u = \left(P_u(\mathbf{g}) : \mathbf{g} \in \mathbb{G}; \sum_{\mathbf{g} \in \mathbb{G}} P_u(\mathbf{g}) = 1 \right) \quad \text{or}$$

$$\left(P_u(\mathbf{m}) : \mathbf{m} \in \mathbb{G}; \sum_{\mathbf{m} \in \mathbb{M}} P_u(\mathbf{m}) = 1 \right) \tag{2.1}$$

A *conditional* model, $P_c : (\mathbb{Q} \times \mathbb{L})^{|\mathbb{R}|} \to [0,1]$, describes the distribution of images $\mathbf{g}$, given a map, $\mathbf{m}^\circ$, or of maps $\mathbf{m}$, given an image, $\mathbf{g}^\circ$, respectively:

$$\mathbf{P}_c = \begin{cases} \left(P_c(\mathbf{g} \mid \mathbf{m}^\circ) : \mathbf{g} \in \mathbb{G}; \sum_{\mathbf{g} \in \mathbb{G}} P_c(\mathbf{g} \mid \mathbf{m}^\circ) = 1 \right); & \mathbf{m}^\circ \in \mathbb{M} \\ \left(P_c(\mathbf{m} \mid \mathbf{g}^\circ) : \mathbf{m} \in \mathbb{M}; \sum_{\mathbf{m} \in \mathbb{M}} P_c(\mathbf{m} \mid \mathbf{g}^\circ) = 1 \right); & \mathbf{g}^\circ \in \mathbb{G} \end{cases} \tag{2.2}$$

The conditional probability of an observed image $\mathbf{g}_{obs}$ as a function of a hidden region map $\mathbf{m}$ defines the *likelihood*, $L(\mathbf{m} \mid \mathbf{g}_{obs}) = P_c(\mathbf{g}_{obs} \mid \mathbf{m})$, and *log-likelihood*, $\ell(\mathbf{m} \mid \mathbf{g}_{obs}) = \log P_c(\mathbf{g}_{obs} \mid \mathbf{m})$, of each map, $\mathbf{m}$, for the observed image, $\mathbf{g}_{obs}$.

A *joint* model $P : (\mathbb{Q} \times \mathbb{L})^{|\mathbb{R}|} \to [0,1]$ specifies probabilities of the image and map pairs:

$$\mathbf{P} = \left(P(\mathbf{g}, \mathbf{m}) : \mathbf{g} \in \mathbb{G}; \mathbf{m} \in \mathbb{M}; \sum_{\mathbf{g} \in \mathbb{G}} \sum_{\mathbf{m} \in \mathbb{M}} P(\mathbf{g}, \mathbf{m}) = 1 \right) \tag{2.3}$$

---

* Here and below random variables, U, of probability density or distribution functions, $P(U)$, are omitted in line with the conventional simplified notation and only their values $\mathbf{u}$ are retained, e.g., $P(\mathbf{u})$ stands for $P(U = \mathbf{u})$.

In accord with the classical *Bayes formula*, called also the Bayes theorem, or rule, the joint model, $P(\mathbf{g}, \mathbf{m}) = P_u(\mathbf{m})P_c(\mathbf{g} \mid \mathbf{m})$, combines the prior and conditional ones into a *posterior* probability model of a hidden map, given an observed image, $\mathbf{g}_{obs}$, e.g.,

$$P_p(\mathbf{m} \mid \mathbf{g}_{obs}) = \frac{P_u(\mathbf{m})P_c(\mathbf{g}_{obs} \mid \mathbf{m})}{\sum_{\mathbf{m}' \in \mathbb{M}} P_u(\mathbf{m}')P_c(\mathbf{g}_{obs} \mid \mathbf{m}')} = \frac{P(\mathbf{g}_{obs}, \mathbf{m})}{\sum_{\mathbf{m}' \in \mathbb{M}} P(\mathbf{g}_{obs}, \mathbf{m}')} = \frac{P(\mathbf{g}_{obs}, \mathbf{m})}{P_u(\mathbf{g}_{obs})} \tag{2.4}$$

The posterior or proportional to them joint probabilities, $P_u(\mathbf{m})P_c(\mathbf{g}_{obs} \mid \mathbf{m}) \sim P_p(\mathbf{m} \mid \mathbf{g}_{obs})$, allow for inferring a hidden map, given an observed image, when the map prior and the conditional image model, given a map, are available. The alternative inference exploits the conditional model of maps, given an image, if this model is already known.

2.1.4 Optimal Statistical Inference

Decisions about the goal maps are based on the conditional or posterior models. For a nonnegative cost function evaluating taken vs. true decisions, the *Bayesian decision rules* ensure the minimum expected cost or risk over a parent population.

Let the posterior model of Equation 2.4 together with the costs, $C(\mathbf{m}', \mathbf{m})$, of taking a decision, $\mathbf{m}' \in \mathbb{L}$, about each true map $\mathbf{m} \in \mathbb{L}$ be known for image segmentation, restoring a region map of an observed image, $\mathbf{g}_{obs} \in \mathbb{G}$. The Bayesian rule:

$$\hat{\mathbf{m}} = \arg \min_{\mathbf{m}' \in \mathbb{M}} \mathcal{E} \left\{ C(\mathbf{m}', \mathbf{m}) \mid P_p(\mathbf{m} \mid \mathbf{g}) \right\} \equiv \arg \min_{\mathbf{m}' \in \mathbb{M}} \sum_{\mathbf{m} \in \mathbb{M}} C(\mathbf{m}', \mathbf{m}) P_p(\mathbf{m} \mid \mathbf{g}) \tag{2.5}$$

which minimizes the risk (expected cost) of each decision $\mathbf{m}'$ about the region map for the image $\mathbf{g}$, has two popular scenarios: (1) the maximum *a posteriori* (MAP) and (2) the maximum posterior marginals (MPM)—with the specific cost functions.

The MAP rule assumes the same unit cost, $C(\mathbf{m}', \mathbf{m}) = 1$, of any false decision, $\mathbf{m}' \neq \mathbf{m}$, about the goal map and zero cost of the true one, $C(\mathbf{m}, \mathbf{m}) = 0$. The expected cost of Equation 2.5 is the error probability, which complements to one the posterior probability of the decision $\mathbf{m}'$, i.e., $C_{err}(\mathbf{m}' \mid \mathbf{g}) = 1 - P_p(\mathbf{m}' \mid \mathbf{g})$. The MAP minimizes the error probability by selecting the region map with the maximum posterior probability:

$$\hat{\mathbf{m}} = \arg \max_{\mathbf{m} \in \mathbb{M}} \left\{ P_p(\mathbf{m} \mid \mathbf{g}) \right\} \tag{2.6}$$

The MPM rule assumes the unit cost of each site-wise error and therefore minimizes the expected number of such errors. The goal region map is built by selecting for each lattice site $\mathbf{r} \in \mathbb{R}$ the label with the maximum posterior marginal probability:

$$\widehat{m}(\mathbf{r}) = \arg\max_{\lambda \in \mathbb{L}} \left\{ P_{\text{p:r}}(\lambda \mid \mathbf{g}) = \sum_{\mathbf{s} \in \mathbb{R} \setminus \mathbf{r}} \sum_{m(\mathbf{s}) \in \mathbb{L}} P_{\text{p}}(m(\mathbf{s}) : \mathbf{s} \in \mathbb{R} \setminus \mathbf{r}; \ m(\mathbf{r}) = \lambda) \right\}$$

(2.7)

If the cost ε of taking no decision, i.e., rejecting the decision, is less than the unit cost of error (i.e., $\varepsilon < 1$), the MAP and MPM decisions with rejection are, respectively:

$$\widehat{\mathbf{m}} = \begin{cases} \arg\max\limits_{\mathbf{m} \in \mathbb{M}} \left\{ P_{\text{p}}(\mathbf{m} \mid \mathbf{g}) \right\} & \text{if } \max\limits_{\mathbf{m} \in \mathbb{M}} \left\{ P_{\text{p}}(\mathbf{m} \mid \mathbf{g}) \right\} \geq 1 - \varepsilon; \\ \text{rejection} & \text{otherwise} \end{cases}$$

(2.8)

and, for each $\mathbf{r} \in \mathbb{R}$,

$$\widehat{m}(\mathbf{r}) = \begin{cases} \arg\max\limits_{\lambda \in \mathbb{L}} \left\{ P_{\text{p:r}}(\lambda \mid \mathbf{g}) \right\} & \text{if } \max\limits_{\lambda \in \mathbb{L}} \left\{ P_{\text{p:r}}(\lambda \mid \mathbf{g}) \right\} \geq 1 - \varepsilon; \\ \text{rejection} & \text{otherwise} \end{cases}$$

(2.9)

The *maximum likelihood* (ML) decision, often taken when the prior is unknown, coincides with the Bayesian MAP for the uniform prior, e.g., $P_{\text{u}}(\mathbf{m}) = \frac{1}{|\mathbb{M}|}$:

$$\widehat{\mathbf{m}} = \arg\max_{\mathbf{m} \in \mathbb{M}} \left\{ P_{\text{c}}(\mathbf{g} \mid \mathbf{m}) \right\}$$

(2.10)

2.1.5 Unessential Image Deviations

Generally, all changes of signal values and locations that do not affect visual perception and classification of objects of interest by their appearance and shapes (in particular, preserve homogeneity and continuity of characteristic regions) are unessential. In image modeling, such deviations are mostly restricted to only a few impacts of imaging the same object at different time and/or place, with different modalities or protocols, and under varying external conditions. Ideally, the image probabilities should be invariant to such deviations.

Unessential perceptive (contrast-offset) deviations, $g' = \alpha^{\mathsf{T}} g + \beta$, transform each scalar site-wise intensity $g(\mathbf{r})$ into another intensity, $g'(\mathbf{r}) = \alpha(\mathbf{r})g(\mathbf{r}) + \beta(\mathbf{r})$ within the same dynamic range of intensities. Individual contrast factors, $\alpha(\mathbf{r})$, and offsets, $\beta(\mathbf{r}); \ \mathbf{r} \in \mathbb{R}$, generally vary randomly over the lattice $\mathbb{R}$. To not affect visual appearances of the objects, in the simplest cases such deviations are either constant over the lattice, $g'(\mathbf{r}) = \alpha g(\mathbf{r}) + \beta$, or at least monotonous, i.e., are spatially variant, but preserve ordinal inter-signal relations to within some distance, d_{max}, between the sites:

$$\alpha(\mathbf{r})g(\mathbf{r}) + \beta(\mathbf{r}) \text{ REL } \alpha(\mathbf{r}')g(\mathbf{r}') + \beta(\mathbf{r}') \quad \text{if } g(\mathbf{r}) \text{ REL } g(\mathbf{r}'); \ |\mathbf{r} - \mathbf{r}'| \leq d_{max}$$

where REL $\in \{<, =, >\}$ stands for a fixed ordinal relation.

The global (lattice-wide) constant or monotonous perceptive deviations can be eliminated by normalizing an image, i.e., stretching its dynamic intensity range to the maximal limits or equalizing its cumulative marginal probability distribution of intensities, respectively. More general monotonous deviations, preserving ordinal relations only in the vicinity of each site, are sometimes taken into account by using deviation-invariant image models.

Unessential geometric deviations move each intensity $g(\mathbf{r})$ to another site, $\mathbf{r}'$, while preserve visually perceived shapes of the objects. Global deviations, including spatially uniform translations, rotations, scaling, or more general affine coordinate transformations, affect the whole image, whereas local deviations are confined to only a particular and rather small region, such as, e.g., object boundary. To model spatially variant visual appearances or shapes of similar medical objects (e.g., lungs or kidneys), multiple images of these objects are spatially co-registered (co-aligned) by translation, rotation, and uniform scaling in order to exclude mutual global geometric deviations.

Translations, rotations, and scaling are particular cases of the affine transformation, which is specified in the 2D/3D cases by 6/12 parameters, respectively:

$$\begin{cases} x' = a_1 x + a_2 y + a_3 \\ y' = a_4 x + a_5 y + a_6 \end{cases} \quad \text{or} \quad \begin{cases} x' = a_1 x + a_2 y + a_3 z + a_4 \\ y' = a_5 x + a_6 y + a_7 z + a_8 \\ z' = a_9 x + a_{10} y + a_{11} z + a_{12} \end{cases}$$

In the 2D case, the separate scaling by coefficients (s_x, s_y) along the coordinate axes, followed by the counter-clockwise rotation by angle ω around the coordinate origin, followed by the relative translation by increments (ξ, η) result in the transformation:

$$\begin{cases} x' = (s_x \cos \omega)x - (s_y \sin \omega)y + \xi \\ y' = (s_x \sin \omega)x + (s_y \cos \omega)y + \eta \end{cases}$$

Generally, parameters a_i of these deviations may (slowly) vary in space and/or time. Projective 3D-to-2D or 3D-to-3D geometric transformations are rare in medical imaging.

Image registration excludes unessential geometric deviations of a *target* image with respect to a fixed *reference* image by geometric mapping (transformation) of the target. To obtain the required accuracy, the mapping usually maximizes similarity between both the images or minimizes the registration error after establishing point-to-point correspondences between the images. The registration techniques differ in the accuracy criteria, optimization techniques, admissible transformations, and resampling methods. The *feature-based registration* relies on detecting and extracting salient local structural image descriptors, which are associated with objects of interest. The *area-based registration* replaces feature extraction with direct point-to-point matching of intensity patterns. Unfortunately, typical similarity scores for matching have many local maxima that hinder any local, e.g., gradient search.

Most of the geometric transformations, except of the pure translation with integer increments, (ξ, η), result in real-valued (noninteger) pixel or voxel coordinates. To perform such a transformation, the target is converted back to a continuous image; transformed geometrically, and then resampled to be supported by the same lattice. The resampling outputs the pixel/voxel-wise signals of the transformed continuous target restored from the signals in the corresponding adjacent pixels or voxels of the initial digital target. Actually, only the positions to be re-sampled are to be known after the continuous transformation.

Forward resampling, which directly applies each mapping step to the initial target pixel or voxel coordinates, might cause signal holes and/or overlaps in the lattice supporting the transformed target. *Backward resampling* escapes these problems due to inverse mapping of the transformed target sites to the initial lattice. After the inverse mapping, the signals in the locations of the continuous transformed 2D/3D target are restored from the adjacent initial target signals using, e.g., the nearest-neighbor (n), bilinear or trilinear (l), or cubic-spline (c) interpolation with the following weighting factors:

$$\beta_l(u) = \begin{cases} 1 - |u| & \text{if } 0 \le |u| < 1 \\ 0 & \text{if } 1 \le |u| \end{cases} \quad \text{and}$$

$$\beta_c(u) = \begin{cases} 1 - 2u^2 + |u|^3 & \text{if } 0 \le |u| < 1 \\ 4 - 8|u| + 5u^2 - |u|^3 & \text{if } 1 \le |u| < 2 \\ 0 & \text{if } 2 \le |u| \end{cases}$$

for the digital image signals in the lattice sites with integer coordinates:

$$g_n(x, y) = g(\lfloor x + 0.5 \rfloor, \lfloor y + 0.5 \rfloor)$$

$$g_l(x, y) = \sum_{\xi=0}^{1} \sum_{\eta=0}^{1} \beta_l(\xi - \varepsilon_x)\beta_l(\eta - \varepsilon_y)g(\lfloor x \rfloor + \xi, \lfloor y \rfloor + \eta)$$

$$g_c(x, y) = \sum_{\xi=-1}^{2} \sum_{\eta=-1}^{2} \beta_c(\xi - \varepsilon_x)\beta_c(\eta - \varepsilon_y)g(\lfloor x \rfloor + \xi, \lfloor y \rfloor + \eta)$$

and

$$g_n(x,y,z) = g(\lfloor x + 0.5 \rfloor, \lfloor y + 0.5 \rfloor, \lfloor z + 0.5 \rfloor)$$

$$g_l(x,y,z) = \sum_{\xi=0}^{1} \sum_{\eta=0}^{1} \sum_{\zeta=0}^{1} \beta_i(\xi - \varepsilon_x)\beta_i(\eta - \varepsilon_y)$$

$$\beta_i(\zeta - \varepsilon_z)g(\lfloor x \rfloor + \xi, \lfloor y \rfloor + \eta, \lfloor z \rfloor + \zeta)$$

$$g_c(x,y,z) = \sum_{\xi=-1}^{2} \sum_{\eta=-1}^{2} \sum_{\zeta=-1}^{2} \beta_c(\xi - \varepsilon_x)\beta_c(\eta - \varepsilon_y)$$

$$\beta_c(\zeta - \varepsilon_z)g(\lfloor x \rfloor + \xi, \lfloor y \rfloor + \eta, \lfloor z \rfloor + \zeta)$$

where x, y, z are the continuous coordinates and $\lfloor u \rfloor$ and $\varepsilon_u = u - \lfloor u \rfloor$ denote the integer and fractional part of a real number u, respectively.

Most of the image registration techniques perform uniform parametric global and limited spatially variant local transformations of the target. The global transformations include rigid (translation and rotation), similarity (translation, rotation, and scaling), affine, and projective mappings of image coordinates, whereas the local coordinate mappings are nonrigid and based on thin-plate spline, radial basis, and above piecewise-linear or cubic coordinate functions. Finding the mapping that minimizes the total coordinate mismatch or maximizes the total similarity between the target and reference is a complex multivariate optimization problem that typically has multiple local optima in the space of the mapping parameters. An exhaustive search to guarantee the global optimum is computationally infeasible, unless the transformation is limited to only relative translations or at most rigid mapping. More complex target-to-reference transformations are mostly found by searching for a local optimum of the alignment score in the parameter space using, e.g., the gradient ascent or descent algorithms. Heuristic genetic algorithms or stochastic simulated annealing are used sometimes to find the globally optimum alignment faster than with the exhaustive search.

2.2 Pixel/Voxel Interactions and Neighborhoods

The simplest way of stochastic modeling is to consider an image a sample from an *independent random field* (IRF). All signals, $g(\mathbf{r})$, on the lattice sites $\mathbf{r} \in \mathbb{R}$ are statistically independent, and the image probability is factored over the sites:

$$P(\mathbf{g}) = \prod_{\mathbf{r} \in \mathbb{R}} P_{\mathbf{r}}(g(\mathbf{r})) \tag{2.11}$$

the factors being marginal signal probabilities for each site. Generally, the marginal distributions, $\mathbf{P_r} = (P_r(q) : q \in Q; \sum_{q \in Q} P_r(q) = 1)$, may differ for different sites.

The model with the same marginal, $\mathbf{P_r} = (P(q) : q \in Q)$, for all the sites has the least descriptive power, but is the easiest for learning—by collecting an empirical marginal probability distribution of signals over a given set G° of training images in the supervised mode or over a given image, $\mathbf{g}$, in the unsupervised mode.

Different for each site $\mathbf{r} \in R$ marginal distributions can be learned only in the supervised mode, provided that the training set G° of co-aligned samples $\mathbf{g}^\circ$ from the goal IRF is sufficiently large to use empirical signal probabilities in each site as accurate statistical estimates of the required marginal probabilities, $P_r(q); q \in Q$.

Mostly, an IRF model assumes that the image lattice is split into K homogeneous regions, $R_k; k = 1, \ldots, K$, which are possibly disjoint and do not intersect:

$$R_k \subseteq R; \bigcup_{k=1}^{K} R_k = R; R_k \bigcap R_\mathbf{J} = \emptyset \quad \text{if } k \neq j; \; k, j \in \{1, \ldots, K\}$$

The marginal signal distributions, $\mathbf{P}_k = (P_k(q) : q \in Q)$, are the same for all sites of each region R_k. Given the region map, the image probability for the IRF model with K homogeneous regions is

$$P(\mathbf{g}) = \prod_{k=1}^{K} \prod_{\mathbf{r} \in R_k} P_k(g(\mathbf{r})) = \prod_{k=1}^{K} \prod_{q \in Q} (P_k(q))^{n_{k:q}} \tag{2.12}$$

where

$$n_{k:q} = |\{\mathbf{r} : \mathbf{r} \in R_k; \; g(\mathbf{r}) = q\}| \equiv \sum_{\mathbf{r} \in R_k} \delta(g(\mathbf{r}) - q)$$

is the number of sites in the region R_k that support the signal q.

The supervised learning of such IRF model needs the region map and one or more corresponding training images with the same regions. The unsupervised learning has to both recover the distinct regions and estimate the marginal distributions, $\mathbf{P}_k$, for each region. Typically, the distribution is represented with a certain parametric function, $\varphi_k(q; \theta_k)$, of signal values, e.g., a single Gaussian in the simplest case, with unknown parameters θ_k, and an image is considered a sample from the homogeneous IRF having the same mixed marginal distribution of signals over the lattice sites:

$$\mathbf{P}_\Theta = \left(P_\Theta(q) = \sum_{k=1}^{J} \pi_k \varphi_k(q \mid \theta_k) : q \in Q \right) \tag{2.13}$$

where π_k is the prior probability of sites from the region $\mathbb{R}_k$; $\sum_{k=1}^{K} \pi_k = 1$. The parameters $\Theta = \{(\pi_k, \theta_k) : k = 1, \ldots, K\}$, including, if necessary, the number of regions K, are estimated from a given image $\mathbf{g}$. This process will be detailed in Chapter 3.

2.2.1 Markov Random Field (MRF)

In most cases the pixel/voxel signals are by no means independent, so that images have to be considered samples of *Markov random fields* that account for mutual dependences, called *interactions*, between the lattice sites and associate a joint probability of the pixel/voxel-wise image signals, $P(\mathbf{g}) \equiv P(g(\mathbf{r}) : \mathbf{r} \in \mathbb{R})$, with geometric structure and quantitative strengths of interactions. In MRF models, probabilities of signal co-occurrences in particular lattice sites conditionally depend on co-occurrences in interacting, or neighboring sites.

Definition 2.3

An undirected interaction graph, $\Gamma = (\mathbb{R}, \mathbb{A})$, describing structure of spatial or spatiotemporal interactions between the lattice sites, $\mathbf{r} \in \mathbb{R}$, has the lattice, $\mathbb{R}$ as the set of nodes. The set of arcs, or edges, $\mathbb{A}$, contains all interacting, i.e., interdependent, or neighboring pairs, $(\mathbf{r}, \mathbf{r}') \in \mathbb{A} \subseteq \mathbb{R} \times \mathbb{R}$, of the nodes.

For the IRFs, the set $\mathbb{A}$ is empty. In line with Definition 2.2, a node $\mathbf{r}$ interacts with, i.e., is the neighbor of the node $\mathbf{r}^\circ$ if the signal value $g(\mathbf{r}^\circ)$ affects the conditional probability, $P(g(\mathbf{r}) \,|\, g(\mathbf{r}^\circ)) : \mathbf{r}^\circ \in \mathbb{R}; \mathbf{r}^\circ \neq \mathbf{r})$, of the signal value $g(\mathbf{r})$, given the signal value $g(\mathbf{r}^\circ)$.

Definition 2.4

The neighborhood, $\mathbb{N}_\mathbf{r}$; $\mathbb{N}_\mathbf{r} \subset \mathbb{R}$, of each node $\mathbf{r}$; $\mathbf{r} \in \mathbb{R}$, consists of all its neighbors: $\mathbb{N}_\mathbf{r} = \{\mathbf{r}^\circ : \mathbf{r}^\circ \in \mathbb{R}; (\mathbf{r}, \mathbf{r}^\circ) \in \mathbb{A}\}$, i.e., all the nodes connected to $\mathbf{r}$ by the arcs from the set $\mathbb{A}$ of the interaction graph, Γ.

The neighborhood relation is symmetric: if $\mathbf{r}^\circ \in \mathbb{N}_\mathbf{r}$, then $\mathbf{r} \in \mathbb{N}_{\mathbf{r}^\circ}$; in other words, if $\mathbf{r}$ is the neighbor of $\mathbf{r}^\circ$, then $\mathbf{r}^\circ$ is the neighbor of $\mathbf{r}$. But two sites from the same neighborhood are not necessarily the neighbors by themselves: the neighborhood relations $(\mathbf{r}, \mathbf{r}^\circ) \in \mathbb{A}$ and $(\mathbf{r}, \mathbf{r}') \in \mathbb{A}$ do not imply the relation $(\mathbf{r}^\circ, \mathbf{r}') \in \mathbb{A}$.

Definition 2.5

An image probability distribution or density, $\mathbf{P} = \{P(\mathbf{g}) : \mathbf{g} \in \mathbb{G}\}$, defines a Markov random field with respect to the neighborhood system, $\mathbb{N} = \{\mathbb{N}_\mathbf{r} : \mathbf{r} \in \mathbb{R}\}$, specified by an interaction graph, Γ, if each marginal conditional probability of the site-wise signal, $g(\mathbf{r})$, depends for all $\mathbf{r} \in \mathbb{R}$ and $\mathbf{g} \in \mathbb{G}$ only on the signals in the neighboring sites:

$$P(g(\mathbf{r})|g(\mathbf{r}^{\circ}) : \mathbf{r}^{\circ} \in \mathbb{R}; \ \mathbf{r}^{\circ} \neq \mathbf{r}) \equiv P(g(\mathbf{r})|g(\mathbf{r}^{\circ}) : \mathbf{r}^{\circ} \in \mathbb{N}_{\mathbf{r}})$$

The Markov property means that the neighborhoods, $\mathbb{N}_{\mathbf{r}}$, of each site $\mathbf{r}$ are proper subsets of, or contain less sites than the remaining lattice. To make the models computationally feasible, the neighborhoods in practice are rather small: $|\mathbb{N}_{\mathbf{r}}| \ll |\mathbb{R}|$.

Definition 2.6

A clique is a complete subgraph of Γ, i.e., a subset of the nodes, such that all their pairs are the neighbors. Its cardinality (the number of nodes) gives its order.

In particular, each individual node and each individual arc of a graph are the first-order and the second-order cliques, respectively.

Definition 2.7

The maximal clique is the largest-order clique that cannot be increased by adding one more node, being the neighbor of all other nodes in that clique.

Each maximal clique embeds multiple lower-order cliques. Generally, each interaction graph, Γ, always contains a set $\mathbb{A}$ of the second-order cliques, which possibly form a number of the higher-order ones, as in a simple example of Figure 2.3.

Importance of cliques in the interaction graph stems from the famous theorem by J. M. Hammersley and P. Clifford defining in general form probability distributions or densities for a very broad class of MRFs.

Theorem 2.1 (Hammersley–Clifford)

A strictly positive probability distribution or density defines a MRF on an interaction graph, Γ, if and only if probabilities or densities of individual samples are factored over cliques of the graph. ■

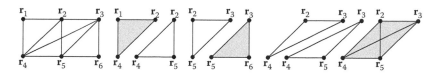

FIGURE 2.3
6-Nodal interaction graph with up to the fourth-order cliques; the maximal ones are shaded.

Let the probabilities or densities, $P(\mathbf{g})$, of all images in a MRF model be positive, $P(\mathbf{g}) > 0; \mathbf{g} \in G$. Given a particular interaction graph, Γ, these probabilities or densities are factored over a subset, C, which is taken from the set of all cliques of the graph Γ and covers the entire lattice $\mathbb{R}$:

$$P(\mathbf{g}) = \frac{1}{Z} \prod_{c \in C} f_c(g(\mathbf{r}) : \mathbf{r} \in c) \text{ where } Z = \sum_{\mathbf{g} \in G} \prod_{c \in C} f_c(g(\mathbf{r}) . \mathbf{r} \in c) \quad (2.14)$$

Each clique $c \in C$ supports its own factor $f_c(\ldots)$, which is generally an arbitrary positive and bounded function, $0 < f_c(\ldots) < \infty$, of signal configurations (co-occurrences) on the clique c. The normalizing constant, Z, called the *partition function*, ensures that the probabilities characterize the whole parent population, $\sum_{\mathbf{g} \in G} P(\mathbf{g}) = 1$.

The factors are often expressed $f_c(g(\mathbf{r}) : \mathbf{r} \in c) = \exp\left(-V_c(g(\mathbf{r}) : \mathbf{r} \in c)\right)$ where the negated exponent $V_c(g(\mathbf{r}) : \mathbf{r} \in c); -\infty < V_c(\ldots) < \infty$, is called a Gibbs *potential*. Each potential quantifies contributions of signals on a relevant clique to the total energy. Summing the potentials over the cliques $c \in C$ gives a total *energy*, $E(\mathbf{g}) = \sum_{c \in C} V_c(g(\mathbf{r}) : \mathbf{r} \in c)$, of signal interactions in the image $\mathbf{g}$ considered as a sample from the MRF. The lesser the potential or the energy, the more probable the corresponding signal configuration (co-occurrence, pattern) over the clique or the entire lattice, respectively.

Definition 2.8

Exponential representation of the probability or density in Equation 2.14 specifying a MRF is called a Gibbs probability distribution (GPD), or sometimes a Boltzmann distribution:

$$P(\mathbf{g}) = \frac{1}{Z} \exp\left(-\sum_{c \in C} V_c(g(\mathbf{r}) : \mathbf{r} \in c)\right) \equiv \frac{\exp\left(-E(\mathbf{g})\right)}{\sum_{\mathbf{g}' \in G} \exp\left(-E(\mathbf{g}')\right)} \quad (2.15)$$

The MRF specified by the GPD is often called the Markov-Gibbs random field (MGRF).

For each particular image, $\mathbf{g}^\circ \in G$, the GPD of Equation 2.15 has the irreducible form:

$$P(\mathbf{g}) = \frac{1}{\sum_{\mathbf{g} \in G} \exp\left(E(\mathbf{g}^\circ) - E(\mathbf{g})\right)} \equiv \frac{1}{1 + \sum_{\mathbf{g} \in G \setminus \mathbf{g}^\circ} \exp\left(E(\mathbf{g}^\circ) - E(\mathbf{g})\right)} \quad (2.16)$$

Given an interaction graph Γ, the order of an MGRF or GPD is up to the maximum order among all the maximal cliques in Γ, but actually may be lower if factors on the maximum-order cliques in Equation 2.14 are in turn products of constituents, supported each by a lower-order clique. Equivalently, the potentials for such maximum-order cliques are sums of terms with the lower numbers of variates, like e.g.,

$$V_c(q_1, q_2) = V(q_1) + V(q_2) \quad \text{for all } (q_1, q_2) \in \mathbb{Q}^2; \quad \text{or}$$

$$V_c(q_1, q_2, q_3)$$

$$= \begin{cases} V(q_1) + V(q_2) + V(q_3) & \text{or} \\ V_{c:1}(q_1, q_2) + V_{c:2}(q_1, q_3) + V_{c:3}(q_1, q_3) & \text{for all } (q_1, q_2, q_3) \in \mathbb{Q}^3 \end{cases}$$

In these cases the order of the MGRF is the maximum order among all the cliques supporting the factors (potentials) that cannot be decomposed further into the products (sums); e.g., a quadratic potential function of K signals, $q_k \in \mathbb{Q}$; $k = 1, \ldots, K$, on a clique of any order K; $K > 2$, with arbitrary finite coefficients, w_k and $w_{k,\kappa}$:

$$V(q_1, \ldots, q_k) = \sum_{k=1}^{K} \left(w_k q_k + w_{k,k} q_k^2 \right) + \sum_{k=1}^{K-1} \sum_{\kappa=k+1}^{K} w_{k,\kappa} q_k q_\kappa$$

decomposes this clique into multiple first- and second-order ones, i.e., K first-order and $\frac{1}{2}(K-1)K$ second-order cliques if all the coefficients are nonzero. Similarly, a polynomial potential function of degree $K_0 < K$ can decompose the same clique into multiple cliques of order up to K_0.

Computational complexity of image analysis based on the MGRF model depends on the average, rather than maximal order of the cliques supporting the Gibbs potentials. Thus, a high-order model with only a few maximum-order cliques might result in almost the same complexity as a low-order model.

2.2.2 Basic Stochastic Modeling Scenarios

Stochastic image modeling that employs MGRFs follows mostly either (1) a mainstream Bayesian or (2) an alternative conditional random field (CRF) scenario. In application, e.g., to image segmentation, the Bayesian scenario starts from building a prior model, $P_u(\mathbf{m}) = \frac{1}{Z_u} \exp(-E_u(\mathbf{m}))$, of the goal region maps and a conditional model, $P_c(\mathbf{g} \mid \mathbf{m}) = \frac{1}{Z_c(\mathbf{m})} \exp(-E_c(\mathbf{g} \mid \mathbf{m}))$, of the observed images, given a map. Both the models sometimes can be prescribed, but basically are learned (in the case of supervised learning—from available training maps and "image–map" pairs, respectively). Then the models are used for building the posterior conditional model of maps, given an image:

$$P_p(\mathbf{m} \mid \mathbf{g}) = \frac{\frac{1}{Z_c(\mathbf{m})} \exp\left(-(E_u(\mathbf{m}) + E_c(\mathbf{g}|\mathbf{m}))\right)}{\sum_{\mathbf{m}' \in \mathbb{M}} \frac{1}{Z_c(\mathbf{m}')} \exp\left(-(E_u(\mathbf{m}') + E_c(\mathbf{g}|\mathbf{m}'))\right)}$$

$$\propto \frac{1}{Z_c(\mathbf{m})} \exp\left(-(E_u(\mathbf{m}) + E_c(\mathbf{g} \mid \mathbf{m}))\right)$$

where the map-dependent normalizer, $Z_c(\mathbf{m}) = \sum_{\mathbf{g} \in \mathbb{G}} \exp\left(-E_c(\mathbf{g} \mid \mathbf{m})\right)$, is most often computationally infeasible.

This posterior, which is not an MGRF in a majority of cases, allows (at least, in principle) for the Bayesian or other statistically optimal inference, e.g., for the Bayesian MAP decision:

$$\mathbf{m}^* = \arg \max_{\mathbf{m} \in \mathbb{M}} \log P_p(\mathbf{m} \mid \mathbf{g}) = \arg \min_{\mathbf{m} \in \mathbb{M}} \{\ln Z_c(\mathbf{m}) + E_u(\mathbf{m}) + E(\mathbf{g} \mid \mathbf{m})\}$$

Because the normalizer, $Z_c(\mathbf{m})$, is mostly unknown, the approximate decision is obtained by energy minimization:

$$\mathbf{m}^* \approx \arg \min_{\mathbf{m} \in \mathbb{M}} \{E_u(\mathbf{m}) + E(\mathbf{g}|\mathbf{m})\}$$

The CRF scenario selects and/or learns directly a conditional MGRF model of maps, given an image (in the supervised case—from the training "image–map" pairs):

$$P_{crf}(\mathbf{m} \mid \mathbf{g}) = \frac{1}{Z_{crf}(\mathbf{g})} \exp\left(-(E_u(\mathbf{m}) + E_{crf}(\mathbf{m}|\mathbf{g}))\right)$$

Then the model learnt is used for the statistical inference, e.g.,

$$\mathbf{m}^* = \arg \max_{\mathbf{m} \in \mathbb{M}} \{\log P_{crf}(\mathbf{m} \mid \mathbf{g})\} = \arg \min_{\mathbf{m} \in \mathbb{M}} \{E_u(\mathbf{m}) + E_{crf}(\mathbf{m} \mid \mathbf{g})\}$$

The learning often involves only the image $\mathbf{g}$ to be segmented.

2.2.3 Invariance to Unessential Deviations

To make a stochastic shape or appearance model invariant to unessential geometric and perceptive image deviations, all the images to be used for model learning and model-based image analysis can be co-registered, or aligned. Ultimately, the alignment unifies global positions, orientations, and scales of objects-of-interest with respect to the lattice; excludes local unessential deviations, and normalizes contrast and offset deviations. But reaching these goals

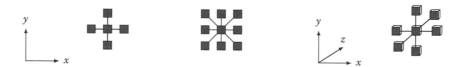

FIGURE 2.4
The nearest 2D 4- and 8-neighborhoods and 3D 6-neighborhood.

in practice is by itself a big challenge, which also requires image modeling. A more frequent alternative is to build and employ the MGRF models with deviation-invariant cliques and potentials.

Translation-invariant MGRFs are in most common use in stochastic image modeling. The set $\mathbb{A}$ of arcs, or *second-order clique families* in the interaction graph, Γ, is stratified into $N = |\mathbf{N}|$ subsets: $\mathbb{A} = \{\mathbb{C}_\mathbf{v} : \mathbf{v} \in \mathbf{N}\}$, where $\mathbf{N}$ is a list of coordinate offsets, $\mathbf{v} = (\xi, \eta)$ or (ξ, η, ζ), for interacting pixel or voxel pairs, respectively. Each family contains the second-order cliques with the same fixed offset: $\mathbb{C}_\mathbf{v} = \{c_\mathbf{v} = (\mathbf{r}, \mathbf{r} + \mathbf{v}) : (\mathbf{r}, \mathbf{r} + \mathbf{v}) \in \mathbb{R}^2\}$. Higher-order translation-invariant models involve the families of the higher-order cliques built from the second-order ones in $\mathbb{A}$.

The translation-invariant geometry is often described by a fixed neighborhood, $\mathbb{N}$, of each site on the infinite lattice: $\mathbb{N} = \{\mathbf{v}; -\mathbf{v} : \mathbf{v} \in \mathbf{N}\}$. The neighborhood is cut off at borders of a finite lattice; however, the model uniformity is typically preserved by one or another lattice padding that extends signals across the borders, e.g., by mirroring, using a fixed signal, or twisting the lattice into the torus. Figure 2.4 exemplifies the nearest 4- and 8-neighborhoods for a 2D lattice and the nearest 6-neighborhood for a 3D lattice.

Each approximately translation-rotation invariant clique family includes all nearly equidistant pixel/voxel pairs, e.g., $\mathbb{C}_d = \{(\mathbf{r}, \mathbf{r} + \mathbf{v}); d - 0.5 \leq |\mathbf{v}| < d + 0.5\}; d \in \{1, 2, \ldots\}$.

2.2.3.1 Multiple Second- and Higher-Order Interactions

Signal dependencies in medical images are rarely limited to only the nearest neighbors or rectangular neighborhoods, which are typical for a majority of common translation invariant MGRFs. Generally, the interaction geometry varies over the lattice and thus is too complex for modeling. Even when an exact or at least approximate translational invariance holds, accurate MGRF models may require high-order cliques with multiple short- and long-range arcs. These cliques and corresponding pixel or voxel neighborhoods may be discontinuous and considerably more intricate, than two simple examples in Figure 2.5.

Nonetheless, the translation or translation-rotation invariant models remain of major interest for modeling various medical objects or their parts. Even the simplest MGRFs with only the nearest-neighbor interactions

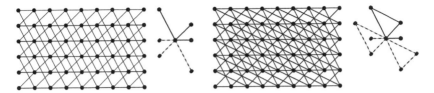

FIGURE 2.5
Multiple translation-invariant second- and second/third-order interactions.

proved their practical usefulness for describing uniform spatial or spatiotemporal binary ("object–background") region maps.

2.2.3.2 Contrast/Offset-Invariant MGRFs

Arbitrary spatially variant perceptive (contrast-offset) deviations preserve relative ordering of uniquely indexed clique's sites by their signal values. In particular, let the sites, $\mathbf{r}$ and $\mathbf{r} + \mathbf{v}$, of a second-order clique be indexed 1 and 2, respectively, i.e., $g(\mathbf{r}) = q_1$ and $g(\mathbf{r} + \mathbf{v}) = q_2$). To be invariant to the perceptive deviations, the second-order potentials, $V_{\mathbf{v}}(q_1, q_2)$, may depend only on the three ordinal signal configurations: $q_1 < q_2, q_1 = q_2$, and $q_1 > q_2$, or, what is the same, on the signs of the clique-wise signal differences: $\text{sign}(q_1 - q_2) \in \{-1, 0, 1\}$.

The numbers of all higher-order ordinal configurations (see, e.g., Table 2.1) grow much slower than of all signal co-occurrences, e.g., 13, 75, and 541 ordinal configurations for a clique of order $k = 3, 4$, and 5, respectively, comparing to the numbers $|\mathbb{Q}|^k$ of signal co-occurrences, e.g., 4,096; 65,536; and 1,048,576 for $|\mathbb{Q}| = 16$. As a result, accurate and computationally feasible learning of the higher-order ordinal models is considerably simplified. In particular, the detailed in Chapter 4 framework for fast approximate learning of generic MGRFs with multiple second-order interactions can be extended to up to the fifth-order models if numbers of distinct signal configurations on the cliques in each translation-invariant family is constrained to 500–600. Accounting for only partial ordinal relations in generalized local binary (LBP) or ternary (LTP) patterns of signals on cliques of arbitrary shapes and

TABLE 2.1

Ordinal Signal Configurations for Second- and Third-Order Cliques

Second-Order Clique: $V_{\mathbf{v}}(q_1, q_2)$

$q_1 < q_2$	$q_1 = q_2$	$q_2 < q_1$			

Third-Order Clique: $V_{\mathbf{c}}(q_1, q_2, q_3)$

$q_1 < q_2 < q_3$	$q_2 < q_1 < q_3$	$q_3 < q_1 < q_2$	$q_1 < q_2 = q_3$	$q_2 = q_3 < q_1$	$q_2 < q_1 = q_3$
$q_1 < q_3 < q_2$	$q_2 < q_3 < q_1$	$q_3 < q_2 < q_1$	$q_1 = q_2 < q_3$	$q_1 = q_3 < q_2$	$q_3 < q_1 = q_2$
$q_1 = q_2 = q_3$					

sizes extends the same learning framework under the same constraint to the MGRFs with multiple up to tenth-order interactions. The higher-order ordinal dependencies compensate for the loss of descriptive and discriminative abilities of the MGRFs, accounting for only the ordinal signal relations, and also allow for modeling more diverse object appearances and shapes than the lower-order models.

2.3 Exponential Families of Probability Distributions

A majority of popular MRF image models, including, e.g., auto-binomial (Potts), Gauss, and auto-regressive (Gauss-Markov) random fields, MGRFs with multiple second-order interactions, and higher-order FoE (Field of Experts) and FRAME (Filters, Random Fields, and Maximum Entropy) models, belong to exponential families of probability distributions. For digital images, an exponential family is defined in the simplest case as

$$P_{\mathbf{V}}(\mathbf{g}) = \frac{1}{Z_{\mathbf{V}}} \exp\left(-\mathbf{V}^{\mathsf{T}}\mathbf{S}(\mathbf{g})\right) \equiv \frac{1}{Z_{\mathbf{V}}} \exp\left(-\sum_{i=1}^{n} V_i S_i(\mathbf{g})\right) \qquad (2.17)$$

where the exponent is a negated linear combination of scalar parameters (factors, or weights), $\mathbf{V} = [V_1, \ldots, V_n]^{\mathsf{T}}$, and values of scalar functions, $\mathbf{S}(\mathbf{g}) = [S_1(\mathbf{g}), \ldots, S_n(\mathbf{g})]^{\mathsf{T}}$, summarizing signal properties in each individual image $\mathbf{g}$. The normalizer, $Z_{\mathbf{V}} = \sum_{\mathbf{g} \in \mathrm{G}} \exp\left(-\mathbf{V}^{\mathsf{T}}\mathbf{S}(\mathbf{g})\right)$, ensuring that $\sum_{\mathbf{g} \in \mathrm{G}} P_{\mathbf{V}}(\mathbf{g}) = 1$, is mostly intractable. The functions, $\mathbf{S}_i(\mathbf{g})$; $i = 1, \ldots, n$, called *sufficient statistics*, completely define the image probabilities.

Due to the exponential form of Equation 2.17, just the same sufficient statistics, $\mathbf{S}(\mathbf{g})$, summarize the properties of a subset $\mathrm{G}_J^\circ = \{\mathbf{g}_j^\circ : j = 1, \ldots, J\}$, of images, sampled independently from the distribution of Equation 2.17. Joint probability of these images:

$$P_{\mathbf{V}}(\mathrm{G}_J^\circ) \equiv P_{\mathbf{V}}(\mathbf{g}_1^\circ, \ldots, \mathbf{g}_J^\circ) = \prod_{j=1}^{J} P_{\mathbf{V}}(\mathbf{g}_j^\circ) = \frac{1}{(Z_{\mathbf{V}})^J}$$

$$\exp\left(-\mathbf{V}^{\mathsf{T}} \sum_{j=1}^{J} \mathbf{S}(\mathbf{g}_j^\circ)\right) \equiv [P_{\mathbf{V}}(\bar{\mathbf{g}}^\circ)]^J$$

can be associated with an imaginary "average" image, $\bar{\mathbf{g}}^\circ$, having the mean sufficient statistics $\mathbf{S}(\bar{\mathbf{g}}^\circ) = \frac{1}{J}\sum_{j=1}^{J} \mathbf{S}(\mathbf{g}_j^\circ)$ for the subset G_J°.

Informativeness of a distribution, $\mathbf{P} = \{P(\mathbf{g}) : \mathbf{g} \in \mathrm{G}; \sum_{\mathbf{g} \in \mathrm{G}} P(\mathbf{g}) = 1\}$, is evaluated by its entropy, defined as the negated expected logarithm of probability:

$$H(\mathbf{P}) = \mathcal{E}\left\{-\ln P(\mathbf{g}) \mid \mathbf{P}\right\} \equiv -\sum_{g \in G} P(\mathbf{g}) \ln P(\mathbf{g}) \tag{2.18}$$

Lemma 2.1 (The Maximum Entropy Property)

Distributions, $\mathbf{P_V}$, from the exponential family of Equation 2.17 have the maximum entropy, $\mathbf{P_V} = \arg\max_{\mathbf{P}}\{H(\mathbf{P})\}$, among all the distributions, $\mathbf{P} = (P(\mathbf{g}) : \mathbf{g} \in G); \sum_{g \in G} P(\mathbf{g}) = 1)$, such that mathematical expectations of the same sufficient statistics are constrained to the prescribed values, $\mathbf{s}^\circ = [s_1^\circ, \ldots, s_n^\circ]^\mathsf{T}$:

$$\begin{aligned}
\mathcal{E}\{\mathbf{S}(\mathbf{g}) \mid \mathbf{P}\} &\equiv \sum_{g \in G} \mathbf{S}(\mathbf{g})P(\mathbf{g}) = \mathbf{s}^\circ; \text{ i.e.} \\
\mathcal{E}\{S_i(\mathbf{g}) \mid \mathbf{P}\} &\equiv \sum_{g \in G} S_i(\mathbf{g})P(\mathbf{g}) = s_i^\circ; \; i = 1, \ldots, n
\end{aligned} \tag{2.19}$$

Proof. The constrained maximization finds a stationary point, $\mathbf{P_V}$, of the Lagrangian:

$$\begin{aligned}
\mathcal{L}(\mathbf{P}, \mathbf{\Lambda}) = &- \sum_{g \in G} P(\mathbf{g}) \log P(\mathbf{g}) - \lambda \left(\sum_{g \in G} P(\mathbf{g}) - 1 \right) \\
&- \mathbf{V}^\mathsf{T} \left(\sum_{g \in G} \mathbf{S}(\mathbf{g}) P(\mathbf{g}) - \mathbf{s}^\circ \right)
\end{aligned}$$

with the $n+1$ Lagrange coefficients $\mathbf{\Lambda} = (\lambda, \mathbf{V})$. This point sets to zero the gradient vector of the Lagrangian, $\nabla\mathcal{L}(\mathbf{P}, \mathbf{\Lambda}) \equiv \frac{\partial \mathcal{L}(\mathbf{P}, \mathbf{\Lambda})}{\partial \mathbf{P}} = \left[\frac{\partial \mathcal{L}(\mathbf{P}, \mathbf{\Lambda})}{\partial P(\mathbf{g})} : \mathbf{g} \in G \right]$, so that

$$\left. \frac{\partial \mathcal{L}(\mathbf{P}, \mathbf{\Lambda})}{\partial P(\mathbf{g})} \right|_{\mathbf{P}=\mathbf{P_\Lambda}} = -\log P_\Lambda(\mathbf{g}) - 1 - \lambda - \mathbf{V}^\mathsf{T}\mathbf{S}(\mathbf{g}) = 0$$

or $P_\Lambda(\mathbf{g}) = \exp\left(-1 - \lambda - \mathbf{V}^\mathsf{T}\mathbf{S}(\mathbf{g})\right) \geq 0$ for $\mathbf{g} \in G$.

The Hessian matrix of the second derivatives of the Lagrangian is diagonal and nonpositive definite: $\frac{\partial^2 \mathcal{L}(\mathbf{P}, \mathbf{\Lambda})}{\partial^2 P(\mathbf{g})} = -\frac{1}{P(\mathbf{g})} \leq 0$ and $\frac{\partial^2 \mathcal{L}(\mathbf{P}, \mathbf{\Lambda})}{\partial P(\mathbf{g})\partial P(\mathbf{g}')} = 0$ for $\mathbf{g}, \mathbf{g}' \in G$. Thus, the distribution $\mathbf{P_\Lambda} = (P_\Lambda(\mathbf{g}) : \mathbf{g} \in G)$ is the unique constrained entropy maximizer.

Excluding the coefficient λ by normalization, $\sum_{g \in G} P(\mathbf{g}) = 1$, yields the exponential family $\mathbf{P_V}$ of Equation 2.17 with the weights, $\mathbf{V}$, satisfying the constraints of Equation 2.19. ∎

The maximum entropy property makes the exponential families the most informative and "random," i.e., the least restricted, among all the distributions with the same constrained statistics of Equation 2.19. Loosely speaking, the exponential family of Equation 2.17 restricts the uniform distribution with equal image probabilities, $P_0(\mathbf{g}) = \frac{1}{|G|}$, by constraining n particular sufficient statistics, $\mathbf{S}(\mathbf{g})$. The core uniform distribution maximizes the entropy of Equation 2.18 if no constraints of Equation 2.19 are imposed, i.e., if all the weights have zero values: $\mathbf{V} = \mathbf{0}$.

The system of constraints in Equation 2.19 may have no solution for the parameters $\mathbf{V}$ if the expected right-side values, $s_i^\circ; i = 1, \ldots, n$, contradict each other. But for the mutually consistent constraints, the exponential family of Equation 2.17 does exist, and its parameters can be found, at least, in principle, by solving the system of constraints. However, the exact solution of this system is mostly computationally infeasible.

To ensure a nonempty solution space for Equation 2.19, the expectations of the statistics $S_i(\mathbf{g}); i = 1, \ldots, n$, are often equated to their empirical mean (average) values for a training subset $\mathbf{G}_j^\circ = \left\{ \mathbf{g}_j^\circ : j = 1, \ldots, J \right\}$ of samples; $J \geq 1$, i.e., to the statistics of an "average" image, $\bar{\mathbf{g}}^\circ$, for the subset $\mathbf{G}_m^\circ$:

$$s_i^\circ = \frac{1}{J} \sum_{j=1}^{J} S_i(\mathbf{g}_j^\circ) \equiv S_i(\bar{\mathbf{g}}^\circ); \quad i = 1, \ldots, n \tag{2.20}$$

This choice coincides with the maximum likelihood estimates (MLE) of the parameters, $\mathbf{V}$, of the model in Equation 2.17 from the training data, $\mathbf{G}_j^\circ$. The likelihood, $L(\mathbf{V}|\mathbf{G}_j^\circ) = P_\mathbf{V}(\mathbf{G}_j^\circ)$, of the parameters $\mathbf{V}$ of distributions from the exponential family in Equation 2.17, is usually replaced with the *log-likelihood* function, $\ell(\mathbf{V}|\bar{\mathbf{g}}^\circ) = \frac{1}{J} \log P_\mathbf{V}(\mathbf{G}_j^\circ)$:

$$\ell(\mathbf{V}|\bar{\mathbf{g}}^\circ) = -\mathbf{V}^\mathsf{T}\mathbf{S}(\bar{\mathbf{g}}^\circ) - \log Z_\mathbf{V} \equiv -\mathbf{V}^\mathsf{T}\mathbf{S}(\bar{\mathbf{g}}^\circ) - \log \sum_{\mathbf{g} \in G} \exp\left(-\mathbf{V}^\mathsf{T}\mathbf{S}(\mathbf{g})\right) \tag{2.21}$$

having just the same stationary points in the parameter space.

Lemma 2.2

The log-likelihood, $\ell(\mathbf{V}|\bar{\mathbf{g}}^\circ)$, is concave down in the space of parameters $\mathbf{V}$. Its unique maximizer, i.e., the MLE of the parameters, $\mathbf{V}^* = \arg\max_\mathbf{V} \{\ell(\mathbf{V}|\bar{\mathbf{g}}^\circ)\}$, if exists, solves the constraining system of Equation 2.19 with the empirical right-side values of Equation 2.20.

Proof. The gradient vector, $\nabla_{\ell:\mathbf{V}}(\bar{\mathbf{g}}^\circ)$, and the Hessian matrix, $\mathbf{H}_{\ell:\mathbf{V}}$, of the second partial derivatives of the log-likelihood of Equation 2.21 are, respectively,

$$\nabla_{\ell:V}(\bar{\mathbf{g}}^\circ) \equiv \tfrac{\partial}{\partial V}\ell\left(V|\bar{\mathbf{g}}^\circ\right) = -\mathbf{S}(\bar{\mathbf{g}}^\circ) - \tfrac{\partial}{\partial V}Z_V \equiv -\mathbf{S}(\bar{\mathbf{g}}^\circ) + \mathcal{E}\left\{\mathbf{S}(\mathbf{g})|\mathbf{P}_V\right\}$$

$$\mathbf{H}_{\ell:V} \equiv \tfrac{\partial^2}{\partial V \partial V^\mathsf{T}}\ell(V|\bar{\mathbf{g}}^\circ) \equiv \tfrac{\partial}{\partial V^\mathsf{T}}\nabla_{\ell:V}(\bar{\mathbf{g}}^\circ) = \tfrac{\partial}{\partial V^\mathsf{T}}\mathcal{E}\left\{\mathbf{S}(\mathbf{g})|\mathbf{P}_V\right\}$$

$$= -\mathcal{E}\left\{\mathbf{S}(\mathbf{g})\mathbf{S}^\mathsf{T}(\mathbf{g})|\mathbf{P}_V\right\} + \mathcal{E}\left\{\mathbf{S}(\mathbf{g})|\mathbf{P}_V\right\}\mathcal{E}\left\{\mathbf{S}^\mathsf{T}(\mathbf{g})|\mathbf{P}_V\right\}$$

$$(2.22)$$

This Hessian matrix is always nonpositive definite because it is equal to the negated covariance matrix, $\mathbf{C}_V$, of the statistics $\mathbf{S}(\mathbf{g})$:

$$\mathbf{C}_V = \mathcal{E}\left\{\mathbf{S}(\mathbf{g})\mathbf{S}^\mathsf{T}(\mathbf{g})|\mathbf{P}_V\right\} - \mathcal{E}\left\{\mathbf{S}(\mathbf{g})|\mathbf{P}_V\right\}\mathcal{E}\left\{\mathbf{S}^\mathsf{T}(\mathbf{g})|\mathbf{P}_V\right\} \qquad (2.23)$$

which is always nonnegative definite. Therefore, the log-likelihood, as well as the likelihood, is concave down in the parameter space.

Hence, for a nonsingular (positive definite) covariance matrix, $\mathbf{C}_V$, the log-likelihood, $\ell(V|\bar{\mathbf{g}}^\circ)$, has the unique maximum at the zero-gradient point, i.e., the MLE V^*, defined by the conditions $-\mathbf{S}(\bar{\mathbf{g}}^\circ) + \mathcal{E}\left\{\mathbf{S}(\mathbf{g})|\mathbf{P}_{V^*}\right\} = \mathbf{0}$, or $\mathcal{E}\left\{\mathbf{S}(\mathbf{g})|\mathbf{P}_{V^*}\right\} = \mathbf{S}(\bar{\mathbf{g}}^\circ)$, coinciding with the constraints of Equations 2.19 and 2.20. ∎

Due to the same system of constraints, the MLE is a natural tool for learning the exponential families from the training data. This property suggests a feasible analytical approximation of the MLE, detailed below, in Section 2.3.1.

In the general case, an exponential family is defined as

$$P_V(\mathbf{g}) = \frac{1}{Z_V}\Psi(\mathbf{g})\exp\left(-V^\mathsf{T}\mathbf{S}(\mathbf{g})\right) \equiv \frac{\Psi(\mathbf{g})\exp\left(-V^\mathsf{T}\mathbf{S}(\mathbf{g})\right)}{\sum\limits_{\mathbf{g}\in G}\Psi(\mathbf{g})\exp\left(-V^\mathsf{T}\mathbf{S}(\mathbf{g})\right)} \qquad (2.24)$$

where a tractable positive scalar function of image signals $\Psi(\mathbf{g})$ defines a certain core distribution, $P_0(\mathbf{g}) = \frac{1}{Z_0}\Psi(\mathbf{g})$. The generic exponential family of Equation 2.24 restricts this core by constraining its additional statistics, $\mathbf{S}(\mathbf{g})$. The core may (but not necessarily) belong to an already learned exponential family, specified with the other statistics.

The GPD of Equation 2.15 also belongs to an exponential family at quite general conditions. Let the set, $\mathbb{C}$, of cliques contain A; $A \geq 1$, clique families $\mathbb{C}_a$; $a = 1, \ldots, A$; $\mathbb{C} = \bigcup_{a=1}^A \mathbb{C}_a$, such that cliques of each family $\mathbb{C}_a$ are of the same order K_a, support the same potential function, $V_a : \mathbb{Q}^{K_a} \to \mathbb{V}_a$, of signals with a finite set, $\mathbb{V}_a$, of values, and have the same shape (i.e., the same relative locations of pixels or voxels), invariant to certain geometric transformations, e.g., translation or translation–rotation with respect to the lattice.

Then the GPD of Equation 2.15 can be rewritten as

$$
P(\mathbf{g}) = \frac{1}{Z_{\mathbf{V}}} \exp\left(-\sum_{a=1}^{A} \sum_{\mathbf{c} \in \mathbb{C}_a} V_a(g(\mathbf{r}) : \mathbf{r} \in \mathbf{c})\right)
$$

$$
= \frac{1}{Z_{\mathbf{V}}} \exp\left(-\sum_{a=1}^{A} \sum_{v_a \in \mathbb{V}_a} v_a S_a(v_a | \mathbf{g})\right) \tag{2.25}
$$

$$
= \frac{1}{Z_{\mathbf{V}}} \exp\left(-\sum_{a=1}^{A} \mathbf{V}_a^{\mathsf{T}} \mathbf{S}_a(\mathbf{g})\right) = \frac{1}{Z_{\mathbf{V}}} \exp\left(-\mathbf{V}^{\mathsf{T}} \mathbf{S}(\mathbf{g})\right)
$$

where the vectors $\mathbf{V}$ and $\mathbf{S}(\mathbf{g})$ concatenate, respectively, vectors of the potential values, $\mathbf{V}_a = [v_a : v_a \in \mathbb{V}_a]$, and corresponding *histograms* of their occurrences over the image $\mathbf{g}$:

$$
\mathbf{S}_a(\mathbf{g}) = \left[S_a(v_a | \mathbf{g}) = \sum_{\mathbf{c} \in \mathbb{C}_a} \delta\left(v_a - V_a(g(\mathbf{r}) : \mathbf{r} \in \mathbf{c})\right) : v_a \in \mathbb{V}_a\right] ; \ a = 1, \dots, A
$$

Each histogram component, $S_a(v_a | \mathbf{g})$, is an empirical frequency (unnormalized probability) of the value, v_a, over the family $\mathbb{C}_a$, i.e., the number of cliques $\mathbf{c} \in \mathbb{C}_a$, such that their signal configurations, $(g(\mathbf{r}) : \mathbf{r} \in \mathbf{c})$, result in the potential value v_a. The histograms $\mathbf{S}(\mathbf{g})$ are the sufficient statistics to be constrained by learning the potentials $\mathbf{V}$ of Equation 2.25.

2.3.1 Learning an Exponential Family

The origin, $\mathbf{V} = \mathbf{0}$, of the parameter space of a generic family in Equation 2.24 corresponds to its core distribution, $\mathbf{P}_0 = \left[P_0(\mathbf{g}) = \frac{1}{Z_0} \Psi(\mathbf{g}) : \mathbf{g} \in \mathbb{G}\right]$. The simplest core, $\Psi(\mathbf{g}) = 1$ and $P_0(\mathbf{g}) = \frac{1}{|\mathbb{G}|}$, in Equation 2.17 is the IRF of equiprobable images with uniform marginal signal probabilities, $\mathbf{P}_{\mathbf{r}} = [P_{\mathbf{r}}(q) = \frac{1}{Q} : q \in \mathbb{Q}]$; $\mathbf{r} \in \mathbb{R}$. In this case both the log-likelihood gradient of Equation 2.22, at the origin, $\mathbf{V} = \mathbf{0}$, of the parameter space: $\nabla_{\ell:0}(\bar{\mathbf{g}}^\circ) = -\mathbf{S}(\bar{\mathbf{g}}^\circ) + \mathcal{E}\{\mathbf{S}(\mathbf{g}) | \mathbf{P}_0\}$, depending on the mathematical expectation, $\mathcal{E}\{\mathbf{S}(\mathbf{g}) | \mathbf{P}_0\}$, and the covariance matrix, $\mathbf{C}_0$, of Equation 2.23 for various multivariate statistics, $\mathbf{S}(\mathbf{g})$, of image signals can be either found analytically or approximated with a reasonably high accuracy empirically, from one or more generated samples of this core IRF.

    Similar accurate analytical or, at least, empirical evaluations of the log-likelihood gradients and covariance matrices of certain signal statistics exist also for a number of other core distributions, such as IRFs with arbitrary marginal distributions of the pixel/voxel-wise signals, selected second-order MGRFs, e.g., auto-binomial, Gauss, and Gauss-Markov models, and so forth.

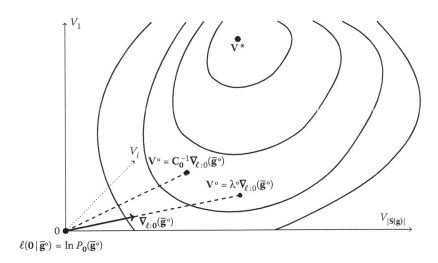

FIGURE 2.6
First approximations, $\mathbf{V}^\circ$, of the MLE, $\mathbf{V}^*$, of parameters $\mathbf{V}$ in a distribution, $P_\mathbf{V}(\mathbf{g})$, of Equation 2.24. The origin, $\mathbf{0}$, of the parameter space defines the core, $P_0(\mathbf{g}) = \frac{1}{Z_0}\Psi(\mathbf{g})$. Curves indicate isolines of the log-likelihood, $\ell(\mathbf{V}\,|\,\bar{\mathbf{g}}^\circ) = \text{const.}$

In all these cases, maximizing the truncated second-order Taylor's series decomposition of the log-likelihood in Equation 2.21 in the close vicinity of the origin $\mathbf{V} = \mathbf{0}$ of the parameter space, as illustrated in Figure 2.6:

$$\ell_{\text{tr}}(\mathbf{V}\,|\,\bar{\mathbf{g}}^\circ) = \ell(\mathbf{0}\,|\,\bar{\mathbf{g}}^\circ) + \mathbf{V}^\mathsf{T}\nabla_{\ell:0}(\bar{\mathbf{g}}^\circ) - \frac{1}{2}\mathbf{V}^\mathsf{T}\mathbf{C}_0\mathbf{V} \qquad (2.26)$$

provides the approximate MLE of parameters $\mathbf{V}$ of a generic family, $\mathbf{P_V}$, in Equation 2.24.

The unconstrained maximization of Equation 2.26 results in the first MLE approximation:

$$\mathbf{V}^\circ = \mathbf{C}_0^{-1}\nabla_{\ell:0}(\bar{\mathbf{g}}^\circ) \qquad (2.27)$$

that involves the inverted covariance matrix, whereas constraining the maximization only along the gradient circumvents the matrix inversion:

$$\mathbf{V}^\circ = \lambda^\circ\nabla_{\ell:0}(\bar{\mathbf{g}}^\circ) \equiv \frac{\nabla_{\ell:0}^\mathsf{T}(\bar{\mathbf{g}}^\circ)\nabla_{\ell:0}(\bar{\mathbf{g}}^\circ)}{\nabla_{\ell:0}^\mathsf{T}(\bar{\mathbf{g}}^\circ)\mathbf{C}_0\nabla_{\ell:0}(\bar{\mathbf{g}}^\circ)}\nabla_{\ell:0}(\bar{\mathbf{g}}^\circ) \qquad (2.28)$$

The unconstrained maximizer, $\mathbf{V}^\circ = \arg\max_{\mathbf{V}}\ell_{\text{tr}}(\mathbf{V}\,|\,\bar{\mathbf{g}}^\circ) = \mathbf{C}_0^{-1}\nabla_{\ell:0}(\bar{\mathbf{g}}^\circ)$, in Equation 2.27 corresponds to the unique stationary, or zero-gradient point of the truncated log-likelihood, $\frac{\partial}{\partial\mathbf{V}}\ell_{\text{tr}}(\mathbf{V}\,|\,\bar{\mathbf{g}}^\circ)\big|_{\mathbf{V}=\mathbf{V}^\circ} = \nabla_{\ell:0}(\bar{\mathbf{g}}^\circ) - \mathbf{C}_0\mathbf{V}^\circ = \mathbf{0}$, due to the negated covariance matrix, $-\mathbf{C_0}$ as the nonpositive definite Hessian. This approximate MLE is feasible for the easily invertible covariance matrices, e.g., for the core IRFs when the covariance matrix is diagonal or is closely approximated by a diagonal matrix.

The alternative approximation in Equation 2.28 requires no matrix inversion and maximizes the truncated log-likelihood of Equation 2.26 just along the gradient direction from the origin. The constrained maximizer, $\mathbf{V}^\circ = \arg\max_\lambda \ell_{\text{tr}}(\lambda\boldsymbol{\nabla}_{\ell:0}(\bar{\mathbf{g}}^\circ)\mid\bar{\mathbf{g}}^\circ) = \lambda^\circ\boldsymbol{\nabla}_{\ell:0}(\bar{\mathbf{g}}^\circ)$, corresponds to the unique stationary point with zero first derivative by λ,

$$\frac{d}{d\lambda}\ell_{\text{tr}}(\lambda\boldsymbol{\nabla}_{\ell:0}(\bar{\mathbf{g}}^\circ)\mid\bar{\mathbf{g}}^\circ)\Big|_{\lambda=\lambda^\circ} = \boldsymbol{\nabla}_{\ell:0}^{\mathsf{T}}(\bar{\mathbf{g}}^\circ)\boldsymbol{\nabla}_{\ell:0}(\bar{\mathbf{g}}^\circ)$$

$$-\lambda^\circ\boldsymbol{\nabla}_{\ell:0}^{\mathsf{T}}(\bar{\mathbf{g}}^\circ)\mathbf{C_0}\boldsymbol{\nabla}_{\ell:0}(\bar{\mathbf{g}}^\circ) = 0$$

due to the nonpositive negated quadratic form as the second derivative,

$$\frac{d}{d\lambda}\ell_{\text{tr}}(\lambda\boldsymbol{\nabla}_{\ell:0}(\bar{\mathbf{g}}^\circ)\mid\bar{\mathbf{g}}^\circ) = -\boldsymbol{\nabla}_{\ell:0}^{\mathsf{T}}(\bar{\mathbf{g}}^\circ)\mathbf{C_0}\boldsymbol{\nabla}_{\ell:0}(\bar{\mathbf{g}}^\circ) \leq 0$$

In some cases, e.g., for the diagonal covariance matrix $\mathbf{C_0} = \sigma^2\mathbf{I}$, where $\mathbf{I}$ is the identity matrix with the unit diagonal and zero nondiagonal components, both the approximate estimates in Equations 2.27 and 2.28 coincide: $\mathbf{V}^\circ = \frac{1}{\sigma^2}\boldsymbol{\nabla}_{\ell:0}(\bar{\mathbf{g}}^\circ)$.

2.4 Appearance and Shape Modeling

Applied stochastic modeling always focuses on probability distributions or densities, which are either tractable $|\mathbb{R}|$-variate functions, or, at least, directly proportional to such functions. Even the IRFs specified by easy-to-learn marginal probability distributions of signals are often used successfully, in spite of their very limited descriptive and discriminative abilities, to model selected medical objects. More powerful MRFs account for conditional dependencies between N-tuples; $N \geq 2$, of adjacent and/or distant pixels or voxels to describe and separate intricate appearances and/or shapes of objects. The lesser the maximal number, N, of interdependent lattice sites, i.e., the lower the model's order N, the more feasible and easier to learn the MRF, but at the expense of the weaker modeling abilities.

Stochastic models describe an image by a collection of sufficient statistics, being each a tractable scalar function of all, $|\mathbb{R}|$, or smaller numbers of variables, and a collection of corresponding weights of these statistics. Images with the same numerical values of these statistics are equiprobable with respect to a particular model with the fixed parameters (weights).

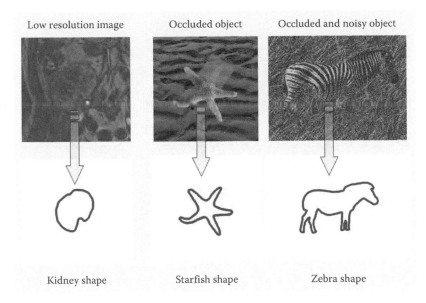

FIGURE 2.7
Noisy, diffuse, and occluded image boundaries vs. contour shape models.

Selecting a set of the sufficient statistics means, to a large extent, just the same as specifying a random field model, provided that the parameters can be easily estimated from the given training data. The most common MGRF models assume spatially homogeneous interactions with repetitive shapes and potential values for cliques over the lattice. Empirical probability distributions of these values for families of the same-shape cliques in an image are the sufficient statistics and allow for the feasible approximate MLE of the model parameters.

Both the IRF and MRF models of visual appearance (texture) mostly fail in separating medical objects with diffuse boundaries under spatially variant geometric and perceptive deviations, mutual occlusions, heavy noise, and poor resolution. But typical medical organs have well-defined 3D shapes, making prior shape models, like, e.g., flexible template contours in Figure 2.7, a very useful addition to the appearance models of the same objects.

To enhance the accuracy of image segmentation and registration, the shape priors describe object boundaries of the same type either by (1) inherent probabilistic variations of boundaries around a mean shape or (2) specific internal and external forces, evolving a deformable model to detect and approximate the goal boundary. The mean shape and its variations are learned from a given set of co-aligned training boundaries, like in Figure 2.8. A flexible prior of such type is often a linear combination of components, obtained by the principal component analysis (PCA) of the co-aligned training boundaries.

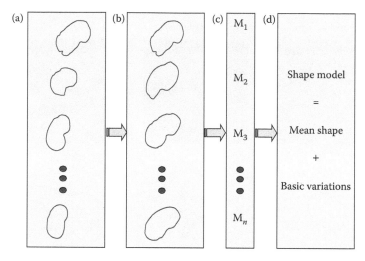

FIGURE 2.8
Shape modeling: (a) training contours; (b) their co-alignment; (c) contour descriptors; and (d) the mean contour and its basic variations.

Definition 2.9

A *deformable model* is a closed elastic 2D curve (contour) or 3D surface, which is moving under internal and external forces toward the boundary of a required 2D image region or a 3D image volume, respectively.

The model is placed first near the goal boundary and then evolves (deforms) iteratively until fitting closely the boundary. The *internal forces* depend on the model itself and try to keep it smoother during the deformation. The *external forces*, pushing the model to the object boundary, mostly depend on image signals inside and outside the model. The forces guide the evolving contour or surface to approach as close as possible the goal boundary.

A *parametric deformable model* is an evolving curve (called an active contour, or snake) on a 2D image plane or surface in a 3D image volume, being explicitly specified with a continuous parametric coordinate function, $\mathbf{b}(u)$. This function relates each model point to a parameter value, u, in a certain domain, $\mathbb{U}$, of values. A *nonparametric*, or *geometric deformable model* specifies an evolving curve or surface implicitly, with a zero level of a specific higher-dimensional function, supported by the image plane or volume, $\mathbb{R}$, respectively. This function is called the level set function.

In particular, let a closed 2D parametric curve $\mathcal{B} = \{\mathbf{b}(u) = (x(u), y(u)) : u \in [0, n]\}$, such that $\mathbf{b}(n)) \equiv \mathbf{b}(0)$, be defined by n control points; $\mathbf{b}_\alpha = \mathbf{b}(\alpha); \alpha = 0, 1, \ldots, n-1$. Interpolating the control coordinates relates all continuous positions, $(x(u), y(u))$, along the snake to a real-valued positional parameter, u, in the interval $[0, n]$; $0 \leq u \leq n$, e.g., for a piecewise-linear snake. $\mathbf{b}(u) = \mathbf{b}_\alpha + \varepsilon(\mathbf{b}_{\alpha+1} - \mathbf{b}_\alpha)$; $\alpha \leq u < \alpha + 1$, where $\alpha = \lfloor u \rfloor$ and $\varepsilon = u - \alpha$; $0 \leq \varepsilon < 1$, are the integer and fractional part of the real number u, respectively.

The curve evolves through the image plane in such a way as to minimize the total energy:

$$E_{tot}(\mathcal{B}) = E_{int}(\mathcal{B}) + E_{ext}(\mathcal{B}) \equiv \int_0^n \zeta_{int}(\mathbf{b}(u)) + \zeta_{ext}(\mathbf{b}(u))\, du \qquad (2.29)$$

where an internal force, $\zeta_{int}(\mathbf{b}(u))$, keeps the snake as a single unit and an external force, $\zeta_{ext}(\mathbf{b}(u))$, guiding the evolution, attracts the model to the goal region boundary.

The internal force frequently accounts for continuity and smoothness of the curve, e.g.,

$$\zeta_{int}(\mathbf{b}(u)) = \lambda_{ten} \left| \frac{d\mathbf{b}(u)}{du} \right|^2 + \lambda_{rig} \left| \frac{d^2\mathbf{b}(u)}{d^2u} \right|^2 \qquad (2.30)$$

where λ_{ten} and λ_{rig} are weights that control the curve's tension and rigidity, respectively.

The classical external force leading a snake toward a step-edge boundary depends on the gradient of the original, $\mathbf{g}$, or smoothed grayscale mage, $\mathbf{g}_\sigma$:

$$\zeta_{ext}(\mathbf{b}(u)) = -\left| \nabla_\mathbf{g}(\mathbf{b}(u)) \right|^2 \quad \text{or} \quad -\left| \nabla_{\mathbf{g}_\sigma}(\mathbf{b}(u)) \right|^2 \qquad (2.31)$$

where $\nabla_\mathbf{g}(x, y)$ denotes the image gradient:

$$\nabla_\mathbf{g}(x, y) = \left[\frac{\partial g(x, y)}{\partial x}; \frac{\partial g(x, y)}{\partial y} \right]^\mathsf{T}$$

and $\mathbf{g}_\sigma$ is the smoothed image, obtained by convolving the original image, $\mathbf{g}$, with a fixed 2D Gaussian filter specified by the variance σ^2:

$$g_\sigma(x, y) = \int_{-\infty}^{\infty} \int_{-\infty}^{\infty} \varphi_\sigma(\xi, \eta) g(x - \xi, y - \eta)\, d\xi d\eta$$

where

$$\varphi_\sigma(\xi, \eta) = \varphi(\xi \mid 0, \sigma)\varphi(\eta \mid 0, \sigma) = \frac{1}{2\pi\sigma^2} \exp\left(-\frac{1}{2\sigma^2}(\xi^2 + \eta^2) \right)$$

The smoothing decreases areas of initially small or zero gradients around a goal boundary where the forces become too small to guide the evolution, but affects the shape of the boundary, too. These and other external forces, exploiting local discontinuities, such as lines or edges, typically cannot guide a deformable model in a large homogeneous region or toward an intricate boundary with concavities.

An alternative external force depending on a gradient vector flow (GVF) needs no preliminary image smoothing, because of diffuse propagation of the original image gradients by themselves. To keep the boundary shape, ensure a larger guidance range, and be able to guide into concavities, the GVF $\mathbf{v} = (\mathbf{v}(x,y) = [v_x(x,y),\, v_y(x,y)]^\mathsf{T} : (x,y) \in \mathbb{R})$ is built as a solution of the variational problem:

$$\min_{\mathbf{v} \in \mathcal{R}^{|\mathbb{R}|}} \iint_{\mathbf{r}=(x,y)\in\mathbb{R}} \left(\gamma \left\| \frac{\partial \mathbf{v}(\mathbf{r})}{\partial \mathbf{r}} \right\|^2 + |\nabla_{\mathbf{g}}(x,y)|^2 \, |\mathbf{v}(x,y) - \nabla_{\mathbf{g}}(x,y)|^2 \right) dx\, dy$$

where γ is a weight of the squared norm of the matrix of the vector GVF derivatives:

$$\left\| \frac{\partial \mathbf{v}(\mathbf{r})}{\partial \mathbf{r}} \right\|^2 = \left(\frac{\partial v_x(x,y)}{\partial x} \right)^2 + \left(\frac{\partial v_x(x,y)}{\partial y} \right)^2 + \left(\frac{\partial v_y(x,y)}{\partial x} \right)^2 + \left(\frac{\partial v_y(x,y)}{\partial y} \right)^2$$

Equivalently, the GVF solves the system of the Euler's partial differential equations (PDE):

$$w \left(\frac{\partial^2 v_x(x,y)}{\partial x^2} + \frac{\partial^2 v_x(x,y)}{\partial y^2} \right) = |\nabla_{\mathbf{g}}(x,y)|^2 \left(v_x(x,y) - \frac{\partial g(x,y)}{\partial x} \right)$$

$$w \left(\frac{\partial^2 v_y(x,y)}{\partial x^2} + \frac{\partial^2 v_y(x,y)}{\partial y^2} \right) = |\nabla_{\mathbf{g}}(x,y)|^2 \left(v_y(x,y) - \frac{\partial g(x,y)}{\partial y} \right)$$

The GVF elements $\mathbf{v}(x,y)$ are close to the image gradients $\nabla_{\mathbf{g}}(x,y)$ having the large magnitudes, $|\nabla_{\mathbf{g}}(x,y)|$, but are decreasing still slowly even if the gradients become abruptly equal or close to zero. However, much higher computational complexity of such external forces decelerates the evolution too much, comparing to other options.

A *geometric deformable model*, unlike the explicit parametric ones, represents an evolving curve or surface implicitly, via a level set function, $W(\mathbf{r})$, which is equal to zero, $W(\mathbf{b}) = 0$ for the model points, $\mathbf{b} \in \mathcal{B}$, and is negative, $W(\mathbf{r}) < 0$, or positive, $W(\mathbf{r}) > 0$, inside or outside the evolving boundary, respectively. One of the most common level set functions on an image lattice provides the signed distances from any lattice site, $\mathbf{r} \in \mathbb{R}$, to the model:

$$W(\mathbf{r}) = \mathrm{sign}(\mathbf{r} \,|\, \mathcal{B}) \left[\min_{\mathbf{b} \in \mathcal{B}} |\mathbf{r} - \mathbf{b}| \right] \tag{2.32}$$

where $\text{sign}(\mathbf{r}\,|\,\mathcal{B}) = -1$ or 1 if the site, $\mathbf{r}$, is inside or outside the boundary specified with zero level set, $\mathcal{B} = \{\mathbf{b} : \mathbf{b} \in \mathbb{R}; W(\mathbf{b}) = 0\}$.

The deformable models have two main advantages: (1) the closed goal boundary in spite of its possible gaps in the image to be segmented and (2) the inbuilt smoothness constraints making the evolution robust to image noise and spurious edges. At the same time, performance of these models depends on proper initialization, efficiency of the energy minimization, and adequate selection of the force functions and energy functionals. In spite of good segmentation results for objects of relatively simple shapes, image segmentation using most of these models is much slower than other segmentation techniques, and the model evolution frequently stops well before approaching a complicated object boundary with concavities. Most of the models typically require human interaction to be placed initially near the goal objects and choose appropriate settings of the forces; are unsuitable for scattered objects, and cannot handle shapes under large geometric deformations. This manual initialization by drawing a close curve interactively near the desired object boundary hinders the use of such models in many medical analysis applications. Nonetheless, the most recent models are considerably less sensitive to their initialization. Many other drawbacks, such as, e.g., poor convergence to concave boundaries, are partially alleviated by selecting the adequate forces and adapting the model topology.

2.5 Bibliographic and Historical Notes

Stochastic modeling and optimal inference by energy minimization are for a long time among the most efficient and successful image processing and analysis tools [29,30,185,297]. Diversity and complexity of natural medical images turned their modeling, analysis, and synthesis into an extremely complex and computational expensive problem, even if only spatially homogeneous or piecewise homogeneous textures are under consideration. Nonetheless, significant achievements in solving the problem have been obtained through the use of MGRF models of grayscale, color, or multi-band images and/or region maps that label areas-of-interest in the images. Stochastic image modeling, originated in the late 1970s [64,134] is under active development up to the present.

The widespread development and use of MGRFs, a.k.a. MRF with GPD, for describing shapes and appearances of objects in 2D, 3D, and 4D images had begun after seminal papers by J. Besag [24] and D. Geman and S. Geman [113]. Their works brought attention of the computer vision and image analysis community to easiness, flexibility, and sound theoretical and practical benefits of MGRFs, stemming from the famous proof by J. M. Hammersley and P. Clifford (Theorem 2.1, Section 2.2.1) that each

GPD is factored over a system of maximal cliques of an undirected interaction graph. The graph links conditionally dependent (called interacting,
or neighboring) lattice sites, and every its maximal clique supports a factor,
being a strictly positive and bounded, but otherwise arbitrary function of signal configurations (co-occurrences or patterns) on the clique. Each potential
function in the GPD is the logarithm of the corresponding factor. The MGRF
modeling, which associates probabilities of images and/or region maps of
objects with negated Gibbs energies, obtained by summing the potentials
over the entire interaction graph, reduces the optimal statistical inference to
minimizing the Gibbs energy functionals.

However, learning, or identification of a MGRF model remains a challenging problem that eludes satisfactory solutions in a majority of cases [185],
especially, when both the characteristic shapes and Gibbs potential functions
of much higher, than second-order signal co-occurrences on cliques are to be
estimated. The cardinality $|\mathbb{Q}^K|$ of the co-occurrences space $\mathbb{Q}^K$ is growing
exponentially with the clique order K, whereas the amount of the training
data is universally limited to n; $n \geq 1$ (at most, a few) training images, e.g.,
to $n|\mathbb{R}|$ training co-occurrences; $n|\mathbb{R}| \ll |\mathbb{Q}|^K$. That the learning has to rely
mostly on a very small, in the statistical sense, training sample sets tight
limits on the choice of feasible models.

Stochastic modeling in medical applications typically relies on human
anatomy, suggesting that most of the close neighbors of every pixel or voxel
belong to the same object. Nonetheless, realistic appearances and shapes
of typical medical objects rarely depend on only the nearest or arbitrarily
prescribed dependencies. Also, the actual dependencies are too intricate to
be selected by hand. To simplify learning in these cases, the clique shapes
and potentials typically presume translation or translation-rotation invariant, yielding spatially repetitive fixed neighborhoods of the lattice sites,
although in reality characteristic signal patterns are not necessarily repetitive
under translations and rotations [137,252]. The assumed repetitiveness of
signal statistics makes the learned translation or translation-rotation invariant MGRF a "homogeneous" model of the actually inhomogeneous training
images. Fortunately, the obtained homogeneous description is often quite
sufficient for detecting, aligning, segmenting, or classifying natural medical
images of certain types.

The generative MGRF models show considerable promise in both
synthesizing spatially homogeneous textures and segmenting piecewise-
homogeneous textures [30,185,297]. The MGRF to model and synthesize
essentially inhomogeneous textured objects, being typical in medical image
analysis, can be learned only if a sufficiently large stack of training
images with co-aligned objects-of-interest is available. Fortunately, often
such images can be aligned, segmented, and analyzed using much less
detailed knowledge about their signal relationships.

Typical unsupervised segmentation of complex images where objects-of-
interest are associated with dominant modes of marginals of pixel/voxel

signals (intensities, colors, etc.) assumes in many cases only piecewise homogeneity, i.e., conditionally independent signals with different marginals in each region (class). Then an image is initially segmented by approximating its mixed empirical marginal with a mixture of class-wise signal marginals and classifying individual pixels or voxels [29,76]. Such very rough, but fast classification is of obvious interest for automated screening of medical CT images, MRI, and MRA.

Even if the conditional IRF models of regions to be segmented are justified, the obtained maps are inaccurate because signal ranges for different classes of objects generally overlap. In the simplest case, regions obtained after the pixel/voxel-wise classification are refined using their MGRF priors. The images and region maps are specified with a joint MGRF combining an unconditional model of interdependent region labels and a conditional model of independent signals in each region [34,185,297], and the initial map is iteratively refined using the joint model.

An alternative *marked point process* (MPP), or the MRF on a stochastic lattice, describes an image as a random pattern formed by multiple texture elements (texels) of given types on an almost arbitrary background. The MPP uses a library of basic elementary shapes of foreground texels and a set of probabilistic rules, which constrain location, pose, scale, and contrast of these elements with respect to each other and an image background. The rules guide mutual placements of the texels under arbitrary translations, rotations and varying scales, but strongly limited overlaps. The texel locations are specified by a joint distribution or density of individual spatial or spatiotemporal sites, r. Sampling of the sites not only changes locations of the current texels, but also may exclude some of them and/or add some new ones. The related joint and conditional distributions control the sampling from the texel library for each site, the admissible adjacency and overlaps between the texels, and their admissible geometric and perceptive deviations.

Comparing to the MRF models, the MPP introduces a more extended notion of homogeneity (repetitiveness), permitting substantial translational, rotational, and scaling variations of geometric shapes, as well as perceptual (contrast/offset) deviations of visual appearances of individual texels. Generally, each texel can be produced also by a hierarchical stochastic process, starting from the most primitive elements and having flexible rules of building each higher-level element from mutually arranged lower-level ones. For example, Figure 2.9 shows a small library of texels in a specific multi-MPP model and obtained with this model descriptions of various 2D textures, being homogeneous in the extended sense. The texels have simple geometric shapes and uniform appearance in contrast to the nearest background.

The MPP-based modeling with a library of basic elements (e.g., in Reference 178) is rarely used at present in the medical image analysis due to considerable difficulties in learning such elements and probabilistic rules guiding their mutual arrangements and unessential geometric and perceptive

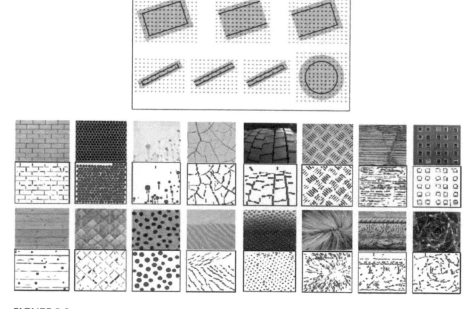

FIGURE 2.9
Texel shape library and texel-based texture descriptions. (Adapted from F. Lafarge, G. Gimel'farb, and X. Descombes. *IEEE Transactions on Pattern Analysis and Machine Intelligence,* 32(9):1597–1609, 2010.)

transformations in the images. Learning frameworks for the MGRFs are more feasible. For example, an easy-learnable generic second-order MGRF, introduced in References 116 and 117 and then developed further in References 119 and 121, allows for learning both multiple arbitrary pairwise interactions and potential functions of signal co-occurrences from the training data on the basis of the approximate MLE of the potentials, generalized in Section 2.3.1. Approximate partial energies are instrumental for selecting, among a large pool of candidates, the clique families describing the most characteristic close- and, if any, long-range interactions. The initial potentials for the learned clique families could be further refined by stochastic approximation of the exact MLEs [117].

2.5.1 Shape Modeling with Deformable Models

Parametric active contours [158,309], introduced first by Kass et al. [158], and geometric models (e.g., [48,234,235]) gave rise to a host of successful edge detection, image segmentation, shape modeling, and visual tracking techniques. Typical external forces designed in Reference 158 led an active contour toward step edges in a grayscale image. However, the original iterative energy minimization in Reference 158, based on a closed-form solution of Eulerian differential equations to specify the desired minimum, was unstable and usually trapped by the local minima. Also, it was difficult to constrain the force or entire energy functions. These shortcomings of the minimization process were addressed and partly overcome in Reference 5 by representing a snake with a linked chain of control points and using discrete dynamic programming to minimize the total energy of the chain. Due to rigid constraints on the energy function, the minimization became more stable, but its control parameters had to be adjusted very carefully, and the process remained too time consuming. Another advanced greedy algorithm proposed in Reference 303 had linear time complexity both by the number of control points and the number of their neighbors taken into account for energy minimization. It was more stable and simultaneously more than an order of magnitude faster than the earlier techniques. Even at present, it is one of the fastest snake-evolving algorithms.

The sensitivity of the standard parametric deformable models to initialization can be considerably decreased [47,200,309]. Other drawbacks, such as poor convergence to concave boundaries, can be partially alleviated through modifying the external force, e.g., by involving the pressure force [309]. Implicit representation instead of explicit parametrization results in adaptive model topology [47,200]. An extensive review on deformable models in medical image analysis can be found in Reference 204.

The geometric models based on the level set paradigm [227] account for no prior shape constraints and search for strong signal discontinuities (grayscale or color edges) in an image. But the evolution, guided only by edges and general continuity and curvature limitations, fails when a goal object is not clearly distinguishable from its background. More accurate results, at the expense of a considerably reduced speed, were obtained by restricting grayscale or color patterns within an evolving surface [51]. Nonetheless, the accuracy remained poor without the prior knowledge of goal shapes. At present, the 2D/3D parametric and geometric deformable models with shape and/or appearance priors learned from a training set of manually segmented images are of the main interest.

The snake model was extended to color regions in Reference 219, as well as it was segmented for better flexibility in Reference 308. The latter snake could handle region boundaries with relatively sharp corners due to recursive split-and-merge procedure of dividing each boundary into segments to approximate them locally. An alternative flexible snake in Reference 299 was based on a B-spline curve representation and multiple-stage energy minimization.

To closely approach a realistic boundary with concavities, the snake evolution was controlled in Reference 126 by simulated annealing, which in principle can eventually reach the global minimum of the energy and escape local traps. Actually, as shown in Reference 35, simulated annealing typically stops very far from the global minimum, whereas alternative min-cut/max-flow graph algorithms guarantee a close approximation of geodesic 2D contours or 3D surfaces having the minimum global energy under an arbitrary set of boundary conditions in the Riemannian geometric metrics. But these minimization processes are quite slow. A faster precise boundary approximation in Reference 309 introduces a GVF as a new external force, and a bidirectional snake in Reference 235 combines the geodesic contour and the GVF. Although both the parametric and geometric deformable models are widely used for image segmentation, in many applications, especially in the medical image analysis, the accurate segmentation with these models is a challenging problem due to noisy or low-contrast 2D/3D images with fuzzy boundaries between the objects (such as anatomical structures) and their background; similar shapes of the objects with different visual appearances, and discontinuous boundaries due to occlusions or similar visual appearances of adjacent parts of the objects of different shapes [289]. Prior knowledge about the goal shape and/or visual appearance helps in resolving such problems.

Initial attempts to involve the prior knowledge of shape were built upon the edges. The evolving curve was described in References 62 and 240 with shape and pose parameters of a set of points matched to strong image gradients. The PCA was used to model variations from an average shape with linear combinations of eigenvectors. More efficient results were obtained by learning the priors from a training set of manually segmented images of goal objects. To segment 3D medical images, a deformable coarse-to-fine medial shape representation was used in References 243 and 283. A level set-based energy function guiding the evolution was augmented in Reference 271 with special terms attracting to more likely shapes specified with the PCA of a training set of objects. A flexible shape prior describes the variability of shapes with a linear combination of characteristic elements (eigenvectors) built by the PCA of the training samples. A family of shape priors with a Gaussian probability distribution was built in Reference 233 from the training data and used then in an external energy component of a level set framework.

The most advanced level set-based geometric model in Reference 289 (see also Section 8.4) represented the desired shape with a linear combination of weighted signed 2D distance maps for a set of mutually aligned training images. The weights were estimated by minimizing a mutual information based dissimilarity score. A multidimensional Gaussian distribution of the weights was used in Reference 311 for describing the shape variations. However, high dimensionality of the distance map space hinders the PCA, and to simplify the model, only a few top-rank principal components were typically included to form their linear combinations. Furthermore, the signed distance space is not closed with respect to linear operations. Therefore, the zero level contour of a linear combination may define either an impossible shape, or a shape that differs much from the training shapes. This is the main limitation of shape modeling with a linear combination of the signed distance maps.

Explicit visual appearance priors are rarely used to guide the evolving deformable models. Typically, the guidance assumes a simple predefined appearance model of significantly different signal means and/or variances for an object and its background [289]. Learning the appearance model looks more promising, although at present in this case the segmentation accounts usually for only pixel/voxel-wise classification [184]. An alternative non-parametric warping of a deformable goal surface to an anatomic atlas in Reference 155 transfers contours from the atlas to the goal volume. However, because of no shape prior, the transferred boundaries need not approach the actual ones. Speed of the iterative warping of an entire image volume is also quite low.

To overcome these problems, joint probabilistic shape-appearance prior models for the goal objects was learned in Reference 234 using the PCA. Simplified variants of such priors have been successful in segmenting complex 3D medical images [160], however, the segmentation was very slow due to setting up model-to-image pixel/voxel-wise correspondences at each step. To accelerate the process, probabilistic appearance priors accounting for only low-order signal statistics were introduced in References 109 and 311. The variability of goal shapes and image signals was modeled in Reference 311 with a joint Gaussian distribution, optimization algorithms having been developed to estimate the model parameters from a set of training images and conduct the Bayesian MAP segmentation. A special level-set function, such that its zero level produces approximately the goal shapes, was derived in Reference 109, as well as empirical marginal signal distributions for the training objects were used as the appearance prior to guide aligning a deformable model to an image to be segmented.

3

IRF Models: Estimating Marginals

The simplest exponential families of distributions—independent random fields (IRF) of signals at the lattice sites—are of limited descriptive power, but due easy learning is often used in image analysis. An IRF is specified by site-wise marginal probability distributions of discrete signals or densities of continuous signals (called *marginals*), which generally vary over the lattice: $\mathbf{P_r} = (P_\mathbf{r}(q) : q \in \mathbb{Q}); \sum_{q \in \mathbb{Q}} P_\mathbf{r}(q) = 1; \mathbf{r} \in \mathbb{R}$. The probability or density $P_{\text{irf}}(\mathbf{g})$ of an image $\mathbf{g}$ sampled from the IRF is factored over the lattice sites:

$$P_{\text{irf}}(\mathbf{g}) = \prod_{\mathbf{r} \in \mathbb{R}} P_\mathbf{r}(g(\mathbf{r})) \equiv \prod_{\mathbf{r} \in \mathbb{R}} \prod_{q \in \mathbb{Q}} [P_\mathbf{r}(q)]^{\delta(g(\mathbf{r}) - q)}$$

$$\equiv \exp \left(\sum_{\mathbf{r} \in \mathbb{R}} \sum_{q \in \mathbb{Q}} \ln P_\mathbf{r}(q) \delta(g(\mathbf{r}) - q) \right) \qquad (3.1)$$

3.1 Basic Independent Random Fields

An *inhomogeneous* IRF with different site-wise marginals has the simplest sufficient statistics, namely, just the signal $g(\mathbf{r})$ at each site, or $|\mathbb{Q}|$ its binary indicators: $\mathbf{S}_{\text{irf}}(\mathbf{g}) = [(\delta(g(\mathbf{r}) - q) : q \in \mathbb{Q}) ; \mathbf{r} \in \mathbb{R}]^\mathsf{T}$. The negated log-marginals, $\mathbf{V}_{\text{irf}} = [- \ln P_\mathbf{r}(q) : q \in \mathbb{Q}; \mathbf{r} \in \mathbb{R}]^\mathsf{T}$, act as weights, or potentials in Equation 2.17: $P_{\text{irf}}(\mathbf{g}) = \exp \left(-\mathbf{V}_{\text{irf}}^\mathsf{T} \mathbf{S}_{\text{irf}}(\mathbf{g}) \right)$.

Piecewise-homogeneous, or *piecewise-uniform IRFs*, which are very popular in image modeling, split the lattice into several regions $\mathbb{R}_l$; $l \in \mathbb{L} = \{1, \dots, L\}$; $L \geq 2$, characterized each by own conditional marginal $\mathbf{P}_l = (P(q \mid l) : q \in \mathbb{Q}); \sum_{q \in \mathbb{Q}} P(q \mid l) = 1$. The regions may be discontinuous and cover the entire lattice with no overlaps: $\bigcup_{l \in \mathbb{L}} \mathbb{R}_l = \mathbb{R}; \mathbb{R}_l \cap \mathbb{R}_k = \emptyset$ if $l \neq k$; $l, k \in \mathbb{L}$.

A conditional piecewise-homogeneous IRF presumes that all images $\mathbf{g} \in \mathbb{G}$ have the same region map $\mathbf{m} = [m(\mathbf{r}) : \mathbf{r} \in \mathbb{R}; m(\mathbf{r}) \in \mathbb{L}]$, so that $\mathbb{R}_l = \{\mathbf{r} : \mathbf{r} \in \mathbb{R}; m(\mathbf{r}) = l\} \subset \mathbb{R}$. The conditional probability or density of an image $\mathbf{g}$, given a map $\mathbf{m}$:

$$P_{\text{irf}}(\mathbf{g} \mid \mathbf{m}) = \prod_{\mathbf{r} \in \mathbb{R}} P(g(\mathbf{r}) \mid m(\mathbf{r})) = \prod_{l \in \mathbb{L}} \prod_{q \in \mathbb{Q}} [P(q \mid l)]^{h_{\mathbf{g}:\mathbf{m}}(q \mid l)} \qquad (3.2)$$

and the log-likelihood of the marginal $\mathbf{P} = \{P_l : l \in \mathbb{L}\}$, given an image $\mathbf{g}$ and a map $\mathbf{m}$:

$$\ell(\mathbf{P} \mid \mathbf{g}, \mathbf{m}) = \sum_{l \in \mathbb{L}} \sum_{q \in Q} h_{\mathbf{g}:\mathbf{m}}(q \mid l) \ln P(q \mid l) \tag{3.3}$$

depend on the conditional signal histogram, or the nonnormalized empirical conditional probability distribution of signals $\mathbf{h}(\mathbf{g} \mid \mathbf{m}) = [h_{\mathbf{g}:\mathbf{m}}(q \mid l) : q \in Q; l \in \mathbb{L}]$. Each component

$$h_{\mathbf{g}:\mathbf{m}}(q \mid l) = \sum_{\mathbf{r} \in \mathbb{R}} \delta(m(\mathbf{r}) - l)\delta(g(\mathbf{r}) - q) \equiv |\mathbb{R}_{q:l}|$$

of this histogram is the cardinality of the subset $\mathbb{R}_{q:l} = \{\mathbf{r} : m(\mathbf{r}) = l; g(\mathbf{r}) = q\} \subseteq \mathbb{R}_l$ of sites supporting the signal q in the region $\mathbb{R}_l$:

$$\sum_{q \in Q} |\mathbb{R}_{q:l}| = |\mathbb{R}_l| \quad \text{and} \quad \sum_{l \in \mathbb{L}} |\mathbb{R}_l| = |\mathbb{R}|$$

Given a map $\mathbf{m}$, the components $h_{\mathbf{g}:\mathbf{m}}(q \mid l)$ are scalar sufficient statistics of the image $\mathbf{g}$ with the potentials $V_{q:l} = -\log P(q \mid l)$ in Equation 2.17.

A *homogeneous (uniform)* IRF has the marginal $\mathbf{P} = (P(q) : q \in Q)$; $\sum_{q \in Q} P(q) = 1$, at all lattice sites. The probability or density of the image $\mathbf{g}$:

$$P_{\text{irf}}(\mathbf{g}) = \prod_{\mathbf{r} \in \mathbb{R}} P(g(\mathbf{r})) = \prod_{q \in Q} P(q)^{h_{\mathbf{g}}(q)} \tag{3.4}$$

and the log-likelihood of the marginal $\mathbf{P}$, given an image $\mathbf{g}$:

$$\ell(\mathbf{P}) = \sum_{q \in Q} h_{\mathbf{g}}(q) \ln P(q) \tag{3.5}$$

depend on the signal histogram:

$$\mathbf{h}(\mathbf{g}) = \left[h_{\mathbf{g}}(q) = \sum_{\mathbf{r} \in \mathbb{R}} \delta(g(\mathbf{r}) - q) : q \in Q; \; \sum_{q \in Q} h_{\mathbf{g}}(q) = |\mathbb{R}| \right]^{\mathsf{T}} \tag{3.6}$$

or, what is the same, on the normalized histogram (the empirical marginal):

$$P_{\text{emp}}(\mathbf{g}) = \frac{1}{|\mathbb{R}|} \mathbf{h}(\mathbf{g}) = \left[P_{\text{emp}:\mathbf{g}}(q) = \frac{1}{|\mathbb{R}|} h_{\mathbf{g}}(q) : q \in Q; \; \sum_{q \in Q} P_{\text{emp}:\mathbf{g}}(q) = 1 \right]^{\mathsf{T}} \tag{3.7}$$

Independent component analysis (ICA) linearly transforms vectors $\mathbf{g}$, sampled from an arbitrary random field, into the vectors $\mathbf{f} = \mathbf{T}_{\text{ica}}\mathbf{g}$, where $\mathbf{T}_{\text{ica}}$ is a full-rank $|\mathbb{R}| \times |\mathbb{R}|$ matrix. The elements $f_{\mathbf{r}}; \mathbf{r} \in \mathbb{R}$, of the transformed vectors should have non-Gaussian probability distributions and be statistically independent. The degree of their independence is measured quantitatively, using, e.g., their mutual information (MI) or higher than second-order moments, like the fourth-order kurtosis. In principle, the ICA can be helpful for reducing to the IRF models more common image analysis cases where spatial or spatiotemporal signal dependencies have to be taken into account because objects of different classes cannot be separated by only pixel- or voxel-wise signal properties.

More conventional linear *whitening*, or *sphering* transformation $\mathbf{f} = \mathbf{T}_{\mathbf{w}}\mathbf{g}$, that decorrelates the vectors $\mathbf{g}$, i.e., converts their second-order moment (the covariance matrix) into the diagonal unit matrix, is generally insufficient for approaching statistical independence. It leads to the IRF only if the vectors $\mathbf{g}$ have a multivariate Gaussian density. However, the whitening is frequently used for data preprocessing before applying the ICA.

3.2 Supervised and Unsupervised Learning

Supervised learning. A homogeneous IRF with the same unknown marginal, $\mathbf{P}$, at all the lattice sites, $\mathbf{r} \in \mathbb{R}$, can be easily learned from a single training image $\mathbf{g}$, which is large enough to obtain from its histogram of Equation 3.6 the accurate classical MLE or Bayesian estimates (if $|\mathbb{R}| \gg |\mathbb{Q}|$) of probabilities of discrete signals:

$$\text{for each } q \in \mathbb{Q} \quad \widetilde{P}(q) = \begin{cases} \dfrac{1}{|\mathbb{R}|} h_{\mathbf{g}}(q) & = P_{\text{emp}:\mathbf{g}}(q) & \text{MLE} \\[3ex] \dfrac{1}{|\mathbb{R}| + |\mathbb{Q}|}\left(h_{\mathbf{g}}(q) + 1\right) = \dfrac{P_{\text{emp}:\mathbf{g}}(q) + \frac{1}{|\mathbb{R}|}}{1 + \frac{|\mathbb{Q}|}{|\mathbb{R}|}} & \text{Bayesian} \end{cases}$$

$$(3.8)$$

or Parzen window-based estimates of probability densities of continuous signals. Otherwise the required histogram $\mathbf{h}$ has to be collected over two or more training images, sampled from the same homogeneous IRF under consideration.

The MLE $\widetilde{\mathbf{P}}$ of the marginal in Equation 3.8 comes from the constrained maximization of the log-likelihood of Equation 3.5 using the Lagrangian $\mathcal{L}(\mathbf{P}) = \ell(\mathbf{P}) - \lambda(\mathbf{P}^{\mathsf{T}}\mathbf{u} - 1)$ where $\mathbf{u} = [u_q = 1 : q \in \mathbb{Q}]^{\mathsf{T}}$ is the vector of unit components: $\frac{d}{d\mathbf{P}}\mathcal{L}(\mathbf{P}) = 0$, i.e.,

$$\frac{\partial \mathcal{L}(\mathbf{P})}{\partial P(q)} = \frac{h_{\mathbf{g}}(q)}{P(q)} - \lambda = 0 \text{ implying } \widetilde{P}(q) = \frac{h_{\mathbf{g}}(q)}{\sum\limits_{q \in \mathbb{Q}} h_{\mathbf{g}}(q)} = \frac{1}{|\mathbb{R}|} h_{\mathbf{g}}(q) \quad (3.9)$$

The Bayesian estimate of Equation 3.8, which assumes the uniform prior distribution of probabilities $P(q); q \in Q$, has a more complicated derivation.

Given a true region map $\mathbf{m}$ with sufficiently large regions $\mathbb{R}_l; l \in \mathbb{L}$, a piecewise-homogeneous IRF can be learned accurately from a single training image $\mathbf{g}$, too, using the like ML or Bayesian estimates of the conditional marginals:

for each $q \in Q$ and $l \in \mathbb{L}$

$$
\tilde{P}(q \mid l) = \begin{cases} \dfrac{h_{\mathbf{g}:\mathbf{m}}(q \mid l)}{|\mathbb{R}_l|} = P_{\mathrm{emp}:\mathbf{g}:\mathbf{m}}(q \mid l) & \text{MLE} \\[3mm] \dfrac{h_{\mathbf{g}:\mathbf{m}}(q \mid l) + 1}{|\mathbb{R}_l| + |Q|} = \dfrac{P_{\mathrm{emp}:\mathbf{g}:\mathbf{m}}(q \mid l) + \frac{1}{|\mathbb{R}_l|}}{1 + \frac{|Q|}{|\mathbb{R}_l|}} & \text{Bayesian} \end{cases}
$$

Otherwise, the conditional histogram for learning a piecewise-homogeneous IRF or the site-wise signal histograms for learning an inhomogeneous IRF are to be built from more than one training image with the known region map(s) or from a large collection of co-aligned images, respectively. The inhomogeneous IRF of binary object/background labels, having been learned from the co-aligned maps for multiple objects of the same type, provides a so-called *stochastic shape portrait* for image alignment.

Unsupervised learning of a piecewise-homogeneous IRF in a majority of applications, including medical image analysis, assumes that each image $\mathbf{g}$ is sampled from a homogeneous IRF, characterized by a mixture of the unknown conditional marginals:

$$
P(q) = \sum_{l \in \mathbb{L}} w_l P(q \mid l); \quad \sum_{l \in \mathbb{L}} w_l = 1 \tag{3.10}
$$

where the mixing weights, $w_l; l \in \mathbb{L}$, are prior probabilities, or *priors* of regions. Then the probability or density of the image $\mathbf{g}$ is specified by Equation 3.4 with the marginal of Equation 3.10:

$$
P_{\mathrm{irf}}(\mathbf{g}) = \prod_{r \in \mathbb{R}} P(g(\mathbf{r})) = \prod_{q \in Q} P(q)^{h_{\mathbf{g}}(q)} = \prod_{q \in Q} \left(\sum_{l \in \mathbb{L}} w_l P(q \mid l) \right)^{h_{\mathbf{g}}(q)} \tag{3.11}
$$

The learning pursues the goal of estimating both the hidden region map, $\mathbf{m}$, and the regional IRF models, namely, the conditional marginals, $\mathbf{P}_l$, and priors, w_l, for all the regions from a given image $\mathbf{g}$ and its empirical marginal $\mathbf{P}_{\mathrm{emp}}(\mathbf{g})$ of Equation 3.7.

Figure 3.1 exemplifies a bimodal empirical marginal for two objects—lungs and surrounding tissues—on a chest CT slice. To classify image signals for segmenting the lattice into the regions occupied by objects-of-interest, the mixture of Equation 3.10 is to be separated into its components, $(w_l, \mathbf{P}_l)$; $l \in \mathbb{L}$. The separation, which is often called *mixture identification*, usually

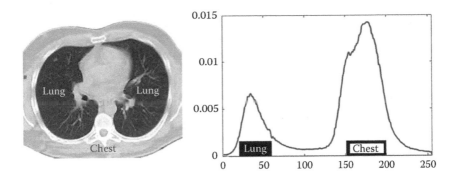

FIGURE 3.1
Bimodal empirical marginal for a CT chest slice (signals in the range of $[0, 255]$).

presumes that each object is associated with a prominent peak, or mode of the histogram in Equation 3.6 and is modeled by an individual mixture component.

Each scalar component $P(q \mid l)$ of the conditional marginal $\mathbf{P}_l$ is often either a continuous Gaussian (normal) probability density $\varphi(q; \theta_l)$ depending on two parameters $\theta_l = (\mu_l, \sigma_l)$ – the mean μ_l and the standard deviation σ_l, having the analytical MLE:

$$P(q \mid l) = \varphi(q; \theta_l) = \frac{1}{\sigma_l \sqrt{2\pi}} \exp\left(-\frac{(q - \mu_l)^2}{2\sigma_l^2}\right) ; \quad \int_{-\infty}^{\infty} \varphi(v; \theta_l) dv = 1 \quad (3.12)$$

or a discrete probability $\psi(q; \theta_l)$; $\sum_{q=0}^{Q-1} \psi(q; \theta_l) = 1$, called the *discrete Gaussian* (DG):

$$P(q \mid l) = \psi(q; \theta_l) = \begin{cases} \Phi(0.5; \theta_l) & \text{if } q = 0 \\ \Phi(q + 0.5; \theta_l) - \Phi(q - 0.5; \theta_l) & \text{if } q = 1, \ldots, Q - 2 \\ 1 - \Phi(Q - 1.5) & \text{if } q = Q - 1 \end{cases}$$

$$(3.13)$$

where $Q = |\mathbb{Q}|$ is the cardinality of the signal set $\mathbb{Q} = \{0, 1, \ldots, Q - 1\}$ and $\Phi(q; \theta_l) = \int_{-\infty}^{q} \varphi_l(v; \theta_l) dv$ is the cumulative Gaussian probability function.

The models in Equations 3.2 or 3.11, approximating unknown actual IRFs, can be combined into the core $\Psi(\mathbf{g})$ of a general-case exponential family in Equation 2.24. It helps to build new exponential families, which restrict the core by imposing additional constraints on multivariate signal statistics and reduce to the core for zero potentials $\mathbf{V} = 0$.

3.2.1 Parametric Versus Nonparametric Models

The unknown signal probability distributions or densities are learned from training data using either parametric or nonparametric models. Neither type prevails universally in all the cases. Nonparametric modeling of an arbitrary marginal, e.g., with the Parzen windows, increases its accuracy after observing more training data, but at the expense of the growing computational complexity of the model. The unsupervised separation of a nonparametric mixture into individual components associated with different objects-of-interest presents significant difficulties (if possible at all). Thus, the nonparametric models suit better the supervised identification of the mixed empirical data.

Conversely, the complexity of a parametric model is generally fixed or limited in growth, but its accuracy may not improve with more empirical data. The identification of the parametric models is more feasible due to the possible ML or Bayesian estimation of parameters and priors for the mixture components. In particular, an empirical marginal for a piecewise-homogeneous IRF can be separated into a mixture of the parametric components, one per individual class of objects, by using powerful *Expectation-Maximization* (EM) techniques.

3.3 Expectation-Maximization to Identify Mixtures

Finding the MLE of parameters $\Theta = [(\theta_l, w_l) : l \in \mathbb{L}]$ of the Gaussian mixture model in Equations 3.10 and 3.12 is computationally infeasible because the log-likelihood function is too complicated:

$$\ell(\Theta) = \ln\left(\prod_{\mathbf{r}\in\mathbb{R}} P(g(\mathbf{r}))\right) = \sum_{\mathbf{r}\in\mathbb{R}} \ln\left(\sum_{l\in\mathbb{L}} w_l\varphi(g(\mathbf{r});\theta_l)\right) \tag{3.14}$$

Adding region indicators, $\delta = (\delta_{\mathbf{r}:l} : \mathbf{r} \in \mathbb{R}; l \in \mathbb{L})$, such that $\delta_{\mathbf{r}:l} = 1$ if the site $\mathbf{r} \in \mathbb{R}_l$ and $\delta_{\mathbf{r}:l} = 0$ otherwise, to the model considerably simplifies its log-likelihood:

$$\begin{aligned}
\ell(\Theta;\delta) &= \sum_{\mathbf{r}\in\mathbb{R}}\sum_{l\in\mathbb{L}} \delta_{\mathbf{r}:l} \ln\left(w_l\varphi(g(\mathbf{r});\theta_l)\right) \\
&= \sum_{l\in\mathbb{L}} \ln(w_l) \sum_{\mathbf{r}\in\mathbb{R}} \delta_{\mathbf{r}:l} + \sum_{l\in\mathbb{L}}\sum_{\mathbf{r}\in\mathbb{R}} \delta_{\mathbf{r}:l} \ln\left(\varphi(g(\mathbf{r});\theta_l)\right) \\
&\equiv \sum_{l\in\mathbb{L}} \ln(w_l)|\mathbb{R}_l| + \sum_{l\in\mathbb{L}}\sum_{\mathbf{r}\in\mathbb{R}_l} \ln\left(\varphi(g(\mathbf{r});\theta_l)\right)
\end{aligned} \tag{3.15}$$

where $|\mathbb{R}_l| = \sum\limits_{r \in \mathbb{R}} \delta_{r:l}$, and provides the conventional MLE of the parameters Θ for $l \in \mathbb{L}$:

$$
\begin{aligned}
\tilde{w}_l &= \frac{1}{|\mathbb{R}|} \sum_{r \in \mathbb{R}} \delta_{r:l} &&\equiv \frac{|\mathbb{R}_l|}{|\mathbb{R}|} \\
\tilde{\mu}_l &= \frac{1}{|\mathbb{R}_l|} \sum_{r \in \mathbb{R}} \delta_{r:l} g(r) &&\equiv \frac{1}{|\mathbb{R}_l|} \sum_{r \in \mathbb{R}_l} g(r) &&(3.16) \\
\tilde{\sigma}_l^2 &= \frac{1}{|\mathbb{R}_l|} \sum_{r \in \mathbb{R}} \delta_{r:l}(g(r) - \tilde{\mu}_l)^2 &&\equiv \frac{1}{|\mathbb{R}_l|} \sum_{r \in \mathbb{R}_l} (g(r) - \tilde{\mu}_l)^2
\end{aligned}
$$

The EM framework replaces the actually unobserved, or latent indicators δ with their computable expectations, $\gamma = (\gamma_{r:l} : l \in \mathbb{L}; r \in \mathbb{R})$, called *responsibilities*, so that the expected log-likelihood remains a relatively simple function of the mixture parameters:

$$
\ell_\gamma(\Theta) = \sum_{l \in \mathbb{L}} \ln(w_l) \sum_{r \in \mathbb{R}} \gamma_{r:l} + \sum_{l \in \mathbb{L}} \sum_{r \in \mathbb{R}} \gamma_{r:l} \ln \left(\varphi(g(r); \theta_l) \right) \qquad (3.17)
$$

The responsibility $\gamma_{r:l}$ of the mixture component $l \in \mathbb{L}$ for the signal $g(r)$ in the site $r \in \mathbb{R}$ is the expected value of the indicator $\delta_{r:l}$, i.e., the probability of the unit indicator, $\delta_{r:l} = 1$, for the signal $g(r)$, given the estimated mixture parameters $\tilde{\Theta}$:

$$
\gamma_{r:l} = \frac{\tilde{w}_l \varphi(g(r); \tilde{\theta}_l)}{\sum\limits_{k \in \mathbb{L}} \tilde{w}_k \varphi(g(r); \tilde{\theta}_k)}; \ 0 \le \gamma_{r:l} \le 1; \ \sum_{l \in \mathbb{L}} \gamma_{r:l} = 1; \ l \in \mathbb{L}; \ r \in \mathbb{R} \qquad (3.18)
$$

The responsibilities are not the posterior region probabilities, given the signals, because the true mixture parameters may differ from their estimates.

Because the responsibilities of Equation 3.18 depend on the signals, rather than their positions in the lattice, the EM-based mixture identification requires only the signal histogram $\mathbf{h}(\mathbf{g})$ of Equation 3.6 or the closely related empirical marginal $\mathbf{P}_{emp}(\mathbf{g})$ of Equation 3.7. Then the responsibilities $\gamma = (\gamma_{q:l} : q \in \mathbb{Q}; l \in \mathbb{L})$ of the mixture components for the signal values and the MLE of the mixture parameters are, respectively,

$$
\gamma_{q:l} = \frac{\tilde{w}_l \varphi(q; \tilde{\theta}_l)}{\sum\limits_{k \in \mathbb{L}} \tilde{w}_k \varphi(q; \tilde{\theta}_k)}; \ q \in \mathbb{Q}; \ l \in \mathbb{L} \qquad (3.19)
$$

and

$$\widetilde{w}_l = \frac{1}{|\mathbb{R}|} \sum_{q \in Q} \gamma_{q:l} h_{\mathbf{g}}(q) \qquad\qquad \equiv \sum_{q \in Q} \gamma_{q:l} P_{\text{emp}:\mathbf{g}}(q);$$

$$\widetilde{\mu}_l = \frac{1}{\widetilde{w}_l |\mathbb{R}|} \sum_{\mathbf{q} \in Q} \gamma_{q:l} q h_{\mathbf{g}}(q) \qquad \equiv \frac{1}{\widetilde{w}_l} \sum_{q \in Q} \gamma_{q:l} q P_{\text{emp}:\mathbf{g}}(q);$$

$$\widetilde{\sigma}_l^2 = \frac{1}{\widetilde{w}_l |\mathbb{R}|} \sum_{q \in Q} \gamma_{q:l} (q - \widetilde{\mu}_l)^2 h_{\mathbf{g}}(q) \equiv \frac{1}{\widetilde{w}_l} \sum_{q \in Q} \gamma_{q:l} (q - \widetilde{\mu}_l)^2 P_{\text{emp}:\mathbf{g}}(q); \;\; l \in \mathbb{L}$$

$$(3.20)$$

The EM Algorithm 1 iteratively updates the responsibilities and the parameter estimates, starting from the initial parameter values, which were found manually or by a separate initialization procedure.

In medical image analysis the number $L = |\mathbb{L}|$ of the prominent modes in the empirical marginal, which relate to objects-of-interest and should be modeled with a Gaussian mixture of Equations 3.10 and 3.12, is mostly specified manually. In some cases it can be also estimated from the available data by searching for a top-quality mixture in line with one or another statistical quality measure, such as, e.g., the Akaike information criterion (AIC).

Algorithm 1 EM Identification of a Gaussian Mixture

---

1. *Initialization* $[t = 0]$:
   Guess the initial parameter estimates $\widetilde{\Theta}_0$, i.e., the parameters $\widetilde{\theta}_{l:0} = (\widetilde{\mu}_{l:0}, \widetilde{\sigma}_{l:0})$ of the Gaussian components $\varphi(q; \widetilde{\theta}_{l:0})$, and their priors $\widetilde{w}_{l:0}; l \in \mathbb{L}$.

2. *Iteration* $[t \leftarrow t + 1]$:
   until the parameters and priors converge to (almost) stationary values, **repeat**:

   a. *E-step:* Find the new responsibilities γ_{t+1} using the estimates $\widetilde{\Theta}_t$ of Equation 3.19:

   $$\gamma_{q:l:t+1} = \frac{\widetilde{w}_{l:t} \varphi(q; \widetilde{\theta}_{l:t})}{\sum_{k \in \mathbb{L}} \widetilde{w}_{k:t} \varphi(q; \widetilde{\theta}_{k:t})}; \;\; q \in Q; \;\; l \in \mathbb{L}$$

   b. *M-step:* Find the new MLE Θ_{t+1} of Equation 3.20 using the responsibilities found for weighting the signal values:

   $$\widetilde{w}_{l:t+1} = \sum_{q \in Q} \gamma_{q:l:t+1} P_{\text{emp}:\mathbf{g}}(q); \;\; \widetilde{\mu}_{l:t+1} = \frac{1}{\widetilde{w}_{l:t+1}} \sum_{q \in Q} \gamma_{q:l:t+1} q P_{\text{emp}:\mathbf{g}}(q);$$

   $$\widetilde{\sigma}_{l:t+1}^2 = \frac{1}{\widetilde{w}_{l:t+1}} \sum_{q \in Q} \gamma_{q:l:t+1} (q - \widetilde{\mu}_{l:t+1})^2 P_{\text{emp}:\mathbf{g}}(q); \;\; l \in \mathbb{L}$$

The AIC compares numerical values of the expected log-likelihoods of the k-component mixtures for $k = 1, 2, \ldots, K$, in order to find the optimal number, $L < K$, of the components. However, such a search meets often with difficulties in the cases when the adjacent modes to be resolved resemble a single expanded peak or a small object associated with a lower mode has to be found in the presence of a number of the higher alternatives.

3.4 Gaussian Linear Combinations Versus Mixtures

Conventional Gaussian mixtures may not be accurate in modeling empirical marginals of complex shape, such as, e.g., in Figure 3.2, even if the number of terms in the mixture is much larger than the number of the actual dominant modes, associated with objects-of-interest. One of possible reasons is that conditional marginals $\mathbf{P}_l = (P(q \,|\, l) : q \in \mathbb{Q})$ in a mixture of Equation 3.10 are strictly nonnegative: $P(q \,|\, l) \geq 0$ for all $l \in \mathbb{L}$ and $q \in \mathbb{Q}$. If this requirement is relaxed, the empirical marginal $\mathbf{P}_{\text{emp}}(\mathbf{g})$ can be approximated more precisely with a *pseudo-marginal* $\mathbf{P}(\mathbf{g})$, mixing conditional pseudo-marginals $\mathbf{P}_l$, one per object-of-interest (a specific image region or a class of signals).

Each pseudo-marginal (either the unconditional, $P(q)$, or the conditional one, $P(q \,|\, l)$) is a linear combination of sign-alternate (i.e., positive and negative) unimodal terms—Gaussians of Equation 3.12 or DG of Equation 3.13. It is abbreviated below linear combination of Gaussians (LCG) or linear combination of DGs (LCDG), respectively. The conventional Gaussian mixture may remain inaccurate even after including much more Gaussians, than the actual number of the dominant modes, as in Figure 3.2. Contrastingly, the LCG or

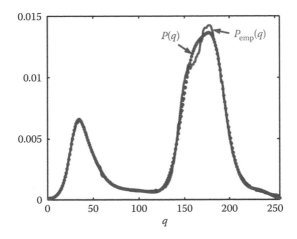

FIGURE 3.2
Modeling the bimodal empirical marginal with a mixture of 12 Gaussians.

LCDG can approximate accurately not only the dominant modes of intricate shapes, but also transitions between the modes. Thus, such models facilitate precise restoration of both the main body and tails of each conditional object model from the empirical marginal $\mathbf{P}_{emp}(\mathbf{g})$.

The LCG or LCDG for each conditional pseudo-marginal $\mathbf{P}_l; l \in \mathbb{L}$, consists of a single positive dominant term, associated with the relevant prominent mode of the empirical marginal, and a number of sign-alternate subordinate terms, accounting for deviations between the dominant term and an arbitrary-shaped conditional object model to be estimated from the empirical data:

$$P(q\,|\,l) = \varphi(q; \theta_{p:l}) + \sum_{i=1}^{N_{p:l}} \upsilon_{p:l:i} f(q; \theta_{p:l:i}) - \sum_{j=1}^{N_{n:l}} \upsilon_{n:l:j} f(q; \theta_{n:l:j}) \qquad (3.21)$$

where $f(q; \ldots)$ stands for the Gaussian $\varphi(q; \ldots)$ or DG $\psi(q; \ldots)$ and $N_{p:l}$ and $N_{n:l}$ are the numbers of the positive and negative subordinate terms with the parameters $(\theta_{p:l:i}, \upsilon_{p:l:i}); i = 1, \ldots, N_{p:l}$, and $(\theta_{n:l:j}, \upsilon_{n:l:j}); j = 1, \ldots, N_{n:l}$, respectively. The strictly positive weighting factors $\upsilon_{p:l:i}; i = 1, \ldots, N_{p:l}$, and $\upsilon_{n:l:j}; j = 1, \ldots, N_{p:j}$ in Equation 3.21 meet the obvious normalizing condition:

$$\sum_{i=1}^{N_{p,l}} \upsilon_{p:l:i} - \sum_{j=1}^{N_{n,k}} \upsilon_{n,k,l} = 0 \qquad (3.22)$$

ensuring the integral unit value $\int_{q \in \mathbb{Q}} P(q\,|\,l) dq = 1$ for the continuous signals in the LCG or $\sum_{q \in \mathbb{Q}} P(q\,|\,l) = 1$ for the discrete signals in the LCDG.

The LCG or LCDG for the pseudo-marginal $\mathbf{P}$, combining the conditional models of Equation 3.21 in accord with the mixture of Equation 3.10, adds to the mixture of $|\mathbb{L}|$ dominant terms the linear combination of the $N_p = \sum_{l \in \mathbb{L}} N_{p:l}$ positive and $N_n = \sum_{l \in \mathbb{L}} N_{n:l}$ negative subordinate terms:

$$P(q) = \sum_{l \in \mathbb{L}} w_l P(q\,|\,l) = \sum_{l \in \mathbb{L}} w_l f(q; \theta_{p:l}) + \sum_{i=1}^{N_p} w_{p:i} f(q; \theta_{p:l})$$

$$- \sum_{j=1}^{N_n} w_{n:j} f(q; \theta_{n:j}); \qquad (3.23)$$

$$\sum_{l \in \mathbb{L}} w_l = 1, \quad \text{and} \quad \sum_{i=1}^{N_p} w_{p:i} - \sum_{i=j}^{N_n} w_{n:j} = 0$$

In contrast to a probability mixture, the weights of the unimodal terms bear no relation to priors, and the model is not, strictly speaking, a true probability density or distribution function. The probability densities (distributions) form a proper subset of all possible LCGs (LCDGs), such that the weights

---

Algorithm 2 EM-Based Identification of an LCG/LCDG Model

---

1. *Sequential model initialization* (Algorithm 3) with the conventional EM Algorithm 1.

2. *Model refinement* (Algorithm 4) with the EM, accounting for the sign-alternate terms.

3. *Model partitioning* into the object models of Equation 3.21, one per the dominant mode.

---

and parameters of the terms are constrained to guarantee the nonnegative densities (probabilities) of signals over the whole signal range Q.

Accounting for such constraints makes the model identification computationally infeasible because the weights and parameters become strongly interdependent. If the interdependence is ignored and the resulting constraints on the weights and parameters are of no concern, the model of Equation 3.23 approximates better than the dominant mixture alone not only main bodies of the dominant empirical modes, but also transitions between the modes.

More accurate approximation of the mixed empirical marginal $\mathbf{P}_{emp}(\mathbf{g})$ is important in many applications of the IRFs to medical image analysis where signal models for individual objects have to be restored to within a limited signal range and used for signal classification. The model parameters are estimated using an EM-based Algorithm 2. Such model identification by maximizing the data likelihood tends to keep the pseudo-marginal of Equation 3.23 positive for all signal values that appear in the log-likelihood function. After the pseudo-marginal is identified from the empirical marginal, it is partitioned into the individual conditional pseudo-marginals of Equation 3.21 for each object $l \in \mathbb{L}$ by associating the subordinate terms with the dominant ones to minimize the total classification error.

3.4.1 Sequential Initialization of an LCG/LCDG Model

To ensure convergence to the most likely model parameters, the search for a pseudo-marginal, approximating accurately a given multimodal empirical marginal, should start in a vicinity of the log-likelihood maximum. An initial approximation toward this goal is obtained by identifying first a mixture of a given number of the dominant terms with the conventional EM Algorithm 1 and searching then for the subordinate terms representing deviations between the empirical marginal and the dominant mixture. Algorithm 3 for sequential initialization estimates both the weights and parameters of the individual terms in the starting pseudo-marginal model including the number of the subordinate components. Each dominant mode of the empirical marginal is roughly approximated with a single term, and its deviations are described by the other terms of the LCG or LCDG in Equation 3.23.

Algorithm 3 Sequential LCG/LCDG Model Initialization

---

1. Using the conventional EM (Algorithm 1), approximate a given empirical marginal, $\mathbf{P}_{emp}(\mathbf{g}) = [P_{emp:g}(q) : q \in \mathbb{Q}]$, with a mixture $\mathbf{P}_L = [P_L(q) : q \in \mathbb{Q}]$ of a given number L of the dominant terms.

2. Split the deviations $\mathbf{\Delta}_L = \mathbf{P}_{emp}(\mathbf{g}) - \mathbf{P}_L$, where $\mathbf{\Delta}_L = [\Delta_L(q) = P_{emp:g}(q) - P_L(q) : q \in \mathbb{Q}]$, into the absolute positive, $\mathbf{\Delta}_p = [\Delta_p(q) = \max\{\Delta(q), 0\} : q \in \mathbb{Q}]$, and negative part, $\mathbf{\Delta}_n = [\Delta_n(q) = \max\{-\Delta(q), 0\} : q \in \mathbb{Q}]$, such that $\Delta(q) = \Delta_p(q) - \Delta_n(q)$.

3. Compute the deviation scale: $\zeta = \int_{-\infty}^{\infty} \Delta_p(q) dq \equiv \int_{-\infty}^{\infty} \Delta_n(q) dq$ for the LCG or $\zeta = \sum_{q \in \mathbb{Q}} \Delta_p(q) \equiv \sum_{q \in \mathbb{Q}} \Delta_n(q)$ for the LCDG.

4. **If** ζ is below a preset accuracy threshold, **then** terminate and return the mixture $\mathbf{P}_L$ as the initial LCG or LCDG model $\mathbf{P}^{[0]}$; i.e., $\mathbf{P}^{[0]} = \mathbf{P}_L$.

5. **Else** build the subordinate LCG or LCDG:

   a. Consider the scaled-up absolute deviations $\frac{1}{\zeta}\mathbf{\Delta}_p$ and $\frac{1}{\zeta}\mathbf{\Delta}_n$ as two new "empirical marginals."

   b. Use iteratively the conventional EM (Algorithm 1) to find sizes N_p and N_n of the Gaussian or DG mixtures, $\mathbf{P}_p$ and $\mathbf{P}_n$, respectively, which closely approximate the scaled-up deviations.

      i. The size of each mixture corresponds to the minimum of the integral absolute error between the scaled-up absolute positive or negative deviation and its mixture model, the number of the mixture terms increasing sequentially by one, while the error decreases.

      ii. Due to multiple local optima, such a search may be repeated several times with different initial parameter values in order to select the best approximation.

   c. Scale down the subordinate mixtures $\mathbf{P}_p$ and $\mathbf{P}_n$, i.e., scale down the mixing weights of their components.

   d. Add the scaled-down sign-alternate difference of the subordinate mixtures to the dominant mixture to build the goal pseudo-marginal, $\mathbf{P} = \mathbf{P}_L + \zeta(\mathbf{P}_p - \mathbf{P}_n)$, with $L + N_p + N_n$ unimodal terms.

6. Terminate and return the pseudo-marginal $\mathbf{P}$ as the initial LCG or LCDG model $\mathbf{P}^{[0]}$; i.e., $\mathbf{P}^{[0]} = \mathbf{P}$.

Because the EM algorithm converges to a local maximum of the log-likelihood, each stage of the initialization may be repeated several times, starting from different parameter values, in order to choose the best approximation. Moreover, in principle, the initialization can be iterated to approximate more closely the residual absolute deviations between the empirical marginal $\mathbf{P}_{\text{emp}}(\mathbf{g})$ and the current initial LCG or LCDG $\mathbf{P}$. Because each new term added to the latter model impacts all the values $P(q)$, the iterations should terminate when the approximation quality begins to decrease. But the single-iteration initialization with Algorithm 3 is mostly sufficient in practice.

One of the possible quality measures is the Levy distance, $\rho(\mathbf{F}, \mathbf{F}_{\text{emp}}(\mathbf{g}))$, between the cumulative probability distributions $\mathbf{F} = [F(q) : q \in \mathbf{Q}]$ and $\mathbf{F}_{\text{emp}}(\mathbf{g}) = [F_{\text{emp}:\mathbf{g}}(q) : q \in \mathbf{Q}]$ for the estimated pseudo-marginal $\mathbf{P}$ and the empirical marginal $\mathbf{P}_{\text{emp}}(\mathbf{g})$, respectively:

$$\rho(\mathbf{F}, \mathbf{F}_{\text{emp}}(\mathbf{g})) = \min_{\alpha > 0; q \in \mathbf{Q}} \{F(q - \alpha) - \alpha \leq F_{\text{emp}:\mathbf{g}}(q) \leq F(q + \alpha) + \alpha\}$$

(3.24)

where $F(q) = \sum_{\kappa \in \mathbf{Q}; \kappa \leq q} P(\kappa)$ and $F_{\text{emp}:\mathbf{g}}(q) = \sum_{\kappa \in \mathbf{Q}; \kappa \leq q} P_{\text{emp}:\mathbf{g}}(\kappa)$. The probability models provably converge to each other when their Levy distance tends to zero.

3.4.2 Refinement of an LCG/LCDG Model

The found by Algorithm 3 pseudo-marginal $\mathbf{P}^{[0]}$ of Equation 3.23 with L dominant and $N_{\text{p}} + N_{\text{n}}$ subordinate terms and starting parameter values

$$\tilde{\boldsymbol{\Theta}}_0 = \left[\tilde{w}_{l:0}; \tilde{\boldsymbol{\theta}}_{i:0}; \ l \in \mathbb{L} = \{1, \ldots, L\}; \ \tilde{w}_{\text{p}:i:0}; \tilde{\boldsymbol{\theta}}_{\text{p}:i:0}; \ i = 1, \ldots, N_{\text{p}};\right.$$

$$\left.\tilde{w}_{\text{n}:j:0}; \tilde{\boldsymbol{\theta}}_{\text{n}:j:0}; \ j = 1, \ldots, N_{\text{n}}\right]$$

is assumed strictly positive for all values $q \in \mathbf{Q}$. This condition usually holds in practice in the limited range $\mathbf{Q}$ of signals, e.g., for the discrete signals $\mathbf{Q} = \{0, 1, \ldots, Q - 1\}$ and LCDG models. The initial numbers of the terms do not change during the model refinement, searching for the closest local maximum of the log-likelihood of the empirical data.

Let $\mathbf{P}^{[t]} = \left[P_{[t]}(q) : q \in \mathbf{Q}\right]$ denote the pseudo-marginal in Equation 3.23 at iteration t of refinement, i.e.,

$$P_{[t]}(q) = \sum_{l=1}^{L} \tilde{w}_{l:t} f\left(q; \tilde{\boldsymbol{\theta}}_{l:t}\right) + \sum_{i=1}^{N_{\text{p}}} \tilde{w}_{\text{p}:i:t} f\left(q; \tilde{\boldsymbol{\theta}}_{\text{p}:i:t}\right) - \sum_{j=1}^{N_{\text{n}}} \tilde{w}_{\text{n}:j:t} f\left(q; \tilde{\boldsymbol{\theta}}_{\text{n}:j:t}\right);$$

$$\sum_{l=1}^{L} \tilde{w}_{l:t} + \sum_{i=1}^{N_{\text{p}}} \tilde{w}_{\text{p}:i:t} - \sum_{j=1}^{N_{\text{n}}} \tilde{w}_{\text{n}:j:t} = 1 \qquad (3.25)$$

The conventional EM framework, such as, e.g., Algorithm 1, can be equivalently conceived as a block relaxation, or "maximization–maximization" process of finding the responsibilities, given the parameters of the terms, and the parameters, given the responsibilities, by conditional maximization of the log-likelihood function. Such a view of the model identification is more reasonable for the pseudo-marginals. Given the current estimates $\widetilde{\Theta}_t$ of the model parameters, the new responsibilities of each term for the signal values:

$$
\gamma_{q:l:t+1} = \frac{\widetilde{w}_{i:t} f\left(q; \widetilde{\Theta}_{l:t}\right)}{P^{[t]}(q)}; \qquad q \in Q; \quad l \in \mathbb{L}
$$

$$
\gamma_{q:p:i:t+1} = \frac{\widetilde{w}_{p:i:t} f\left(q; \widetilde{\Theta}_{p:i:t}\right)}{P^{[t]}(q)}; \qquad q \in Q; \quad i = 1,\ldots,N_p \qquad (3.26)
$$

$$
\gamma_{q:n:j:t+1} = \frac{\widetilde{w}_{p:j:t} f\left(q; \widetilde{\Theta}_{n:j:t}\right)}{P^{[t]}(q)}; \qquad q \in Q; \quad j = 1,\ldots,N_n
$$

result in the next parameter estimates:

$$
\widetilde{\Theta}_{t+1} = \left[\left(\widetilde{w}_{l:t+1} = \sum_{q\in Q} \gamma_{q:l:t+1} P_{\text{emp}}(q); \; \widetilde{\mu}_{l:t+1} = \frac{1}{\widetilde{w}_{l:t+1}} \sum_{q\in Q} \gamma_{q:l:t+1} q P_{\text{emp}}(q); \right. \right.
$$

$$
\widetilde{\sigma}^2_{l:t+1} = \frac{1}{\widetilde{w}_{l:t+1}} \sum_{q\in Q} \gamma_{q:l:t+1} (q - \widetilde{\mu}_{l:t+1})^2 P_{\text{emp}}(q) \left. \right) ; \; l \in \mathbb{L};
$$

$$
\left(\widetilde{w}_{p:i:t+1} = \sum_{q\in Q} \gamma_{q:p:i:t+1} P_{\text{emp}}(q); \; \widetilde{\mu}_{p:i:t+1} = \frac{1}{\widetilde{w}_{p:i:t+1}} \sum_{q\in Q} \gamma_{q:p:i:t+1} q P_{\text{emp}}(q); \right.
$$

$$
\widetilde{\sigma}^2_{p:i:t+1} = \frac{1}{\widetilde{w}_{p:i:t+1}} \sum_{q\in Q} \gamma_{q:p:i:t+1} (q - \widetilde{\mu}_{p:i:t+1})^2 P_{\text{emp}}(q) \left. \right) ; \; i = 1,\ldots,N_p;
$$

$$
\left(\widetilde{w}_{n:j:t+1} = \sum_{q\in Q} \gamma_{q:n:j:t+1} P_{\text{emp}}(q); \; \widetilde{\mu}_{n:j:t+1} = \frac{1}{\widetilde{w}_{n:j:t+1}} \sum_{q\in Q} \gamma_{q:n:j:t+1} q P_{\text{emp}}(q); \right.
$$

$$
\left. \widetilde{\sigma}^2_{n:j:t+1} = \frac{1}{\widetilde{w}_{n:j:t+1}} \sum_{q\in Q} \gamma_{q:n:j:t+1} (q - \widetilde{\mu}_{n:j:t+1})^2 P_{\text{emp}}(q) \right) ; \; j = 1,\ldots,N_n \left. \right]
$$

$$(3.27)$$

The EM refinement (Algorithm 4) of the pseudo-marginal is valid until the responsibilities of Equation 3.26 are strictly positive, and the initial model $P^{[0]}$ should comply with this constraint. The iterations are terminated when the log-likelihood begins to decrease, e.g., in Figure 3.3. Generally, the initial pseudo-marginal has to closely approximate the empirical marginal, because if the initialization is incorrect, the refinement may diverge from the very beginning. Experiments have shown the refinement notably decreases an initially large Levy distance between the empirical marginal and its estimated LCG or LCDG model. A few examples of such modeling are sketched in Section 3.5.

Algorithm 4 Refinement of an Initial LCG/LCDG

---

1. *Initialization* $t = 0$: the pseudo-marginal $\mathbf{P}^{[0]}$ with the parameter estimates $\widetilde{\Theta}_0$ after the model initialization stage of Algorithm 2.

2. *Iteration* $t \leftarrow t + 1$ – **while** the likelihood $\ell(\mathbf{P}^{[t]}) = \sum_{q \in Q} P_{\text{emp}}(q)$ $\ln\left(P_{[t]}(q)\right)$ increases, **repeat**:

   a. Find the responsibilities γ_{t+1} using the parameter estimates $\widetilde{\Theta}_t$ of Equation 3.26.

   b. Find the parameter estimates $\widetilde{\Theta}_{t+1}$ of Equation 3.27 using the responsibilities γ_{t+1} found.

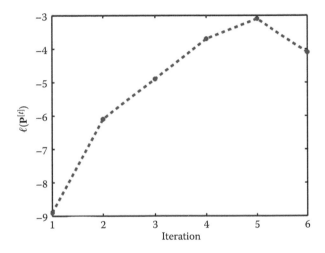

FIGURE 3.3
Changes of the log-likelihood during the LCG refinement.

The accuracy of the parameter estimates for an LCG may be affected by tails of the continuous Gaussian density beyond the limited range $[0, Q - 1]$ of the observed signals, i.e., by areas from $-\infty$ to 0 and from $Q - 1$ to ∞ shaded in Figure 3.4. The LCDGs overcome this drawback, but at the expense of only the approximate parameter MLE of Equation 3.27.

3.4.3 Model Partitioning by Allocating Subordinate Terms

The refined pseudo-marginal $\mathbf{P}$ is then partitioned into the L object models $\mathbf{P}(l) = [P(q \mid l) : q \in Q]$, one per dominant mode $l \in \mathbb{L}$. Each subordinate term is allocated to the conditional object models as to decrease the expected signal classification error due to overlaps between the adjacent models.

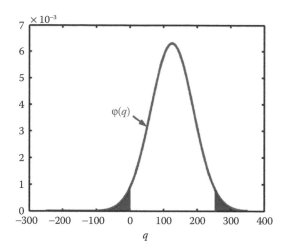

FIGURE 3.4
Gaussian density limitations in modeling image signals.

To illustrate this process, let us consider a bimodal pseudo-marginal with the two dominant terms, having the means μ_1 and μ_2; $0 \leq \mu_1 < \mu_2 \leq Q - 1$. After ordering all subordinate terms by their means, the means smaller than μ_1 and greater than μ_2 allocate the terms to the object model 1 and 2, respectively. When the means are in the range $[\mu_1, \mu_2]$, the terms are associated with the objects by simple thresholding that allocates the terms with the means below the threshold, τ, to the object 1 and minimizes overlaps between the models:

$$\tau = \arg\min_{\kappa \in Q} \left\{ \sum_{q=0}^{\kappa-1} P(q\,|\,2) + \sum_{q=\kappa}^{Q-1} P(q\,|\,1) \right\} \qquad (3.28)$$

The like successive thresholding with obvious modifications can associate the subordinate terms with each of the L dominant modes; $L > 2$.

3.5 Pseudo-Marginals in Medical Image Analysis

Robustness and feasibility of modeling empirical marginals with pseudo-marginals (LCGs or LCDGs), rather than mixtures of strictly positive Gaussians or DGs, are illustrated below on a synthetic image in Figure 3.5 and five real medical images: axial slices of human chest and head by spiral-scan low-dose computer tomography (LDCT); computed tomographic angiography (CTA); time-of-flight magnetic resonance angiography (TOF-MRA); phase-contrast MRA (PC-MRA), and magnetic resonance imaging (MRI).

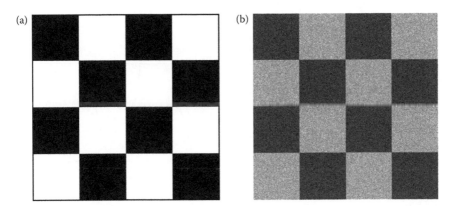

FIGURE 3.5
The checkerboard region map (a) and a checkerboard image (b) sampled from a conditional IRF specified by the pseudo-marginals in Figure 3.6.

The TOF-MRA, PC-MRA, and MRI slices were acquired with the Picker 1.5T Edge MRI scanner. The 512 × 512 PC-MRA, CTA, LDCT and TOF-MRA, and 256 × 256 MRI slices were 1 mm thick. The 8 mm thick LDCT slices were built every 4 mm with the scanning pitch of 1.5 mm. In these examples the number of objects (dominant modes) in the empirical marginal is specified by the user, whereas all other model parameters are estimated by the EM-based algorithms described in Section 3.4.

3.5.1 Synthetic Checkerboard Images

Synthetic checkerboard images, sampled form the known conditional IRF of image intensities (gray levels) in the range of $Q = \{0, 1, \ldots, 255\}$, permit comparing the estimated pseudo-marginals and true pseudo-marginals, including the numbers, means, variances, and mixing weights of their positive and negative terms. Each true region (object) model in this particular case consists of one dominant and four subordinate terms shown in Figure 3.6a. Bimodal grayscale samples, such as in Figure 3.5b, are generated in accord with the region map in Figure 3.5a and the true pseudo-marginals in Figure 3.6b, which are strictly positive for all signal values $q \in Q = [0, 255]$.

Figure 3.7 illustrates Steps 1 through 3 of Algorithm 3. The initial pseudo-marginal to estimate the empirical marginal $\mathbf{P}_{emp}$ for the simulated checkerboard image in Figure 3.5b is built by finding first the dominant mixture $\mathbf{P}_2$ of Gaussians or DGs representing the two objects—the darker and brighter regions of the checkerboard. Then the sign-alternate deviations of the dominant mixture from the empirical marginal are converted into the absolute deviations and scaled up to build the additional subordinate pseudo-marginals because of the large Levy distance of 0.1; see

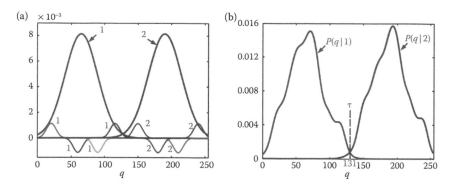

FIGURE 3.6
Dominant and sign-alternate subordinate terms (a) of the true pseudo-marginals (b) for the dark (1) and bright (2) regions of the checkerboard map in Figure 3.5 supporting the conditional IRF specified by these pseudo-marginals.

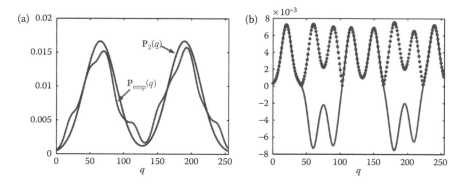

FIGURE 3.7
The empirical marginal $\mathbf{P}_{emp}$ vs. the dominant mixture $\mathbf{P}_2$ (a) and their sign-alternate and absolute mutual deviations (b).

Equation 3.24, indicating a considerable mismatch between the empirical marginal $\mathbf{P}_{emp}$ and the dominant mixture $\mathbf{P}_2$.

The search for the number of the subordinate terms by minimizing the approximation error at Step 5 of Algorithm 3 (the eight terms in this example), and the initial pseudo-marginal after the subordinate linear positive and negative terms are, respectively, added to and subtracted from the dominant mixture at Step 5d are illustrated in Figure 3.8.

Figure 3.9 shows the initial estimated pseudo-marginal $\mathbf{P}^{[0]}$ and its partitioning into the conditional object models. The separation threshold $\tau = 126$ in Equation 3.28 gives the minimum misclassification rate of 0.0028 between these two objects. In this case the subordinate terms 3–6 and 7–10 relate to the objects 1 and 2, respectively.

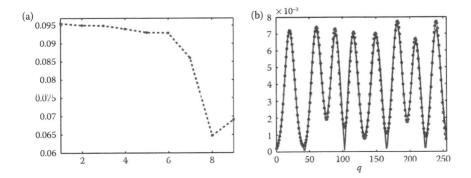

FIGURE 3.8
Mixture modeling of the scaled absolute deviation in Figure 3.7: the approximation error (a) in function of the number n of the mixed terms and the most accurate mixture (b) giving the eight subordinate terms of the initial pseudo-marginal.

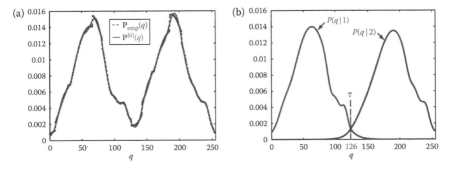

FIGURE 3.9
The empirical marginal $\mathbf{P}_{emp}$ for the image in Figure 3.5b vs. the initial estimated pseudo-marginal $\mathbf{P}^{[0]}$ with 10 terms (a) and the initial conditional object models (b) for the separation threshold $\tau = 126$ giving the minimum misclassification rate of 0.0028.

Figure 3.10 shows the final pseudo-marginal $\mathbf{P}$ after refining the initial model $\mathbf{P}^{[0]}$ in Figure 3.9a by Algorithm 4; the estimated 10 terms of this linear combination, and the final conditional object models obtained by partitioning the final pseudo-marginal using the refined separation threshold $\tau = 131$. The initial Levy distance of 0.1 between the empirical marginal and its bimodal mixture model is decreased to 0.0012 for the obtained pseudo-marginal, indicating the close approximation. Successive changes of the log-likelihood of Equation 3.17 during the refining iterations are shown in Figure 3.10b. The first five iterations increase the log-likelihood of Equation 3.17 from -9.0 to -2.1. Then the refinement is terminated since the log-likelihood begins to decrease. The final estimated parameters for both the LCG and LCDG based pseudo-marginals are listed in Table 3.1.

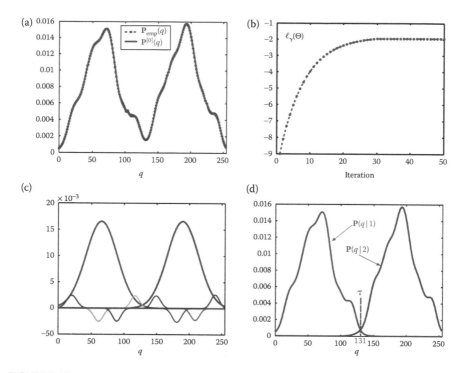

FIGURE 3.10

The refined pseudo-marginal (a); changes (b) of its log-likelihood at successive iterations of Algorithm 4; the final two dominant and eight subordinate terms (c); and the final conditional object models (d) for the separation threshold $\tau = 131$.

TABLE 3.1

True and Estimated Parameters of the Dominant (1, 2) and Positive (p) and Negative (n) Subordinate Terms (3–10) of the LCDG and LCG Models of the Empirical Marginal for the Synthetic Image

Term	p/n	Weight			Mean			Variance		
		True	LCDG	LCG	True	LCDG	LCG	True	LCDG	LCG
1	p	0.500	0.506	0.530	65.0	64.8	66.3	600	590	581
2	p	0.500	0.494	0.470	190.0	189.7	185.1	600	582	581
3	p	0.020	0.021	0.017	20.0	19.1	21.8	50	55	59
4	n	0.020	0.019	0.020	60.0	62.1	63.4	50	57	61
5	n	0.020	0.017	0.020	90.0	89.2	92.1	50	49	45
6	p	0.020	0.020	0.019	116.0	117.0	119.1	50	47	42
7	p	0.020	0.019	0.023	150.0	151.1	148.2	50	51	54
8	n	0.020	0.019	0.018	180.0	179.9	182.0	50	48	53
9	n	0.020	0.021	0.023	210.0	207.1	207.0	50	52	57
10	p	0.020	0.021	0.018	240.0	243.0	244.6	50	49	56

3.5.2 Modeling Lungs on Spiral LDCT Chest Scans

The pseudo-marginals appear promising to model LDCT chest images, having two dominant regions-of-interest and thus bimodal empirical marginals. The darker regions correspond primarily to lung tissues, whereas the brighter regions relate for the most part to surrounding, or background anatomical structures, such as the chest, ribs, and liver. Accurate estimation of the conditional pseudo-marginals for both the regions by applying Algorithm 2 to the empirical marginal is an efficient preliminary step for separating the lung region from its background.

The empirical marginal for the LDCT chest slice in Figure 3.11 together with the bimodal dominant mixture of the DGs and the scaled deviations between these two marginals are shown in Figure 3.12. The notable mismatch between the marginals is evident from the large Levy distance of 0.09 in Equation 3.24.

The search for a mixture approximating the absolute deviations with the minimum error and the found mixture of 10 subordinate DGs are illustrated in Figure 3.13.

The threshold $\tau = 108$ for the estimated initial pseudo-marginal in Figure 3.14 yields the minimum misclassification rate of 0.004 between the conditional LCDG models of the lung and chest tissues in Equation 3.28.

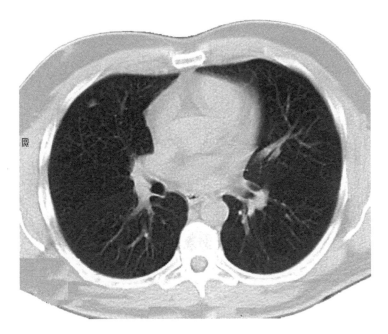

FIGURE 3.11
Typical chest slice produced by spiral LDCT scanning.

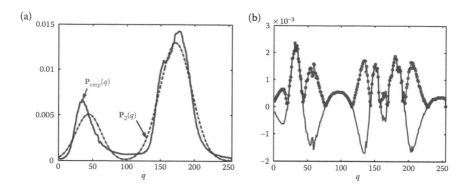

FIGURE 3.12
The empirical marginal $\mathbf{P}_{emp}$ vs. the dominant mixture $\mathbf{P}_2$ (a) and their sign-alternate and absolute mutual deviations (b).

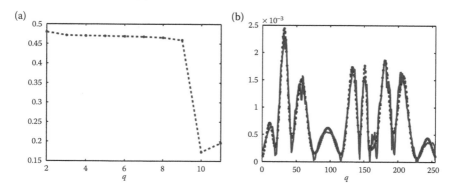

FIGURE 3.13
Mixture modeling of the scaled absolute deviation in Figure 3.12: the approximation error (a) in function of the number of the mixed terms and the most accurate mixture (b) providing the 10 subordinate terms of the initial pseudo-marginal.

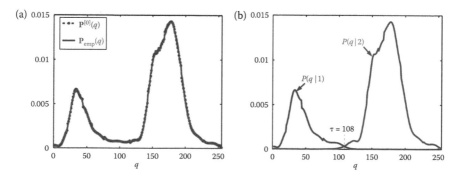

FIGURE 3.14
The empirical marginal $\mathbf{P}_{emp}$ for the LDCT slice in Figure 3.11 vs. the initial estimated pseudo-marginal $\mathbf{P}^{[0]}$ with the 12 terms (a) and the conditional pseudo-marginals (b) for the lung and chest tissues in Figure 3.11 giving the minimum misclassification rate of 0.004 for the separation threshold $\tau = 108$.

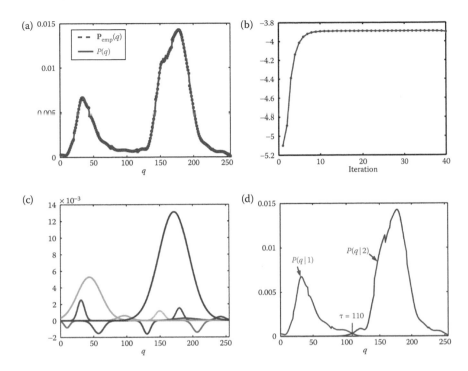

FIGURE 3.15
The refined pseudo-marginal (a); changes (b) of its log-likelihood at successive iterations of Algorithm 4; the final two dominant and 10 subordinate terms (c); and the final conditional object models (d) for the separation threshold $\tau = 110$.

Here, the first four and the remaining six subordinate DGs correspond to the lung and chest models, respectively, shown in Figure 3.14.

The final pseudo-marginal, which is obtained after refining the initial model in Figure 3.14 with Algorithm 4 is shown in Figure 3.15, its dominant DGs having the following parameters: $w_1 = 0.26$; $\mu_1 = 40.8$; $\sigma_1^2 = 242.5$; $w_2 = 0.74$; $\mu_2 = 170.8$; and $\sigma_2^2 = 296.0$. The decreased to 0.02 Levy distance indicates that the estimated final pseudo-marginal more closely approximates the empirical marginal.

Figure 3.15 shows also how the log-likelihood is changing during the model refinement. Also, Figure 3.15 demonstrates the 12 terms of the final LCDG and the final conditional models of each object for the best separation threshold $\tau = 110$. The refinement increases the log-likelihood of Equation 3.17 from -5.1 to -3.9 for the first few iterations, but then this process terminates since the log-likelihood begins to decrease.

The advantages of the LCG and LCDG models as pseudo-marginals are highlighted by approximating the same empirical marginal with a conventional mixture of 12 positive Gaussians. The resulted mixture model in Figure 3.16 has more than three times higher misclassification rate (0.013),

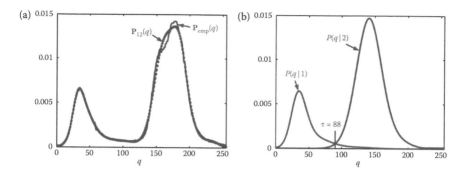

FIGURE 3.16
Modeling the empirical marginal $\mathbf{P}_{emp}$ for the lung and chest tissues in Figure 3.11 with a conventional mixture $\mathbf{P}_{12}$ of 12 positive Gaussians (a): the minimum misclassification rate of 0.013 for the separation threshold $\tau = 88$ (b).

because one of its terms combines the overlapped separate tails of both the objects and actually should not be assigned to only one dominant mode. This principal drawback of the mixture partitioning is the basic motivation behind applying the pseudo-marginals to build more accurate conditional object models.

3.5.3 Modeling Blood Vessels on TOF-MRA Images

By the same procedure, conditional models for three dominant objects in a TOF-MRA image: dark bones and fat; gray brain tissues, and bright blood vessels—are estimated for accurate separation of the blood vessels. Figure 3.17 shows a typical MRA image and its three-modal empirical

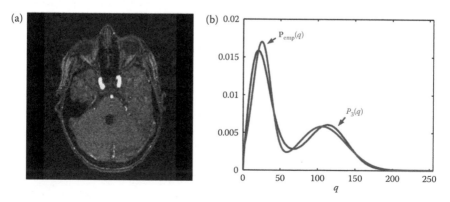

FIGURE 3.17
Typical TOF-MRA scan slice (a) and its empirical marginal $\mathbf{P}_{emp}$ vs. the dominant mixture P_3 (b).

TABLE 3.2

Parameters of the Initial Dominant Terms for the
MRA Image in Figure 3.17

Bones and Fat			Brain Tissues			Blood Vessels		
w_1	μ_1	σ_1^2	w_2	μ_2	σ_2^2	w_3	μ_3	σ_3^2
0.52	23	116	0.45	103	335	0.03	208	256

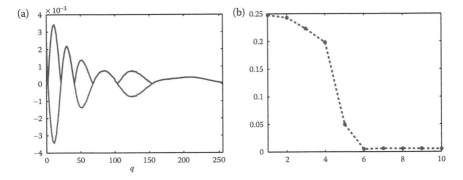

FIGURE 3.18

Sign-alternate and absolute deviations (a) and the approximation error (b) in function of the
number of mixed subordinate terms.

marginal approximated with the dominant three-term mixture, the estimated
parameters (w_i, μ_i, σ_i^2); $i = 1, 2, 3$, of its terms being listed in Table 3.2.

The Levy distance of 0.08 indicates a big mismatch between this dominant
mixture and the empirical marginal. Their scaled deviations and the search
for the six subordinate terms giving the minimum approximation error are
illustrated in Figure 3.18.

Figure 3.19 presents the estimated initial pseudo-marginal and the conditional LCDG models for each object. The minimum classification error of
0.01 on the intersecting tails of these conditional models is obtained for the
separation thresholds $\tau_1 = 56$ and $\tau_2 = 190$, allocating the subordinate components 1–3, 4–5, and 6 to the first (bones and fat), second (brain tissues), and
third (blood vessels) object, respectively.

Figures 3.20 and 3.21 present the final pseudo-marginal after refining the
initial model in Figure 3.19; successive changes of the log-likelihood at the
refining iterations, the nine terms of the final LCDG, and the final conditional
pseudo-marginals for each object for the best separation thresholds $\tau_1 = 54$
and $\tau_2 = 188$. The resulting Levy distance between the empirical marginal
and the final model decreases to 0.01 from the initial 0.08. The first nine iterations of the refinement increased the log-likelihood of Equation 3.17 from
-5.8 to -3.8.

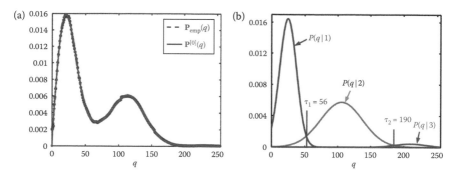

FIGURE 3.19
Empirical marginal vs. the initial pseudo-marginal (a) with the three dominant and six subordinate terms for the MRA image in Figure 3.17 and the initial conditional LCDG models (b) of the objects "Bones," "Brain tissues," and "Blood vessels."

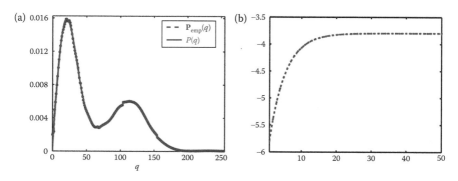

FIGURE 3.20
Refined pseudo-marginal **P** with the three dominant terms vs. the empirical marginal **P**emp (a) and the log-likelihood changes (b) during the refinement.

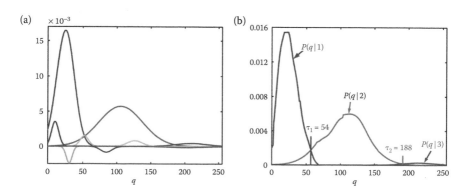

FIGURE 3.21
Dominant and subordinate terms of the refined model (a), and the final conditional object models (b).

3.5.4 Modeling Brain Tissues on MRI

To accurately separate the main objects: dark bones and fat, gray matter, white matter, and cerebrospinal fluid (CSF), on a weighted T2 MRI in Figure 3.22, its empirical marginal is approximated by a dominant mixture of four Gaussians with parameters in Table 3.3.

The Levy distance of 0.11 between these marginals indicates a large mis match, and the search for the mixture of the 16 subordinate terms minimizing the absolute deviations between the marginals is shown in Figure 3.23.

Figure 3.24 presents the estimated initial pseudo-marginal with four dominant DGs and 16 sign-alternate subordinate DGs, as well as the initial conditional LCDGs, which model the chosen four objects. The minimum classification error of 0.01 due to the intersecting tails of the conditional models is obtained for the thresholds $\tau_1 = 53$, $\tau_2 = 110$, and $\tau_3 = 179$ that assign the subordinate DGs 1–3, 4–8, 9–12, and 13–16 the first (bones and fat), second (white matter), third (gray matter), and fourth (CSF)) objects, respectively.

After refining this initial model, the Levy distance between the empirical marginal and the final LCDG model decreases to 0.02 from the initial 0.11. Successive changes of the log-likelihood at the refining iterations; the 20 terms of the final LCDG, and the final conditional LCDG models of each object for the best separation thresholds $\tau_1 = 51$; $\tau_2 = 107$; and $\tau_3 = 184$ are

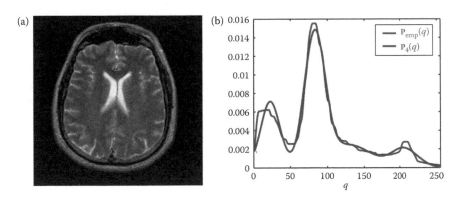

FIGURE 3.22
Typical T2 weighted MRI (a) and its empirical marginal vs. the dominant 4-term mixture (b).

TABLE 3.3

Parameters of the Final Dominant Terms for the MRI in Figure 3.22

Bones and Fat			White Matter			Gray Matter			CSF		
w_1	μ_1	σ_1^2	w_2	μ_2	σ_2^2	w_3	μ_3	σ_3^2	w_4	μ_4	σ_4^2
0.23	23	181	0.50	85	206	0.19	127	793	0.09	207	306

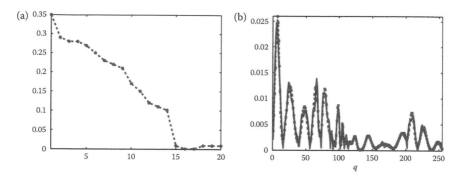

FIGURE 3.23
Approximation error (a) in function of the number of mixed subordinate terms and the Gaussian 16-term mixture (b) that closely approximates the scaled-up absolute deviation between the empirical and dominant marginals in Figure 3.22.

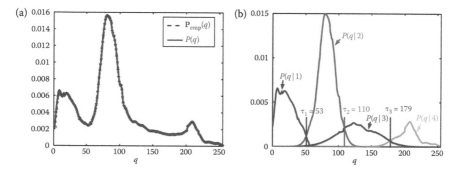

FIGURE 3.24
Empirical marginal vs. the initial pseudo-marginal (a) with the four dominant and 16 subordinate terms for the MRI in Figure 3.22 and the initial conditional LCDG models (b) of the objects "Bones," "Gray matter," "White matter," and "CSF."

shown in Figures 3.25 and 3.26. The first three refining iterations increase the log-likelihood of Equation 3.17 from -9.5 to -7.55.

3.5.5 Modeling Brain Blood Vessels on PC-MRA Images

Figure 3.27 shows a PC-MRA image with three main objects: dark bones, gray brain tissues, and bright blood vessels—and illustrates the initialization, refinement, and partitioning of the corresponding LCDG model. The empirical marginal is approximated first with the dominant mixture of three DGs with parameters in Table 3.4. Then the search for the closest mixture model of the scaled-up absolute deviations between the empirical and dominant marginals provides the 12-term initial pseudo-marginal (LCDG model) with the nine subordinate DGs associated with the three dominant DGs. Finally, the goal LCDG model is obtained after the seven refining iterations, which

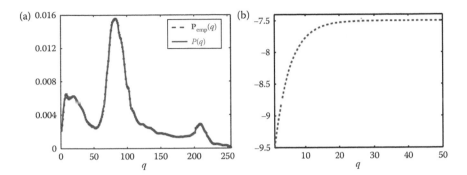

FIGURE 3.25
Refined pseudo-marginal **P** (a) vs. the empirical marginal **P**_emp and the log-likelihood changes (b) during the refinement.

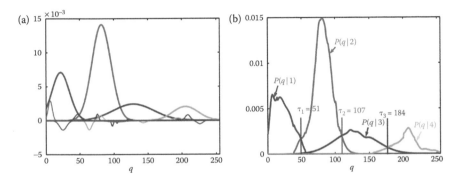

FIGURE 3.26
Dominant and subordinate terms of the refined model (a) and the final conditional object models (b).

increase the model log-likelihood from -5.45 to -4.40 before the refinement terminates.

3.5.6 Aorta Modeling on CTA Images

The last example in Figure 3.28 illustrates the estimation of a pseudo-marginal that approximates the empirical marginal for a CTA image containing four main objects: the dark background and colon tissues, gray liver and kidney, light gray aorta blood vessels, and bright bones. The modeling goal is to accurately separate the aorta vessels from the three surrounding objects.

Parameters of the initial dominant mixture are given in Table 3.5. The initialization returns the 13-term LCDG model, and the 16 refining iterations before the process terminates increase the log-likelihood of the pseudo-marginal from -6.2 to -5.1.

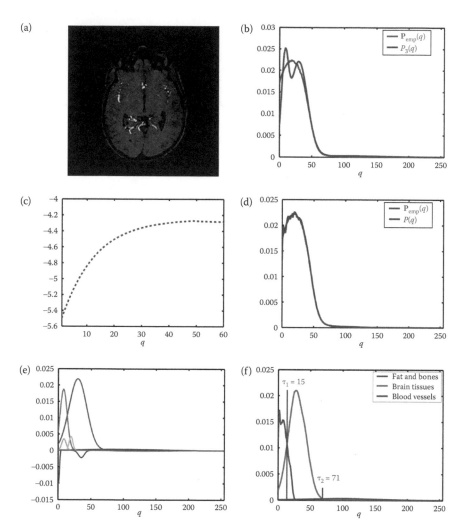

FIGURE 3.27

Typical PC-MRA image (a); its empirical marginal vs. the dominant mixture of three DGs (b); the log-likelihood changes during the refinement of the initial pseudo-marginal (c); the refined LCDG model (d); and its sign-alternate terms (e); and the final conditional object models (f).

TABLE 3.4

Parameters of the Initial Dominant Terms for the PC-MRA Image in Figure 3.27

Bones and Fat			Brain Tissues			Blood Vessels		
w_1	μ_1	σ_1^2	w_2	μ_2	σ_2^2	w_3	μ_3	σ_3^2
0.25	8.2	28	0.73	30	178	0.02	99	3013

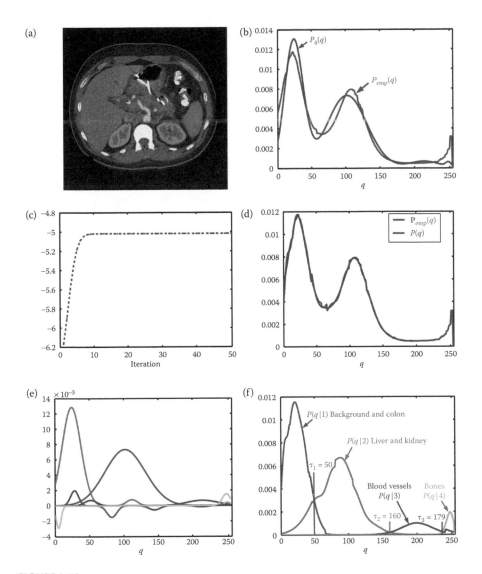

FIGURE 3.28
Typical CTA image (a); its empirical marginal vs. the dominant mixture of four DGs (b); the log-likelihood changes during the refinement of the initial pseudo-marginal (c); the refined LCDG model (d); its sign-alternate terms (e); and the final conditional object models (f).

TABLE 3.5

Parameters of the Initial Dominant Terms for the CTA Image in Figure 3.28

Background and Colon			Liver and Kidney			Blood Vessels			Bones		
w_1	μ_1	σ_1^2	w_2	μ_2	σ_2^2	w_3	μ_3	σ_3^2	w_4	μ_4	σ_4^2
0.44	22	182	0.49	99	902	0.04	216	4703	0.03	243	17

3.6 Bibliographic and Historical Notes

Learning an IRF of scalar or low-dimensional signals by optimal statistical, e.g., the ML or Bayesian estimation of a marginal probability distribution or density from a collection of independent samples is a well-established and active area of applied statistics and engineering, widely covered in the literature over many years; see References 69,114,124,236, and 265 to cite only a few. Given a single training image, $\mathbf{g}°$ or a subset $\mathbf{G}_J° = \{\mathbf{g}_j° : j = 1, \dots, J\}$ of J images; $J > 1$, sampled from an IRF under consideration, parametric or nonparametric estimates of one or more unknown marginals, specifying the IRF are learned from a collected empirical marginal, i.e., the normalized histogram of the site-wise image signals.

A parametric model of the unknown marginal is known up to a few parameters, e.g., a Gaussian, or normal density of Equation 3.12 or its discrete analogue—a DG of Equation 3.13 with unknown mean values and/or variances to be estimated. A nonparametric model, which is not constrained to a particular functional form, is more flexible. Its accuracy increases when more training data could be observed, but at the expense of growing computational complexity of the model [291]. The parametric model, such as a conventional mixture of the positive Gaussian terms or a pseudo-marginal (the LCG or LCDG), is of limited complexity. However, its accuracy may not improve after using more empirical data. The LCGs and LCDGs, introduced in References 84 and 101, approximate the empirical marginals more accurately, than the conventional mixtures with the same numbers of individual parametric terms.

Nonparametric estimates of probability densities of continuous scalar signals account conventionally for distances from each signal value to all the training values or to a fixed number of its nearest neighbors in the training data set. A kernel-based estimator, called often a *Parzen window* [236,265], models an unknown one-dimensional density as

$$\widehat{P}_{\alpha_n}(q) = \frac{1}{n\alpha_n} \sum_{i=1}^{n} \mathcal{K}\left(\frac{q - q_i°}{\alpha_n}\right)$$

where α_n is a common scaling factor and $\mathcal{K}(s)$ is a symmetric and nonnegative kernel function, such that $\mathcal{K}(s) \geq 0$ and $\int_{s=-\infty}^{\infty} \mathcal{K}(s)ds = 1$ implying $\frac{1}{\alpha}\int_{s=-\infty}^{\infty} \mathcal{K}\left(\frac{s}{\alpha}\right) ds = 1$. In some cases the kernels are even not necessarily strictly nonnegative. Each kernel is centered on one of the n available training signal values, $q_i°; i = 1, \dots, n; q_i° \in \mathbb{Q}$. The scale α_n depends inversely on the number n of the training samples: the larger the data size n, the smaller the scaling factor, i.e., the closer the kernel to the delta-function: $\lim_{n\to\infty} \alpha_n = 0$ and $\lim_{n\to\infty} n\alpha_n = \infty$.

To reduce the computational load, a representative subset of the training intensities is selected, e.g., by maximizing an entropy-based similarity between the densities $P_{\alpha_n}(q)$ and $P_{\alpha_v}(q)$; $v < n$, estimated from the full and reduced training data, respectively [110]. Nonetheless, such nonparametric estimators are more suitable for supervised learning of conditional object models because the separation of a nonparametric model of mixed training data into individual object models meets with significant difficulties.

Univariate Parzen estimates of probability density for equispaced discrete signals are found efficiently with the fast Fourier transform (FFT); in this case, the Fourier spectrum of the estimate is the direct product of the kernel and data spectra. Data spacing can be modified to reduce data-related errors, but the FFT cannot be applied to the irregularly spaced signals (e.g., when a nonparametric signal classifier employs the Parzen density estimates). A fast Parzen estimator with a reduced training data set was proposed in Reference 122.

The kernel-based estimates are often used for the d-dimensional signals; $d > 1$, too:

$$\widehat{P}_{\alpha_n}(\mathbf{q}) = \frac{1}{n\alpha_n^d} \sum_{i=1}^{n} \mathcal{K}\left(\frac{\mathbf{q}-\mathbf{q}_i^\circ}{\alpha_n}\right) \tag{3.29}$$

where $\mathbf{q} = [q_1, \ldots, q_d]^\mathsf{T}$. In this case the kernel is often the Gaussian zero-mean and unit-variance density $\mathcal{K}(\mathbf{q}) = (2\pi)^{-\frac{d}{2}} \exp\left(-\frac{1}{2}\mathbf{q}^\mathsf{T}\mathbf{q}\right)$. Such multidimensional kernels effectively make the estimates parametric and similar to probability mixtures of Equation 3.10.

Parametric estimates of probability densities or distributions of scalar measurements are widely used in the today's advanced data analysis [76]. Typically, an empirical marginal is modeled as in Equation 3.10 with a mixture of parametric terms, such as, e.g., Gaussians [125,245], representing individual objects. The mixture models are identified using the Bayesian or ML parameter estimates.

EM algorithms for computing the MLE of the parameters for either a Gaussian, or a general-case mixture were introduced first as early as in the 1950s–1960s and independently by Ceppellini e.a. [49], Day [65], Hartley [133], and Schlesinger [263]. The widely known Baum-Welch forward-backward algorithm for learning hidden Markov models, which belongs to a family of the so-called generalized EM (GEM) algorithms, also appeared at the end of the 1960s [16]. However, the EM received its current name and became very popular almost a decade later, after a pivotal paper by Dempster, Laird, and Rubin [66] had reintroduced this algorithm and extended it to a general problem of statistical inference and parameter estimation from an incomplete training data set. At present, a rich variety of the EM or similar algorithms exist for identifying the probability mixtures [205,214,251].

The multidimensional kernel-density estimates of Equation 3.29 are often built after applying the principal component analysis (PCA) to the training data set [265] in order to find a linear transformation that decorrelates the centered training data vectors and unifies data variances along the coordinate axes. After modeling the transformed data, the estimate returns to the initial data vectors. Generally, the PCA is justified for a Gaussian data distribution, making independence equivalent to zero covariances of the coordinate axes. By minimizing these covariances, the PCA-based transformation yields the more accurate density estimates.

The alternative *independent component analysis* (ICA), which was introduced mainly at the mid-1990s [146,183,255], is justified for the more frequent non-Gaussian data because it minimizes the mutual information (MI) or kurtosis (the fourth-order moment) of the coordinate axes. At present the ICA is a popular technique for converting vectors of interdependent scalar signals sampled from an arbitrary random field or chain into a linear combination of vectors with statistically independent elements, having the non-Gaussian probability distributions.

The Levy distance (or more correctly, Lévy distance) of Equation 3.24; see, e.g., [180], which was introduced by French mathematician Paul Lévy and is referred to by his name, is one of popular statistical measures of closeness between two probability distributions. Let $\mathbf{P} = (P(u) : u \in \mathbb{U})$ and $\mathbf{P_e} = (P_c(u) : u \in \mathbb{U})$ denote these distributions, e.g., a theoretical and an empirical distributions, respectively, of a random scalar variable, u, with a set $\mathbb{U}$ of values. The Levy distance in the range from 0 to 1 separates the two corresponding cumulative distributions,

$$\mathbf{F} = \left(F(u) = \sum_{t \leq u;\, t \in \mathbb{U}} P(u) : u \in \mathbb{U} \right);$$

$$\mathbf{F_e} = \left(F_e(u) = \sum_{t \leq u;\, t \in \mathbb{U}} P_e(u) : u \in \mathbb{U} \right);$$

and is measured with the linear size of the largest square, which can be placed between these curves:

$$D_{\text{Levy}}(\mathbf{P}, \mathbf{P_e}) = \arg \min_{\varepsilon \geq 0} \{ F(u - \varepsilon) - \varepsilon \leq F_e(u) \leq F(u + \varepsilon) + \varepsilon : u \in \mathbb{U} \}$$

When this distance tends to zero, the distributions $\mathbf{P}$ and $\mathbf{P_e}$ weakly converge one to another.

4

Markov-Gibbs Random Field Models: Estimating Signal Interactions

Descriptive power of a Markov random field (MRF) of signals at the lattice sites is considerably higher than of any IRF because interdependencies, or interactions between different signals are taken into account. As was already detailed in Chapter 2; Equations 2.14 and 2.15, the probability or density $P(\mathbf{g})$ of an image $\mathbf{g}$ sampled from a certain MRF, such that the positivity condition $P(\mathbf{g}) > 0$ holds for all the images, is factored over a system $\mathbb{C}$ of selected subsets $\mathbf{c}$ of the lattice sites (cliques of an interaction graph, Γ). Thus it is represented in the exponential form as the GPD:

$$P(\mathbf{g}) = \frac{1}{Z} \prod_{\mathbf{c} \in \mathbb{C}} f_{\mathbf{c}}(g(\mathbf{r}) : \mathbf{r} \in \mathbf{c}) \equiv \frac{1}{Z} \exp\left(- \sum_{\mathbf{c} \in \mathbb{C}} V_{\mathbf{c}}(g(\mathbf{r}) : \mathbf{r} \in \mathbf{c}) \right)$$

defining the corresponding Markov-Gibbs random field (MGRF). The largest clique cardinality, $k = \max_{\mathbf{c} \in \mathbb{C}} |\mathbf{c}|$, specifies the order of the MGRF. One of basic difficulties of using and learning a vast majority of the MGRF image models is that their normalizer, or partition function $Z = \sum_{\mathbf{g} \in \mathbb{G}} \exp\left(- \sum_{\mathbf{c} \in \mathbb{C}} V_{\mathbf{c}}(g(\mathbf{r}) : \mathbf{r} \in \mathbf{c}) \right)$ is computationally infeasible.

Each factor $f_{\mathbf{c}}(\mathbf{q}_{\mathbf{c}})$ is a bounded positive scalar function, $0 < f_{\mathbf{c}}(\mathbf{q}_{\mathbf{c}}) < \infty$, of $|\mathbf{c}|$ variables $\mathbf{q}_{\mathbf{c}} = [q_1 = g(\mathbf{r}_1), \ldots, q_{|\mathbf{c}|} = g(\mathbf{r}_{|\mathbf{c}|})]$, which quantifies inherent clique-wise interaction strengths of signal configurations, or co-occurrences $\mathbf{q}_{\mathbf{c}} \in \mathbb{Q}^{|\mathbf{c}|}$ on the clique $\mathbf{c}$, given a fixed ordering $\mathbf{r}_1, \ldots, \mathbf{r}_{|\mathbf{c}|}$ of the sites $\mathbf{r} \in \mathbf{c}$. The relevant potentials $V_{\mathbf{c}}(\mathbf{q}_{\mathbf{c}}) = -\ln f_{\mathbf{c}}(\mathbf{q}_{\mathbf{c}})$ are also bounded $|\mathbf{c}|$-variate scalar functions: $|V_{\mathbf{c}}(\mathbf{q}_{\mathbf{c}})| < \infty; \mathbf{c} \in \mathbb{C}; \mathbf{q}_{\mathbf{c}} = (q_1, \ldots, q_{|\mathbf{c}|}) \in \mathbb{Q}^{|\mathbf{c}|}$.

Estimation (learning) of an MGRF to describe visual appearances of objects of interest on images and/or shapes of these objects on region maps is often called *model identification*. A characteristic system $\mathbb{C}$ of cliques and a collection $\mathbf{V}_{\mathbb{C}} = (V_{\mathbf{c}}(\mathbf{q}_{\mathbf{c}}) : \mathbf{q}_{\mathbf{c}} \in \mathbb{Q}^{|\mathbf{c}|}; \mathbf{c} \in \mathbb{C})$ of their potentials, specifying the model, are either selected by hand, or identified (at least, in part) from one or more training samples.

4.1 Generic Kth-Order MGRFs

Generally, the cliques $\mathbf{c} \in \mathbb{C}$ supporting an MGRF may be of arbitrary shape varying over the interaction graph Γ. To account for spatial or spatiotemporal homogeneity of local object appearances and shapes, the cliques are stratified into $|\mathbb{A}|$ transformation-invariant families, where $\mathbb{A}$; $|\mathbb{A}| \geq 1$, denotes an index set. Cliques of each family $\mathbb{C}_a$; $a \in \mathbb{A}$, are of the same order K_a; support the same potential $\mathbf{V}_a = [V_a(\mathbf{q}_a) : \mathbf{q}_a \in \mathbb{Q}^{K_a}]$, and are invariant to certain geometric transformations on the lattice. The transformational invariance means that the K_a sites of each clique $\mathbf{c} \in \mathbb{C}_a$ keep one-to-one correspondence to the K_a arguments $\mathbf{q}_a = (q_1, \ldots, q_{K_a})$ of the potential function $V_a(\mathbf{q}_a)$. Medical image modeling presumes mostly either purely translational, or translational-rotational invariance of the cliques.

Definition 4.1

An arbitrary-shaped translation-invariant clique of order K is specified by a linearly ordered set $\mathbb{N} = \{\mathbf{v}_k : k = 1, \ldots, K-1\}$ of coordinate offsets of the origin, $\mathbf{0}$, from the other $K-1$ lattice sites. Given a set $\mathbb{N}$, the translation-invariant clique with the origin at a site $\mathbf{r} \in \mathbb{R}$, such that all its neighbors $\mathbf{r} + \mathbf{v} \in \mathbb{R}$; $\mathbf{v} \in \mathbb{N}$, is an ordered subset of the sites: $\mathbf{c_r} = \{\mathbf{r}, \mathbf{r} + \mathbf{v}_1, \ldots, \mathbf{r} + \mathbf{v}_{K-1}\}$.

Definition 4.2

A translation-invariant clique family $\mathbb{C}$ of order K is a set of all translation-invariant cliques, $\mathbf{c_r}$, specified on the lattice by a fixed set $\mathbb{N}$; $|\mathbb{N}| = K$, of the coordinate offsets and located entirely within the lattice: $\mathbb{C} = \{\mathbf{c_r} : \mathbf{r} \in \mathbb{R}; \mathbf{c_r} \subset \mathbb{R}\}$.

Because the offsets $\mathbf{v}$ and $-\mathbf{v}$ define just the same translation-invariant second-order clique family, possible duplicates are excluded by replacing the offset $\mathbf{v} = (\xi, \eta)$ with $(\xi, |\eta|)$ if $\eta \neq 0$ or $(|\xi|, 0)$ if $\eta = 0$.

Definition 4.3

A translation/rotation-invariant clique family $\mathbb{C}$ of order K is a set of all cliques, specified by rotating a fixed set $\mathbb{N}$; $|\mathbb{N}| = K$, of the coordinate offsets around its origin and rounding to the closest lattice positions. Each rotation preserves the ordering of the K clique sites, and all the rotated cliques have the same potential function.

Translation/rotation-invariant pairwise interactions can be useful for spatial modeling of central-symmetric textured objects, such as lung nodules, and spatiotemporal modeling of a texture turning slowly from one to another frame in a video sequence.

Let $\mathbb{A} = \{1, 2, 3, \ldots\}$ denote an index set for successive semi-open intervals of characteristic inter-pixel distances specifying central-symmetric pixel

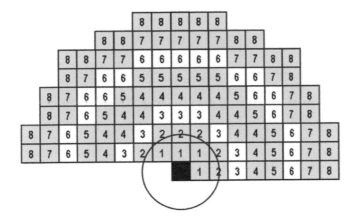

FIGURE 4.1
Central-symmetric coordinate offsets $\mathbf{v}$ for the eight inter-pixel distance ranges $|\mathbf{v}| \in (a - 0.5, a + 0.5]; a \in \mathbb{A} = \{1, 2, \ldots, 8\}$.

neighborhoods $\mathcal{N}_a$. Each neighborhood contains the coordinate offsets $\mathbf{v} = (\xi, \eta)$ between each pixel $\mathbf{r}$ and its neighbor $\mathbf{r} + \mathbf{v}$, such that $d_{a:\min} < |\mathbf{v}| = \sqrt{(\xi^2 + \eta^2)} \leq d_{a:\max}$. Because both the offsets (ξ, η) and $(-\xi, -\eta)$ specify the same second-order clique family, only one of them (with the offsets $\eta > 0$ and $\xi > 0$ for $\eta = 0$) is shown in Figure 4.1 presenting the offsets for the uniform distance intervals $(d_{a:\min} = a - 0.5, d_{a:\max} = a + 0.5)$; $a \in \mathbb{A} = \{1, 2, \ldots, 8\}; d_{a+1:\min} = d_{a:\max}$.

To keep the high-order MGRFs computationally feasible, the exponentially growing space $\mathbb{Q}^K$ of clique-wise signal co-occurrences is mapped for each clique family $\mathbb{C}_a$ to a certain space $\mathbb{U}_a$ of much lower cardinality, $|\mathbb{U}_a| \ll |\mathbb{Q}|^K$. Generally, the mappings $\mathbf{W}_a : \mathbb{Q}^K \to \mathbb{U}_a; a \in \mathbb{A}$ decrease descriptive and discriminant abilities, but facilitate the usage and learning of the models due to a significantly reduced variety of distinct arguments, $\mathbf{u}_a = \mathbf{W}(\mathbf{q}) \in \mathbb{U}_a$, of each potential $\mathbf{V}_a = [V_a(\mathbf{u}_a) : \mathbf{u}_a \in \mathbb{U}_a]$. For the most common grayscale images with $|\mathbb{Q}| = 256$, such mappings become a necessity starting already from the third-order MGRFs ($K \geq 3$).

Given a set of the transformation-invariant Kth-order clique families $\mathbb{C}_a$, defined by the coordinate offsets $\mathbb{N}_a$; the clique-wise signal mapping functions $\mathbf{W}_a$, and the potentials $\mathbf{V}_a; a \in \mathbb{A}$, the MGRF of order K is specified by the GPD $\mathbf{P} = [P(\mathbf{g}) = \frac{1}{Z} \exp(-E(\mathbf{g})) : \mathbf{g} \in \mathbb{G}]$ depending on the interaction energy:

$$
\begin{aligned}
E(\mathbf{g}) &= \sum_{a \in \mathbb{A}} \sum_{\substack{\mathbf{r} \in \mathbb{R}; \\ c_{a:\mathbf{r}} \subset \mathbb{R}}} V_a \left(\mathbf{W}_a \left(g(\mathbf{r}); \{g(\mathbf{r} + \mathbf{v}) : \mathbf{v} \in \mathbb{N}_a\}\right)\right) \\
&= \sum_{a \in \mathbb{A}} \sum_{\mathbf{u}_a \in \mathbb{U}_a} V_a(\mathbf{u}_a) h_a(\mathbf{u}_a \mid \mathbf{g}) \equiv |\mathbb{R}| \sum_{a \in \mathbb{A}} \rho_a \sum_{\mathbf{u}_a \in \mathbb{U}_a} V_a(\mathbf{u}_a) F_a(\mathbf{u}_a \mid \mathbf{g})
\end{aligned}
\tag{4.1}
$$

where $\rho_a = \frac{|C_a|}{|\mathbb{R}|}$ is the relative family size and the histograms $\mathbf{h}_{a:\mathbf{g}} = [h_a(\mathbf{u}_a) : \mathbf{u}_a \in \mathbb{U}_a]$, or empirical probabilities $\mathbf{F}_{a:\mathbf{g}} = \frac{1}{|C_a|}\mathbf{h}_{a:\mathbf{g}} \equiv [F_a(\mathbf{u}_a \,|\, \mathbf{g}) : \mathbf{u}_a \in \mathbb{U}_a]$ of the K-wise co-occurrences reduced by the chosen functional mappings are the sufficient statistics of the images.

4.1.1 MCMC Sampling of an MGRF

A Markov chain of samples is built by a random choice of each next sample with probabilities depending only on the current sample. The chains are irreducible and aperiodic if each sample can eventually appear in any chain starting from an arbitrary initial sample.

Definition 4.4

A homogeneous Markov chain is specified by a distribution $\mathbf{P}_0 = [P_0(\mathbf{g}) : \mathbf{g} \in G]$ of its initial samples $\mathbf{g}_0$ and a transition matrix $\mathbf{P}_{\mathrm{tr}} = [P_{\mathrm{tr}}(\mathbf{g} \,|\, \mathbf{g}') : \mathbf{g}, \mathbf{g}' \in G]$ of conditional probabilities of samples $\mathbf{g}$ at position $t+1$ for each sample $\mathbf{g}'$ at position t; $t = 0, 1, \ldots$; $\sum_{\mathbf{g} \in G} P_{\mathrm{tr}}(\mathbf{g} \,|\, \mathbf{g}') = 1$; $\mathbf{g}' \in G$.

The transition matrix determines how a current distribution $\mathbf{P}_t$ of the samples $\mathbf{g}_t$ is changing at the next position $t+1$ of the chain: $P_{t+1}(\mathbf{g}) = \sum_{\mathbf{g}' \in G} P_{\mathrm{tr}}(\mathbf{g} \,|\, \mathbf{g}')P_t(\mathbf{g}')$; $\mathbf{g} \in G$.

Definition 4.5

Markov chain Monte Carlo (MCMC) sampling produces an irreducible and aperiodic homogeneous chain $(\mathbf{g}_t : t = 0, 1, 2, \ldots)$ of samples from the population G, which have a prescribed probability distribution $\mathbf{P} = [P(\mathbf{g}) : \mathbf{g} \in G]$ if the chain is in equilibrium.

Lemma 4.1

Homogeneous Markov chains produced by the MCMC sampling with a transition matrix $\mathbf{P}_{\mathrm{tr}}$ tend to the equilibrium where the limiting, or stationary probability distribution $\mathbf{P} = [P(\mathbf{g}) : \mathbf{g} \in G]$ of the samples is uniquely determined by the conditions:

$$P(\mathbf{g}) = \sum_{\mathbf{g}' \in G} P_{\mathrm{tr}}(\mathbf{g} \,|\, \mathbf{g}')P(\mathbf{g}'); \quad \mathbf{g} \in G \tag{4.2}$$

Proof. The absolute distance $d(\mathbf{P}_t, \mathbf{P}) = \sum_{\mathbf{g} \in G} |P_t(\mathbf{g}) - P(\mathbf{g})|$ between the current and stationary distributions does not increase along the chain:

$$d(\mathbf{P}_{t+1}, \mathbf{P}) = \sum_{\mathbf{g} \in G} \left| \sum_{\mathbf{g}' \in G} P_{\text{tr}}(\mathbf{g} \mid \mathbf{g}') P_t(\mathbf{g}') - P(\mathbf{g}) \right|$$

$$= \sum_{\mathbf{g} \in G} \left| \sum_{\mathbf{g}' \in G} P_{\text{tr}}(\mathbf{g} \mid \mathbf{g}') \left(P_t(\mathbf{g}') - P(\mathbf{g}') \right) \right|$$

$$\leq \sum_{\mathbf{g} \in G} \sum_{\mathbf{g}' \in G} P_{\text{tr}}(\mathbf{g} \mid \mathbf{g}') |P_t(\mathbf{g}') - P(\mathbf{g}')| = d(\mathbf{P}_t, \mathbf{P})$$

Provided that the transition probabilities at each step are positive, $P_{\text{tr}}(\mathbf{g} \mid \mathbf{g}') > 0$, for all the sample pairs, both positive and negative deviations $P_t(\mathbf{g}) - P(\mathbf{g})$ of the probabilities always exist while $\mathbf{P}_t \neq \mathbf{P}$. Therefore, the strict inequality $d(\mathbf{P}_{t+1}, \mathbf{P}) < d(\mathbf{P}_t, \mathbf{P})$ holds unless the produced Markov chains have already approached the equilibrium where $\mathbf{P}_t = \mathbf{P}_{t+1} = \mathbf{P}$. ■

The $|G|$ constraints of Equation 4.2 allow for a host of different $|G| \times |G|$ transition matrices leading to the same limiting distribution. The most popular sufficient (but not necessary) conditions

$$P_{\text{tr}}(\mathbf{g} \mid \mathbf{g}') P(\mathbf{g}') = P_{\text{tr}}(\mathbf{g}' \mid \mathbf{g}) P(\mathbf{g}); \quad \mathbf{g}, \mathbf{g}' \in G \qquad (4.3)$$

trivialize Equation 4.2:

$$P(\mathbf{g}) = \sum_{\mathbf{g}' \in G} P_{\text{tr}}(\mathbf{g} \mid \mathbf{g}') P(\mathbf{g}') = \sum_{\mathbf{g}' \in G} P_{\text{tr}}(\mathbf{g}' \mid \mathbf{g}) P(\mathbf{g}) = P(\mathbf{g})$$

Although the theoretical length bound of $|G|^2$ for a Markov chain to closely approximate the stationary probability distribution is too high to be practicable, the MCMC samplers are often used to simulate (generate) images described with the MGRF models.

4.1.2 Gibbs and Metropolis-Hastings Samplers

The MCMC sampling of the GPD of Equation 2.15 employs a computationally feasible *site-wise stochastic relaxation*, which updates at each step only a single lattice site. The transition probabilities, $P_{\text{tr}}(\mathbf{g} \mid \mathbf{g}')$, are positive for all pairs $(\mathbf{g}, \mathbf{g}')$, which differ at most in one site, and are equal to zero otherwise, i.e., if the pairs differ in two or more sites.

Produced by stochastic relaxation successive samples of a Markov chain differ at most by a single signal in a site $\mathbf{r}$, varying from one adjacent pair of samples to another along the chain. Let $\mathbf{g}^{\mathbf{r}:q} = (g(\mathbf{r}) = q; \mathbf{g}^{\mathbf{r}})$ denote a sample $\mathbf{g}$, such that its site $\mathbf{r}$ supports the signal q and the signals $\mathbf{g}^{\mathbf{r}}$ at all other sites are fixed. If the sample $\mathbf{g}_t = \mathbf{g}^{\mathbf{r},q}$, then the next sample $\mathbf{g}_{t+1} = \mathbf{g}^{\mathbf{r}:q'}; q, q' \in \mathbb{Q}$, and the equilibrium conditions of Equation 4.3 can be rewritten as

$$P_{tr}(g(\mathbf{r}) = q | \mathbf{g}^{\mathbf{r}:q'}) P(g(\mathbf{r}) = q' | \mathbf{g}^{\mathbf{r}})$$
$$= P_{tr}(g(\mathbf{r}) = q' | \mathbf{g}^{\mathbf{r}:q}) P(g(\mathbf{r}) = q | \mathbf{g}^{\mathbf{r}}); \quad q, q' \in \mathbb{Q} \qquad (4.4)$$

where $P(g(\mathbf{r}) = q | \mathbf{g}^{\mathbf{r}})$ is the conditional probability of the signal $q \in \mathbb{Q}$ at the site $\mathbf{r}$, given the fixed signals $\mathbf{g}^{\mathbf{r}}$ at all other sites.

The site-wise stochastic relaxation is easily performed for an MGRF because its GPD provides consistent conditional probabilities in Equation 4.4, which depend for each site $\mathbf{r}$ only on the neighboring signals and do not involve the partition function:

$$P(g(\mathbf{r}) = q | \mathbf{g}^{\mathbf{r}}) \equiv P(g(\mathbf{r}) = q | g(\mathbf{r}') : \mathbf{r}' \in \mathbb{N}_{C:\mathbf{r}})$$

$$= \frac{\exp\left(\sum\limits_{c \ni \mathbf{r}; \, c \in C} V_c\left(g(\mathbf{r}') : \mathbf{r}' \in c; \, g(\mathbf{r}) = q\right)\right)}{\sum\limits_{q' \in \mathbb{Q}} \exp\left(\sum\limits_{c \ni \mathbf{r}; \, c \in C} V_c\left(g(\mathbf{r}') : \mathbf{r}' \in c; \, g(\mathbf{r}) = q'\right)\right)} \qquad (4.5)$$

where $\mathbb{N}_{C:\mathbf{r}}$ is the neighborhood of the site $\mathbf{r}$, or the union of all cliques $c \in C$ containing the site $\mathbf{r}$. In a Markov chain $\mathbf{g}_t; t = 0, 1, 2, \ldots,$ of images obtained by stochastic relaxation each current image $\mathbf{g}_t$ is formed from the preceding one, $\mathbf{g}_{t-1}$, by randomly choosing the signal $g(\mathbf{r}_t) = q_t \in \mathbb{Q}$ in a site $\mathbf{r}_t \in \mathbb{R}$ in accord with the easy computable probabilities of Equation 4.5.

Definition 4.6

A macrostep of the site-wise stochastic relaxation is a random sequence of the sites $\mathbf{r}_t; t = 0, 1, \ldots,$ tracing the entire lattice $\mathbb{R}$ without repetition.

Due to the positivity condition for the GPD: $P(\mathbf{g} > 0; \mathbf{g} \in \mathbb{G}$, all the site-wise transition probabilities of Equation 4.5 are nonzero for all signal co-occurrences over the neighborhoods $\mathbb{N}_{C:\mathbf{r}}$. The $|\mathbb{R}|$-step transition probabilities $P_{tr}(\mathbf{g} | \mathbf{g}')$ become first nonzero for all the image pairs $\mathbf{g}, \mathbf{g}' \in \mathbb{G}$ after the macrostep. Therefore, the Markov chain of samples generated at each macrostep has in the limit ($t \to \infty$) the equilibrium joint probability distribution of Equation 2.15 specifying the site-wise transition probabilities in Equation 4.5. The stochastic relaxation Algorithm 5 forms the Markov chain of images by iterative random tracing of the lattice and forming the next image from a current one at each macrostep. The stopping condition is

---

Algorithm 5 MCMC Sampling of Images

---

1. *Initialization* [$t = 0$]: Select an initial sample g_0.

2. *Iteration* [$t \leftarrow t + 1$]: Until complying with a stopping condition, repeat the macrostep forming the next sample g_{t+1} from the current one g_t as follows:

   a. *Routing*: Choose an arbitrary route (called a lattice *coloring* or *visiting scheme*) of tracing all the lattice sites without repetitions.

   b. *Updating*: Use either the *Gibbs sampler* or the *Metropolis-Hastings sampler* to update the current signal at each site along a chosen route.

---

selected empirically because statistical criteria verifying that a Markov chain of images has already approached the equilibrium are absent and theoretical estimates result in combinatorial sizes of the chains.

The two most popular stochastic relaxation techniques: the Gibbs sampler and the computationally simpler Metropolis-Hastings sampler—differ in how the transition probabilities are used for updating each current signal. In both cases the candidate is picked up randomly from the set Q according to the site-wise transition probabilities. The conditional probabilities of Equation 4.5 specify the site-wise transition probabilities in Equation 4.4, which depend in this case only on the neighbors of the current site.

The Gibbs sampler chooses a new signal q in each site according to the conditional probabilities of Equation 4.4: $P_{tr}(g(\mathbf{r}) = q \mid \mathbf{g}_{\mathbf{r}:q'}) = P(g(\mathbf{r}) = q \mid \mathbf{g}^{\mathbf{r}}); q, q' \in Q$, i.e., it uses the conditional probabilities of Equation 4.5 as the transition ones. The $|Q|$ probabilities of the possible signals $q \in Q$ are computed at each current site $\mathbf{r}$ for the fixed configuration of its neighboring signals, and the new signal, chosen randomly in accord with these probabilities, replaces the current signal in this site.

The Metropolis-Hastings sampler chooses first a candidate signal q from the set Q with equal probabilities and then substitutes it for the current signal $g(\mathbf{r}) = q'$ with the probability that depends on the ratio of the two conditional probabilities:

$$P(g(\mathbf{r}) = q \mid \mathbf{g}_{\mathbf{r}:q'}) = \min \left\{ 1, \alpha = \frac{P(g(\mathbf{r}) = q \mid \mathbf{g}^{\mathbf{r}})}{P(g(\mathbf{r}) = q' \mid \mathbf{g}^{\mathbf{r}})} \right\}$$

Thus, comparing to the Gibbs sampler, computations per site are reduced from $|Q|$ to only two conditional probabilities.

Let $E_{\mathbf{r}}(g(\mathbf{r}) = q \mid \mathbf{g}[\mathbb{N}_{\mathbf{r}:C}]; \mathbf{V})$ denote a conditional site-wise interaction energy for a signal $g(\mathbf{r}) = q$ at the site $\mathbf{r}$ with the fixed neighboring signals

$$\mathbf{g}[\mathbb{N}_{r:C}] = (g(\mathbf{r}') : \mathbf{r}' \in \mathbb{N}_{r:C}):$$

$$E_{\mathbf{r}}(g(\mathbf{r}) = q \,|\, \mathbf{g}[\mathbb{N}_{r:C}]; \mathbf{V}) = \sum_{c \in C; \, c \ni \mathbf{r}} V_{c}(g(\mathbf{r}') : \mathbf{r}' \in c; \, g(\mathbf{r}) = q)$$

The Metropolis-Hastings sampler replaces the current signal with a new one in the two steps: (1) a candidate value q is selected from Q with the equal probabilities $\frac{1}{|Q|}$ of each choice and (2) if the candidate q is conditionally more probable than the current signal q':

$$P(g(\mathbf{r}) = q \,|\, \mathbf{g}[\mathbb{N}_{r:C}]) > P(g(\mathbf{r}) = q' \,|\, \mathbf{g}[\mathbb{N}_{r:C}]) \text{ or, similarly,}$$

$$E_{\mathbf{r}}(g(\mathbf{r}) = q \,|\, \mathbf{g}[\mathbb{N}_{r:C}]; \mathbf{V}) < E_{\mathbf{r}}(g(\mathbf{r}) = q' \,|\, \mathbf{g}[\mathbb{N}_{r:C}]; \mathbf{V})$$

then the current signal q' is replaced with q, otherwise the candidate q is accepted with the probability

$$\alpha = \exp\left(E_{\mathbf{r}}(g(\mathbf{r}) = q' \,|\, \mathbf{g}[\mathbb{N}_{r:C}]; \mathbf{V}) - E_{\mathbf{r}}(g(\mathbf{r}) = q \,|\, \mathbf{g}[\mathbb{N}_{r:C}]; \mathbf{V})\right)$$

decreasing exponentially fast with the growing difference between the current and candidate conditional energies.

The visiting scheme is arbitrary at each macrostep, but a fully random choice of each site along the route is unnecessary. When the interaction structure is known, the lattice $\mathbb{R}$ is stratified into several conditionally independent sublattices $\mathbb{R}_{j}; \; j \in \mathbb{J}$, which cover the whole lattice and do not intersect: $\mathbb{R} = \bigcup_{j \in \mathbb{J}} \mathbb{R}_{j}$. Each site in a sublattice $\mathbb{R}_{j}$ has the neighbors only in the other sublattices $\mathbb{R}_{i}; \; i \neq j$.

This stratification is uniquely defined by a given neighborhood graph Γ. Because each sublattice contains no neighbors, it may be traced in any order with no impact on the sampled images. Therefore, every new arbitrary visiting scheme is formed by randomizing only the choices of the successive sublattices and implementing a few regular routes through each sublattice to be randomly chosen for a current macrostep.

4.2 Common Second- and Higher-Order MGRFs

Generic K-order GPDs $\mathbf{P}_{\mathbf{V}} = \left[P_{\mathbf{V}}(\mathbf{g}) = \frac{1}{Z_{\mathbf{V}}} \exp(-E_{\mathbf{V}}(\mathbf{g}) : \mathbf{g} \in \mathbf{G}\right]$ with the interaction energies $E_{\mathbf{V}}(\mathbf{g})$ of Equation 4.1 belong to the exponential family of probability distributions, which restricts the uniform IRF of equiprobable signals by constraining empirical probabilities of the reduced K-wise signal co-occurrences. In a more general case, these GPDs restrict a homogeneous IRF with different signal marginals.

The mathematical expectation of an empirical probability F of a certain stochastic event is the probability P of that event, and the variance of F is $P(1 - P)$. Therefore, given a training sample $\mathbf{g}^\circ$, the potentials for the generic MGRF with a known system of clique families in Equation 4.1 can be approximated analytically in line with Section 2.3.1 and Equation 2.27, as either

$$V_a(\mathbf{u}_a) = \frac{-F_a(\mathbf{u}_a \mid \mathbf{g}^\circ) + P_{\mathrm{irf}}(\mathbf{u}_a)}{P_{\mathrm{irf}}(\mathbf{u}_a)\,(1 - P_{\mathrm{irf}}(\mathbf{u}_a))}; \; \mathbf{u}_a \in \mathbb{U}_a; \, a \in \mathbb{A} \qquad (4.6)$$

or

$$V_a(\mathbf{u}_a) = \lambda \rho_a \left(-F_a(\mathbf{u}_a \mid \mathbf{g}^\circ) + P_{\mathrm{irf}}(\mathbf{u}_a) \right); \; \mathbf{u}_a \in \mathbb{U}_a; \, a \in \mathbb{A} \qquad (4.7)$$

where

$$\lambda = \frac{\sum\limits_{a \in \mathbb{A}} \rho_a^2 \sum\limits_{\mathbf{u}_a \in \mathbb{U}} \left(-F_a(\mathbf{u}_a \mid \mathbf{g}^\circ) + P_{\mathrm{irf}}(\mathbf{u}_a) \right)^2}{\sum\limits_{a \in \mathbb{A}} \rho_a^3 \sum\limits_{\mathbf{u}_a \in \mathbb{U}} \left(-F_a(\mathbf{u}_a \mid \mathbf{g}^\circ) + P_{\mathrm{irf}}(\mathbf{u}_a) \right)^2 P_{\mathrm{irf}}(\mathbf{u}_a)\,(1 - P_{\mathrm{irf}}(\mathbf{u}_a))}$$

The probabilities $\mathbf{P}_a = [P_{\mathrm{irf}}(\mathbf{u}_a) : \mathbf{u}_a \in \mathbb{U}_a]$; $a \in \mathbb{A}$, of the potential arguments (reduced signal co-occurrences) for both the uniform and homogeneous IRFs can be derived analytically or estimated empirically from the chains of images produced by the independent sampling of the site-wise signals in accord with the known signal marginals.

Most of the common MGRF models have hand-picked interaction structures. In some cases, e.g., for the second-order MGRFs with multiple pairwise interactions and some higher-order models, the characteristic structures can also be learned by analyzing the interaction energies for a large search set of clique shapes.

4.2.1 Nearest-Neighbor MGRFs

Classical Potts models of 2D/3D digital images and region maps account only for equality of signals (gray values or region labels) in the nearest pixel/voxel neighborhoods. The 2D 4-neighborhoods (Figure 4.2)

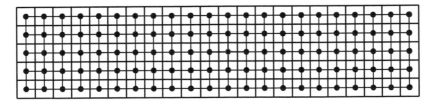

FIGURE 4.2
Interaction structure of a 2D Potts model.

or 3D 6-neighborhoods result in a single second-order clique family: $\mathbb{C} = \{\mathbf{c} = (\mathbf{r}, \mathbf{r} + \mathbf{v}) : \mathbf{v} \in \mathbf{n}; \mathbf{c} \in \mathbb{R}^2\}$ with $\mathbf{n} = \{(1,0),(0,1)\}$ or $\{(1,0,0),$ $(0,1,0),(0,0,1)\}$, respectively. The family is invariant to both translations and step-wise rotations by 90 degrees on the lattice, and its bi-variate potential with a single parameter γ is invariant to arbitrary contrast and offset deviations of the clique-wise signals:

$$V_\gamma(q_1, q_2) = \gamma\,(1 - 2\delta(q_1 - q_2)) = \begin{cases} -\gamma & \text{if } q_1 = q_2 \\ \gamma & \text{if } q_1 \neq q_2 \end{cases}$$

The GPD for the Potts MGRF:

$$P_\gamma(\mathbf{g}) = \frac{1}{Z_\gamma} \exp\left(-\sum_{(\mathbf{r},\mathbf{r}') \in \mathbb{C}} V_\gamma(g(\mathbf{r}), g(\mathbf{r}'))\right) \equiv \frac{1}{Z_\gamma} \exp\left(\gamma\,(2h_{eq}(\mathbf{g}) - |\mathbb{C}|)\right)$$

$$= \frac{1}{Z_\gamma} \exp\left(\gamma|\mathbb{C}|\,(2F_{eq}(\mathbf{g}) - 1)\right)$$

$$(4.8)$$

has the total number $h_{eq}(\mathbf{g}) = \sum_{(\mathbf{r},\mathbf{r}') \in \mathbb{C}} \delta(g(\mathbf{r}) - g(\mathbf{r}'))$ of equal signals over the clique family $\mathbb{C}$, or, what is just the same, their relative number, i.e., the empirical probability $F_{eq}(\mathbf{g}) = \frac{1}{|\mathbb{C}|} h_{eq}(\mathbf{g})$ as a single sufficient statistic of each image $\mathbf{g}$. In spite of its limited descriptive power, this MGRF is frequently used for modeling arbitrary-shaped and possibly discontinuous region maps $\mathbf{m}$. The cardinality, $|\mathbb{C}|$, of the 2D/3D clique family $\mathbb{C}$ on the lattice $\mathbb{R}$, i.e., the total number of all the nearest-neighbor pairs of the sites, is approximately equal to $k|\mathbf{R}|$ with $k = 2$ for the pixel 4-neighborhood and $k = 3$ for the voxel 6-neighborhood.

Obviously, the most probable images are uniform, i.e., contain only equal signals, whereas all the adjacent signal pairs in the least probable images are unequal (Figure 4.3).

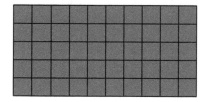 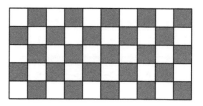

FIGURE 4.3
The most and the least probable images for a 2D binary Potts model.

Given a training image $\mathbf{g}^\circ$, the model in Equation 4.8 has the convenient irreducible form:

$$P_\gamma(\mathbf{g}^\circ) = \frac{1}{1 + \sum\limits_{\mathbf{g} \in G \setminus \mathbf{g}^\circ} \exp\left(2\gamma |\mathbb{C}| \left(F_{eq}(\mathbf{g}) - F_{eq}(\mathbf{g}^\circ)\right)\right)} \qquad (4.9)$$

The log-likelihood of the parameter γ and its first and second derivatives by γ are

$$\ell(\gamma \,|\, \mathbf{g}^\circ) = -\ln\left\{\sum_{\mathbf{g} \in G} \exp\left(2\gamma |\mathbb{C}| \left(F_{eq}(\mathbf{g}) - F_{eq}(\mathbf{g}^\circ)\right)\right)\right\}$$

$$\frac{d}{d\gamma}\ell(\gamma \,|\, \mathbf{g}^\circ) = 2|\mathbb{C}| \left(F_{eq}(\mathbf{g}^\circ) - \mathcal{E}\left\{F_{eq}(\mathbf{g}) \,|\, \gamma\right\}\right)$$

$$\frac{d^2}{d\gamma^2}\ell(\gamma \,|\, \mathbf{g}^\circ) = -4|\mathbb{C}|\mathcal{V}\left\{F_{eq}(\mathbf{g}) \,|\, \gamma\right\}$$

where $\mathcal{E}\left\{F_{eq}(\mathbf{g}) \,|\, \gamma\right\}$ and $\mathcal{V}\left\{F_{eq}(\mathbf{g}) \,|\, \gamma\right\}$ denote, respectively, the expected empirical probability, i.e., the probability $P_{eq:\gamma}$ of equal signals in a clique of the family $\mathbb{C}$ for the MGRF with the parameter γ, and the expected second central moment of the empirical probability, or the variance of the probability of equal clique-wise signals:

$$\mathcal{E}\left\{F_{eq}(\mathbf{g}) \,|\, \gamma\right\} \equiv \sum_{\mathbf{g} \in G} F_{eq}(\mathbf{g})P_\gamma(\mathbf{g}) \qquad\qquad = P_{eq:\gamma}$$

$$\mathcal{V}\left\{F_{eq}(\mathbf{g}) \,|\, \gamma\right\} \equiv \mathcal{E}\left\{F_{eq}^2(\mathbf{g}) \,|\, \gamma\right\} - \left(\mathcal{E}\left\{F_{eq}(\mathbf{g}) \,|\, \gamma\right\}\right)^2 = P_{eq:\gamma}\left(1 - P_{eq:\gamma}\right)$$

The zero parameter $\gamma = 0$ reduces this MGRF to the IRF of equiprobable signals, such that all its samples are equiprobable: $P_0(\mathbf{g}) = \frac{1}{|\mathbb{Q}|^{|\mathbb{R}|}}$, and the probability of equal signals in each pair of sites is $P_{eq:0} = \frac{1}{|\mathbb{Q}|}$.

The partition function Z_γ can be found, but in a fairly complicated analytical form, only for the binary signals, $|\mathbb{Q}| = 2$. Even in this simplest case, let alone more general ones, an exact analytical MLE γ^*, such that $\frac{d\ell(\gamma)}{d\gamma}|_{\gamma=\gamma^*} = 0$, or $P_{eq:\gamma^*} = F_{eq}(\mathbf{g}^\circ)$, is computationally infeasible. The approximate MLE of the parameter γ is obtained, in accord with Equation 2.27, by maximizing the truncated Taylor's decomposition:

$$\ell(\gamma \,|\, \mathbf{g}^\circ) \approx -|\mathbb{R}|\ln\{|\mathbb{Q}|\} + 2\gamma|\mathbb{C}| \left(F_{eq}(\mathbf{g}^\circ) - P_{eq:0}\right) - 2\gamma^2|\mathbb{C}|P_{eq:0}\left(1 - P_{eq:0}\right)$$

of the log-likelihood in the vicinity of the zero origin $\gamma = 0$:

$$\gamma^\circ = \frac{F_{eq}(\mathbf{g}^\circ) - P_{eq:0}}{2P_{eq:0}\left(1 - P_{eq:0}\right)} = \frac{|\mathbb{Q}|}{2}\left(\frac{|\mathbb{Q}|F_{eq}(\mathbf{g}^\circ) - 1}{|\mathbb{Q}| - 1}\right) \qquad (4.10)$$

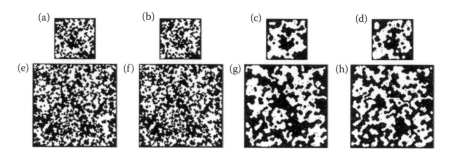

FIGURE 4.4
Training 64×64 and 128×128 images formed by the Gibbs sampler using the prescribed potential (a,e: $\gamma = 0.3$; c,g: $\gamma = 0.6$) vs. the images sampled using the analytical potential MLE (b: $\gamma^\circ = 0.326$; d: $\gamma^\circ = 0.585$; f: $\gamma^\circ = 0.323$; h: $\gamma^\circ = 0.592$).

Obviously, the closer the actual parameter γ to zero, i.e., the closer the training empirical probability $F_{eq}(\mathbf{g}^\circ)$ to $P_{eq:0}$, the more accurate the approximate MLE γ°.

At the same time, for $F_{eq}(\mathbf{g}^\circ) = 1$ the actual MLE $\gamma^* = \infty$, whereas $\gamma^\circ = \frac{1}{2P_{eq:0}} = \frac{|Q|}{2}$. In this case the $|Q|$ terms with $F_{eq}(\mathbf{g}) = 1$ in the denominator in Equation 4.9 do not depend on the parameter γ and all the remaining $|Q|^{|\mathbb{R}|} - |Q|$ terms $\exp\left(\gamma|\mathbb{C}|F_{eq}(\mathbf{g})\right) \xrightarrow[\gamma\to\infty]{} 0$ because $F_{eq}(\mathbf{g}) < 1$.

Similarly, the actual MLE for $F_{eq}(\mathbf{g}^\circ) = 0$ is $\gamma^* = -\infty$, but $\gamma^\circ = -\frac{1}{2(1-P_{eq:0})} = -\frac{|Q|}{2(|Q|-1)}$.

Figure 4.4 shows 64×64 and 128×128 training binary images ($Q = 2$) generated with $\gamma = 0.3$ and $\gamma = 0.6$, respectively, together with the images generated with the approximate parameter MLE γ° of Equation 4.10 obtained for the training images. Similar results for binary images of different size are presented in Figures 4.5 and 4.6. The ML estimator of the true value $\gamma = 0.3$ is compared in Figure 4.7 to a few other known estimators, such as the least square (LS), coding, MCMC, and σ ones, by showing both the estimated parameters and images simulated with these parameters.

A more general, but not contrast/offset-invariant model assumes that the exponential family of Equation 4.8 restricts a homogeneous IRF with the same arbitrary site-wise marginal $\mathbf{P}_0 = [P_0(q) : q \in Q]$. Then the first-order histogram, $\mathbf{h}_0(\mathbf{g}) = [h_0(q \mid \mathbf{g}) = \sum_{\mathbf{r}\in\mathbb{R}} \delta(q - g(\mathbf{r})) : q \in Q]$, of the signals is the additional sufficient statistics:

$$P_\gamma(\mathbf{g}) = \frac{1}{Z_\gamma} \left(\prod_{\mathbf{r}\in\mathbb{R}} P_0(g(\mathbf{r})) \right) \exp\left(-\sum_{(\mathbf{r},\mathbf{r}')\in\mathbb{C}} V_\gamma(g(\mathbf{r}), g(\mathbf{r}')) \right)$$

$$= \frac{1}{Z_\gamma} \exp\left(\sum_{q\in Q} |\mathbb{R}|F_0(q \mid \mathbf{g}) \ln P_0(q) + \gamma|\mathbb{C}|(2F_{eq}(\mathbf{g}) - 1) \right)$$

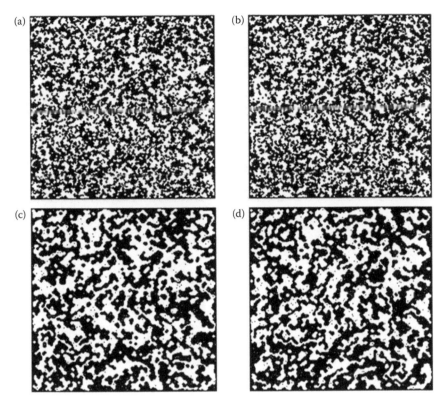

FIGURE 4.5
Training 256×256 images formed with the Gibbs sampler (a: $\gamma = 0.3$; c: $\gamma = 0.6$) vs. the images sampled using the analytical potential MLE (b: $\gamma^\circ = 0.315$; d: $\gamma^\circ = 0.605$).

where $F_0(q \mid \mathbf{g}) = \frac{1}{|\mathbb{R}|} h_0(q \mid \mathbf{g})$ is the empirical probability of the signal q in the image $\mathbf{g}$.

Given a training image $\mathbf{g}^\circ$, the first-order factors are estimated with the empirical marginals $\widetilde{P}_0(q) = F_0(q \mid \mathbf{g}^\circ)$ and the approximate estimate for the parameter γ is the same as in Equation 4.10, but with the probability $P_{\text{eq:0}} = \sum_{q \in \mathbb{Q}} \widetilde{P}_0^2(q)$ of the equal signal pairs in the generic homogeneous IRF. Descriptive abilities of these simple image models can be amplified by adding one or more translation or translation-rotation invariant families of higher-order cliques with potentials that account for ordinal relations between the clique-wise signals.

The translation-rotation-invariant Potts MGRF with the nearest 4- or 8-neighborhood of each pixel or the nearest 6- or 26-neighborhood of each voxel is very popular for a long time as a region map model. Its Gibbs potential is independent of relative orientation of pixel pairs, is the same for all distinct regions, and depends only on whether the pair of labels are equal or not. Under these assumptions, it is the simplest auto-binomial model.

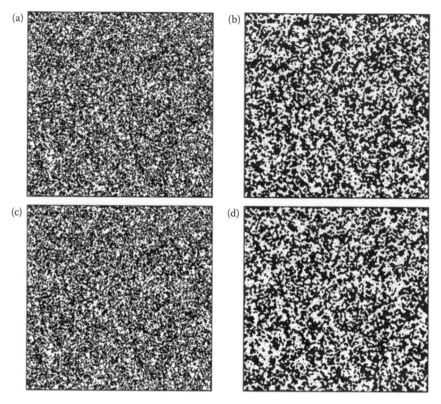

FIGURE 4.6
Training 512×512 images formed by the Gibbs sampler (a: $\gamma = 0.3$; b: $\gamma = 0.6$) vs. the images sampled using the analytical potential MLE (c: $\gamma^\circ = 0.315$; d: $\gamma^\circ = 0.605$).

A simple joint model of piecewise-homogeneous images combines an unconditional Potts model of region maps with different conditional IRF models of image signals for each region:

$$P_\gamma(\mathbf{g}, \mathbf{m})$$

$$= \frac{1}{Z_\gamma} \left(\prod_{r \in \mathbb{R}} P_{\mathrm{irf}}(g(\mathbf{r}) \mid m(\mathbf{r})) \right) \exp \left(- \sum_{(\mathbf{r},\mathbf{r}') \in \mathbb{C}} V_\gamma \left(m(\mathbf{r}), m(\mathbf{r}') \right) \right)$$

$$= \frac{1}{Z_\gamma} \exp \left(|\mathbb{R}| \sum_{l \in \mathbb{L}} F(l \mid \mathbf{m}) \sum_{q \in \mathbb{Q}} F(q \mid l; \mathbf{g}, \mathbf{m}) \ln P(q \mid l) - \gamma |\mathbb{C}| (2F_{\mathrm{eq}}(\mathbf{m}) - 1) \right)$$

where $F(l \mid \mathbf{m}) = \frac{1}{|\mathbb{R}|} \sum_{\mathbf{r} \in \mathbb{R}} \delta(l - m(\mathbf{r}))$ is the empirical probability of the region label l in the map $\mathbf{m}$ and $F(q \mid l; \mathbf{g}, \mathbf{m}) = \frac{1}{|\mathbb{R}_l|} \sum_{\mathbf{r} \in \mathbb{R}}$

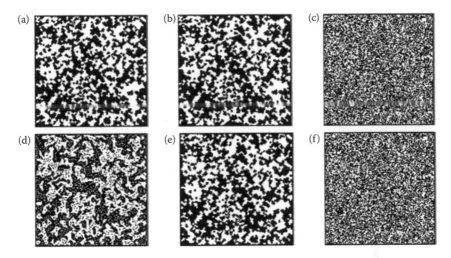

FIGURE 4.7
Training 128×128 image formed by the Gibbs sampler (a: $\gamma = 0.3$) vs. the samples from the models using the analytical MLE (b: $\gamma^\circ = 0.323$) and the least-square (c: $\widehat{\gamma} = 0.115$); coding (d: $\widehat{\gamma} = 0.154$); MCMC (e: $\widehat{\gamma} = 0.348$); and σ (f: $\widehat{\gamma} = 0.027$) estimators.

$\delta(l - m(\mathbf{r}))\delta(q - g(\mathbf{r}))$ is the conditional empirical probability of the image signal q over the region $\mathbb{R}_l = \{\mathbf{r} : \mathbf{r} \in \mathbb{R}; \ m(\mathbf{r}) = l\}$.

4.2.2 Gaussian and Gauss-Markov Random Fields

These second-order models presume continuous (real-valued) pixel- or voxel-wise image signals in the infinite interval $\mathbb{Q} = (-\infty, +\infty)$. A Gaussian random field is specified with a unimodal multivariate Gaussian, or normal probability density:

$$P(\mathbf{g}) = \frac{1}{(2\pi)^{|\mathbb{R}|/2}|\mathbf{C}|^{0.5}} \exp\left(-\frac{1}{2}(\mathbf{g} - \boldsymbol{\mu})^\mathsf{T}\mathbf{C}^{-1}(\mathbf{g} - \boldsymbol{\mu})\right) \tag{4.11}$$

which is centered on the expected "mean" image $\boldsymbol{\mu}$ and has the covariance matrix $\mathbf{C}$. This exponential family is derived by constraining the mean and covariance matrix to their empirical values for one or more training images:

$$\int\limits_{\mathbf{g} \in \mathbb{Q}^{|\mathbb{R}|}} \mathbf{g}P(\mathbf{g})d\mathbf{g} = \boldsymbol{\mu}^\circ; \quad \int\limits_{\mathbf{g} \in \mathbb{Q}^{|\mathbb{R}|}} (\mathbf{g} - \boldsymbol{\mu}^\circ)(\mathbf{g} - \boldsymbol{\mu}^\circ)^\mathsf{T}P(\mathbf{g})d\mathbf{g} = \mathbf{C}^\circ \tag{4.12}$$

The number $|\mathbb{R}| + \frac{1}{2}|\mathbb{R}|(|\mathbb{R}| + 1)$ of the parameters for the general-case Gaussian random field is too large for learning, as well, as such model does not account for spatial or spatiotemporal homogeneity of a majority of textured objects of interest. A particular case, called a simultaneous autoregressive (SAR) model, or a GMRF, was used frequently in early approaches to modeling homogeneous textures. The GMRF excludes excessively long-range pairwise interactions and thus it has much less parameters to be learned from the training data, than the general-case model.

An underlying assumption behind this model is a so-called linear "whitening" of a stochastic process producing the images. It is assumed that pixel/voxel intensities can be predicted by linear filtering of their neighbors and prediction errors are sampled from a "white" Gaussian IRF, i.e., the IRF with the same zero-centered normal distributions of individual errors. In other words, all the signal dependencies are considered deterministic and linear in a fixed rectangular neighborhood (moving window) of a given size around each lattice site.

Let $\mathbf{w}$, $\alpha = [\alpha_{\nu: \nu \in \mathbf{w}}]^{\mathsf{T}}$, and $e_\alpha(\mathbf{r})$ denote an ordered set of relative coordinates, specifying the window, a vector of filter weights, and a prediction error at the filter output, respectively. The set $\mathbf{w}$ represents individual positions (lattice sites) in the window by their coordinate offsets $\nu \in \mathbf{w}$ with respect to the guiding position, e.g., the window center. If the filter output, $e_\alpha(\mathbf{r}) = g(\mathbf{r}) - \sum_{\nu \in \mathbf{w}} \alpha_\nu g(\mathbf{r} + \nu)$, when the window center coincides with a particular lattice site, $\mathbf{r}$, is considered a white Gaussian error, the GPD for the GMRF is

$$P(\mathbf{g}) = \frac{1}{(2\pi)^{|\mathbb{R}|/2} \sigma^{|\mathbb{R}|}} \exp\left(-\frac{1}{2\sigma^2} \sum_{\mathbf{r} \in \mathbb{R}} \left(g\left(\mathbf{r} - \sum_{\nu \in \mathbf{w}} \alpha_\nu g(\mathbf{r} + \nu)\right)\right)^2\right) \quad (4.13)$$

Given one or more training images, $\mathbf{g}^\circ$, the weights α for a fixed-size filter and the noise variance, σ^2, are learned by maximizing the log-likelihood of the training data:

$$\hat{\alpha} = \mathbf{A}^{-1}\mathbf{a}; \quad \hat{\sigma}^2 = \frac{1}{|\mathbb{R}|} \sum_{\mathbf{r} \in \mathbb{R}} e_{\hat{\alpha}}^2(\mathbf{r}) \quad (4.14)$$

where $\mathbf{A} = \left[A_{|\nu-\nu'|} : \nu, \nu' \in \mathbf{w}\right]$ and $\mathbf{a} = [a_\nu : \nu \in \mathbf{w}]^{\mathsf{T}}$ denote the data $|\mathbf{w}| \times |\mathbf{w}|$ matrix and $|\mathbf{w}|$-vector, respectively, with the components

$$A_{|\nu-\nu'|} = \sum_{\mathbf{r} \in \mathbb{R}} g(\mathbf{r} + \nu)g(\mathbf{r} + \nu') \quad \text{and} \quad a_\nu = \sum_{\mathbf{r} \in \mathbb{R}} g(\mathbf{r} + \nu)g(\mathbf{r})$$

Generally, the above whitening process may be considered as producing an IRF with the same symmetric, but not necessarily Gaussian marginal for all the sites. Then not only the filter weights, but also the residual noise distribution have to be learned from the training data. Let $M_Q \{u\}$ denote a mapping of a real-valued filter output $u = e_\alpha(\mathbf{r})$ into Q integer values

$Q = \{0, 1, \ldots, Q-1\}$. Given a particular filter with the quantified outputs, an arbitrary distribution $\mathbf{P}_c = (P_c(q) : q \in Q)$ of the IRF components is estimated by the empirical marginal probabilities $\mathbf{P}_{emp}$ of the filter outputs for training images. The whitened MRF of images is then defined by the distribution

$$P(\mathbf{g}) = \prod_{\mathbf{r} \in \mathbb{R}} P_{emp} \left(M_Q \left\{ g(\mathbf{r}) - \sum_{\mathbf{v} \in \mathbf{w}} \alpha_{\mathbf{v}} g(\mathbf{r} + \mathbf{v}) \right\} \right) \qquad (4.15)$$

4.2.3 Models with Multiple Pairwise Interactions

A generic second-order MGRF is defined by the GPD $\mathbf{P_V} = [P_V(\mathbf{g}) : \mathbf{g} \in \mathbf{G}]$, such that

$$
\begin{aligned}
P_V(\mathbf{g}) &= \frac{1}{Z_V} P_0(\mathbf{g}) \exp \left(- \sum_{a \in \mathbb{A}} \sum_{c_a \in \mathbf{C}_a} V_a(g(\mathbf{r}) : \mathbf{r} \in c_a) \right) \\
&= \frac{1}{Z_V} P_{irf}(\mathbf{g}) \exp \left(- \sum_{a \in \mathbb{A}} |\mathbf{C}_a| \mathbf{V}_a^{\mathsf{T}} \mathbf{F}_a(\mathbf{g}) \right) \qquad (4.16) \\
&\equiv \frac{1}{Z_V} P_{irf}(\mathbf{g}) \exp \left(- |\mathbb{R}| \sum_{a \in \mathbb{A}} \rho_a \mathbf{V}_a^{\mathsf{T}} \mathbf{F}_a(\mathbf{g}) \right)
\end{aligned}
$$

where $P_{irf}(\mathbf{g} = \prod_{\mathbf{r} \in \mathbb{R}} P_{irf}(g(\mathbf{r}))$ is the probability distribution for a homogeneous core IRF; $\rho_a = \frac{|\mathbf{C}_a|}{|\mathbb{R}|}$ is the relative size of the clique family $\mathbf{C}_a$ with respect to the lattice size; $\mathbb{A}$ is an index set of the clique families; $\mathbf{V}_a = [V_a(q, q') : (q, q' \in Q^2]^{\mathsf{T}}$ is the vector of potentials for signal co-occurrences supported by the cliques of the family $\mathbf{C}_a$; $\mathbf{F}_a(\mathbf{g}) = [F_a(q, q' \mid \mathbf{g}) : (q, q' \in Q^2]^{\mathsf{T}}]^{\mathsf{T}}$ is the normalized histogram, or the vector of empirical probabilities of signal co-occurrences over the image $\mathbf{g}$ for the same clique family:

$$F_a(q, q' \mid \mathbf{g}) = \frac{1}{|\mathbf{C}_a|} \sum_{(\mathbf{r}, \mathbf{r}') \in \mathbf{C}_a} \delta(q - g(\mathbf{r})) \delta(q' - g(\mathbf{r}'))$$

and Z_V is the normalizer (partition function), such that $Z_0 = 1$ for the zero potential.

Each clique family $\mathbf{C}_a = \{(\mathbf{r}, \mathbf{r}') : \mathbf{r}, \mathbf{r}' \in \mathbb{R}\}$; $a \in \mathbb{A}$, consists of all pairs $(\mathbf{r}, \mathbf{r}')$ of the sites with a fixed coordinate offset, $\mathbf{r} - \mathbf{r}' = \mathbf{v}_a$, or fixed bounds of the distance, $d_{a:min} < |\mathbf{r} - \mathbf{r}'| \leq d_{a:max}$, between the sites in a translation-invariant or translation/rotation-invariant model, respectively. The set $\mathbb{N} = \{\mathbf{v}_a : a \in \mathbb{A}\}$ of all coordinate offsets in the former model or $\mathbb{N} = \{\mathbf{v} : d_{a:min} < |\mathbf{v} \leq d_{a:max}; a \in \mathbb{A}\}$ in the latter model specifies the characteristic pixel/voxel neighborhood, $\mathcal{N}_{\mathbf{r}} = \{\mathbf{r} \pm \mathbf{v} : \mathbf{v} \in \mathbb{N}\} \cap \mathbb{R}$, which may combine arbitrary close- and long-range pairwise interactions and be continuous or discontinuous (see, e.g., the continuous translation/rotation-invariant neighborhood in Figure 4.1 specified by the bounds: $d_{a:\min} = a - 0.5$; $d_{a:\max} = d_{a+1,\min}$; $\mathbb{A} = \{1, 2, \ldots, 8\}$).

This model restricts the homogeneous core IRF $\mathbf{P}_0$ by constraining the $|\mathbb{A}|$ marginals of the pairwise signal co-occurrences, $\mathbf{P}_{2:a} = [P_{2:a}(q, q') : (q, q') \in \mathbb{Q}^2]^\mathsf{T} \equiv \mathcal{E}\{\mathbf{f}_a(\mathbf{g}) \,|\, \mathbf{P}_V\}$, i.e, the expected empirical marginals for the clique families. In particular, the MLE of the potentials equate these marginals to the corresponding empirical marginals for a given training sample, $\mathbf{g}^\circ$, i.e., $\mathbf{P}_{2:a} = \mathbf{f}_{2:a}(\mathbf{g}^\circ)$.

To analytically identify this MGRF, given a training sample $\mathbf{g}^\circ$, the marginals of the individual signals defining the core IRF are learned from the normalized signal histogram, or the empirical signal marginal: $P_{\text{irf}}^\circ(q) = \frac{1}{|\mathbb{R}|} \sum_{\mathbf{r} \in \mathbb{R}} \delta(q - g(\mathbf{r}))$; $q \in \mathbb{Q}$. Then the approximate MLE of the second-order potentials are obtained (in line with Section 2.3.1) from the truncated Taylor's series decomposition of the log-likelihood:

$$V_a^\circ(q, q') = \frac{P_{\text{irf}}^\circ(q) P_{\text{irf}}^\circ(q') - F_a(q, q' \,|\, \mathbf{g}^\circ)}{P_{\text{irf}}^\circ(q) P_{\text{irf}}^\circ(q') \left(1 - P_{\text{irf}}^\circ(q) P_{\text{irf}}^\circ(q')\right)}; \quad (q, q') \in \mathbb{Q}^2; \ a \in \mathbb{A} \quad (4.17)$$

or, alternatively,

$$V_a^\circ(q, q') = \lambda \rho_V \left(P_{\text{irf}}^\circ(q) P_{\text{irf}}^\circ(q') - F_a(q, q' \,|\, \mathbf{g}^\circ)\right); \quad (q, q') \in \mathbb{Q}^2; \ a \in \mathbb{A} \quad (4.18)$$

with the common scaling factor

$$\lambda = \frac{\displaystyle\sum_{a \in \mathbb{A}} \rho_a^2 \sum_{(q,q') \in \mathbb{Q}^2} \left(P_{\text{irf}}^\circ(q) P_{\text{irf}}^\circ(q') - F_a(q, q' \,|\, \mathbf{g}^\circ)\right)^2}{\displaystyle\sum_{a \in \mathbb{A}} \rho_a^3 \sum_{(q,q') \in \mathbb{Q}^2} \left(P_{\text{irf}}^\circ(q) P_{\text{irf}}^\circ(q') - F_a(q, q' \,|\, \mathbf{g}^\circ)\right)^2 P_{\text{irf}}^\circ(q) P_{\text{irf}}^\circ(q') \left(1 - P_{\text{irf}}^\circ(q) P_{\text{irf}}^\circ(q')\right)}$$

The estimates in Equation 4.18 are almost independent of the lattice size $|\mathbb{R}|$ for the large training images, when the ratios $\rho_a \approx 1$; $a \in \mathbb{A}$.

In the special case of the core IRF with equiprobable signals, $P_{\text{irf}}(q) = \frac{1}{|\mathbb{Q}|}$, the approximate potential MLEs of Equations 4.17 and 4.18 are, respectively,

$$V_a^\circ(q, q') = \frac{\frac{1}{|\mathbb{Q}|^2} - F_a(q, q' | \mathbf{g}^\circ)}{\frac{1}{|\mathbb{Q}|^2} \left(1 - \frac{1}{|\mathbb{Q}|^2}\right)} = \frac{|\mathbb{Q}|^2}{|\mathbb{Q}|^2 - 1} \left(1 - |\mathbb{Q}|^2 f(q, q' | \mathbf{g}^\circ)\right)$$

$$\approx 1 - |\mathbb{Q}|^2 f(q, q' | \mathbf{g}^\circ); \quad (q, q') \in \mathbb{Q}^2; \ a \in \mathbb{A} \quad (4.19)$$

and

$$V_a^\circ(q,q') = \lambda \rho_a \frac{1}{|\mathbf{Q}|^2} \left(1 - |\mathbf{Q}|^2 F_a(q,q'|\mathbf{g}^\circ)\right); \quad (q,q') \in \mathbf{Q}^2; \quad a \in \mathbb{A} \quad (4.20)$$

with

$$\lambda = \frac{|\mathbf{Q}|^4}{|\mathbf{Q}|^2 - 1} \cdot \frac{\sum\limits_{a \in \mathbb{A}} \rho_a^2 \sum\limits_{(q,q') \in \mathbf{Q}^2} \left(1 - |\mathbf{Q}|^2 F_a(q,q'|\mathbf{g}^\circ)\right)^2}{\sum\limits_{a \in \mathbb{A}} \rho_a^3 \sum\limits_{(q,q') \in \mathbf{Q}^2} \left(1 - |\mathbf{Q}|^2 F_a(q,q'|\mathbf{g}^\circ)\right)^2}$$

and hence are almost the same as in Equation 4.19 when $\rho_a \approx \rho \approx 1$; $a \in \mathbb{A}$, and $\lambda \approx |\mathbf{Q}|^2$.

The translation/rotation-invariant MGRF allows for learning visual appearance of objects with no definite shape, position, and pose, e.g., lung nodules (tumors). Typical 2D sections in Figure 4.8 of the training nodules from a database of the 350 3D nodules exemplify variations of the voxel-wise second-order energies for the individual central-symmetric neighborhoods, like those in Figure 4.1, in the learned model of Equation 4.16:

$$E_{2:r}(\mathbf{g}) = \sum_{a \in \mathbb{A}} \sum_{\substack{r \in \{r_1, r_2\}; \\ (r_1, r_2) \in \mathbf{C}_a}} V_a\left(g(\mathbf{r}_1), g(\mathbf{r}_2)\right) \quad (4.21)$$

The same energies specify the voxel-wise conditional probabilities of signals of Equation 4.5 for stochastic relaxation. The characteristic clique families in Figure 4.8 were estimated by thresholding a marginal distribution of family-wise partial interaction energies for a large search set of the candidate

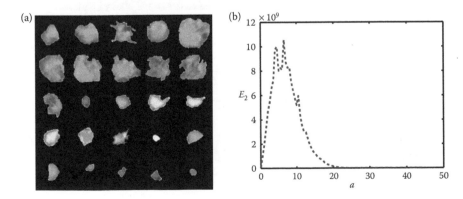

FIGURE 4.8
Typical 2D cross sections (a) of the training nodules and the corresponding gray-coded voxel-wise interaction energies (b) of Equation 4.21 for the central-symmetric neighborhoods $\mathcal{N}_a$; $a \leq 50$, in the training nodules.

families, as detailed below, in Section 4.3. To find the best separating threshold ($\tau = 12$ in this particular case), the latter marginal was approximated by an LCDG with two dominant low- and high-energy components using the modeling algorithms of Chapter 3. Figure 4.9 presents three cross sections of the LDCT image containing lung nodules and the corresponding voxel-wise energies of Equation 4.21. That these energies for the nodules are lower than for all other lung voxels helps in accurate nodule segmentation.

The analytical potential estimates in Equations 4.17 through 4.20 can be further refined by combining the MCMC sampling of the estimated MGRF with simultaneous updates of the potentials. The refinement minimizes the difference between the sufficient statistics, i.e., between the empirical marginals for the sampled and training images by using the approximate

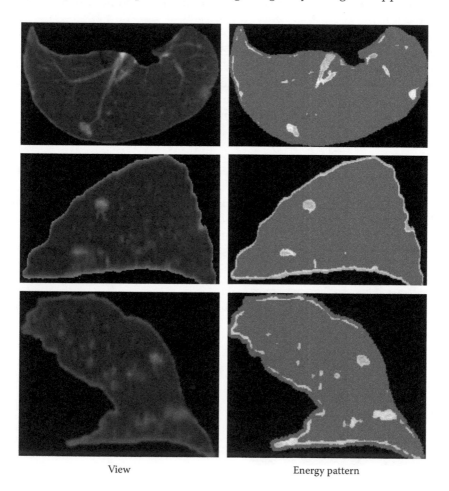

View   Energy pattern

FIGURE 4.9
Original three views (left) and the corresponding gray-coded pixel-wise negated energies (right) for the learned characteristic central-symmetric neighborhoods.

likelihood gradient search. The latter is called sometimes controllable simulated annealing or persistent contrastive divergence.

4.2.4 Higher-Order MGRFs

The approximate MLE of parameters of an exponential family in Section 2.3.1, which have been used to identify the generic second-order MGRFs, exist in principle for any higher-order MGRF with an arbitrary system of the K-order clique families; $K \geq 3$. However, the exponential growth of the number $|Q|^K$ of signal configurations on a K-order clique with respect to a limited number $(J|\mathbb{R}|)$ of their available training samples where $J \geq 1$ is the number of training samples, hinders learning the K-variate potentials from the empirical and expected marginals of the K-ary signal co-occurrences. To remain practicable, the higher-order modeling employs one or another scalar or vectorial mapping $\mathbf{M} : Q^K \to \mathbb{U}$ of the co-occurrence space for each clique family $\mathbb{C}$ to a more tractable space of the transformed signals $\mathbf{u} = \mathbf{M}_a(\mathbf{q}) \in \mathbb{U}$; $\mathbf{q} = [q_1, \ldots, q_K]^\top \in Q^K$.

Moving-window transformations of an image $\mathbf{g}$ with a bank of N co-aligned signal converters, supported by each K-order clique and called *filters*, replace each clique-wise K-ary signal co-occurrence, or configuration $\mathbf{q} = [q_1, \ldots, q_K]^\top \in Q^K$ with a vector $\mathbf{u} = [u_i : i = 1, \ldots, N]^\top$ of N scalar filter outputs: $\mathbf{u}_i = [u_i = M_i(q_1, \ldots, q_K) : i = 1, \ldots, N]^\top$.

Each K-variate filtering function $M_i(\ldots)$ of the clique-wise signals is usually quantified into U; $U \geq 2$, levels, so that the initial space of the $|Q|^K$ signal co-occurrences is projected onto the reduced space of the U^N combinations of outputs of the filters, e.g., $M_i(q_1, \ldots, q_K) = \sum_{k=1}^K w_{i:k} q_k$ for a popular linear mapping where $w_{i:k}$ is the kth weight of the ith filter. The simultaneous linear filtering replaces the clique-wise K-vectors of signals by the lower-dimensional N-vectors $\mathbf{u} = \mathbf{M}\mathbf{q}$ where $\mathbf{M}$ is a rectangular matrix of the coefficients $w_{i:k}$; $i = 1, \ldots, N$; $k = 1, \ldots, K$, for the N linear filters.

Filtering of an IRF with spatially overlapping or nonoverlapping system of the filters produces inter- or independent outputs, respectively. Let the IRF be homogeneous with an arbitrary site-wise marginal $\mathbf{P}_{\text{irf}} = [P_{\text{irf}}(q) : q \in Q]$ having the mean $\mu = \sum_{q \in Q} q P_{\text{irf}}(q)$ and the variance $\sigma^2 = \sum_{q \in Q} q^2 P_{\text{irf}}(q) - \mu^2$. If $K \gg 1$, the marginal of the linear filtering outputs $u_i = \sum_{k=1}^K w_{i:k} q_k$ for this IRF tends to the normal distribution with the mean $\mu_i = \mu \sum_{k=1}^K w_{i:k}$ and the variance $\sigma_i^2 = \sigma^2 \sum_{k=1}^K w_{i:k}^2$.

Conversely, the simultaneous linear or nonlinear filtering is often used to approximate an arbitrary high-order MGRF with a stack of mutually independent, by supposition, IRFs, being combined into a single GPD. The k^2-order FRAME (Filters, Random Fields, and Maximum Entropy) and FoE (Field of Experts) models have square $k \times k$ cliques, centered at each pixel, and perform simultaneous N-channel image filtering to implicitly account for actual interactions between the k^2 signals.

The *FRAME* constrains marginals of quantified outputs of a bank of N linear filters and, possibly, a few nonlinear moving-window filters. The model combines the outputs $u_i(\mathbf{r})$; $u_i \in \mathbb{U}_i$; $\mathbf{r} \in \mathbb{R}$, of all the filters, which are considered mutually independent:

$$P(\mathbf{g}) = \frac{1}{Z} \prod_{\mathbf{r} \in \mathbb{R}} \prod_{i=1}^{N} f_i(u_i(\mathbf{r})) \equiv \frac{1}{Z} \exp\left(-\sum_{\mathbf{r} \in \mathbb{R}} \sum_{i=1}^{N} V_i(u_i(\mathbf{r})) \right)$$

$$= \frac{1}{Z} \exp\left(-|\mathbb{R}| \cdot \sum_{i=1}^{N} \sum_{u \in \mathbb{U}_i} V_i(u) F_i(u|\mathbf{g}) \right) \equiv \frac{1}{Z} \exp\left(-|\mathbb{R}| \sum_{i=1}^{N} \mathbf{V}_i^\mathsf{T} \mathbf{F}_i(\mathbf{g})) \right)$$

Here, $u_i(\mathbf{r})$ denotes the scalar output of the ith filter, centered on the pixel $\mathbf{r}$; every scalar factor $f_i(u_i(\mathbf{r}))$; $u_i(\mathbf{r}) \in \mathbb{U}_i$, evaluates the contribution of this output to the image probability; $\mathbb{U}_i$ is a finite set of the quantified filter outputs; $V_i(u_i(\mathbf{r})) = -\ln f_i(u_i(\mathbf{r}))$ is the potential, or negated logarithm of the factor; $\mathbf{F}_i(\mathbf{g})) = [F_i(u|\mathbf{g}) : u \in \mathbb{U}_i]^\mathsf{T}$ is the marginal of the quantified outputs u of the ith filter over the image $\mathbf{g}$, and $\mathbf{V}_i = [V_i(u) : u \in \mathbb{U}_i]^\mathsf{T}$ is the potential vector for these quantified outputs.

Because the image $\mathbf{g}$ is converted into a stack of N co-aligned filter outputs, every $k \times k$ spatial signal configuration over the clique with the center at the site $\mathbf{r}$ is represented by a site-wise vector, or signature of N elements $\mathbf{u}(\mathbf{r}) = [u_i(\mathbf{r}) : i = 1, \ldots, N]^\mathsf{T}$, being the outputs of the filters. The N marginals $[\mathbf{F}_i(\mathbf{g}) : i = 1, \ldots, N]^\mathsf{T}$ collected over the image $\mathbf{g}$ for the quantified filter outputs are sufficient statistics describing the image. Given a training image, $\mathbf{g}^\circ$, all the FRAME potentials are learned by the approximate likelihood gradient search, starting from the zero or hand-picked potential values. The search goal is to equate the empirical marginals, $F_i(u|\mathbf{g})$; $i = 1, \ldots, N$, of the filter outputs for the images sampled from, i.e., generated with the model to the corresponding training marginals, $F_i(u|\mathbf{g}^\circ)$; $i = 1, \ldots, N$, as was detailed in Section 2.3 (see Equations 2.19 and 2.20).

The linear filters are often symmetric orthogonal 2D Gabor filters with spatially oriented sinusoidal waves of Gaussian-weighted coefficients in the $k \times k$ square window: for $(\xi, \eta) \in \mathbf{w}$; $i = 1, \ldots, N$

$$w_{i:\xi,\eta} = \frac{1}{2\pi\sigma_i^2} \exp\left(-\frac{\xi^2 + \eta^2}{2\sigma_i^2} \right) \cos\left(\frac{2\pi}{r_i}(\xi \cos \phi_i + \eta \sin \phi_i) \right)$$

where σ_i is the Gaussian spatial weight and parameters (r_i, ϕ_i) define the number and orientation of the waves in the window. The filter, or clique size, k^2, is selected manually and usually is small, e.g., $k = 5 \ldots 11$ in known applications, for computational feasibility.

To learn the FRAME, the filters are selected and added to the model sequentially, by comparing their output marginals collected over a training image to the corresponding marginals over an image sampled from the current model. Each step selects a filter from the remaining collection, such that its marginal for the sampled image is the most distant from the training marginal. The process terminates after the next filter insignificantly improves the modeling.

The *FOE* has also the handpicked number, N, and size, k^2, of specific non-linear filters, performing prescribed parametric unimodal nonlinear transformations of outputs of linear filters. Let $\mathbf{w}_i = [w_{i:\mathbf{v}} : \mathbf{v} \in \mathbb{N}]^\mathsf{T}; \sum_{\mathbf{v} \in \mathbb{N}} w_{i:\mathbf{v}}^2 = 1;$ $i = 1, \ldots, N$, denote the vector of normalized filter coefficients with coordinate offsets $\mathbb{N}$ defining the $k \times k$ clique, centered at every pixel $\mathbf{r}$. Let $\zeta_i(v, \alpha_i, \beta_i) - -\alpha_i \log \left(1 + \frac{1}{2}\beta_i^2 v^2\right), v_i(\mathbf{r})$, and $\mathbb{U}_i$ denote non-linear transformation function; the output of the ith linear filter:

$$v_i(\mathbf{r}) = \sum_{\mathbf{v} \in \mathbb{N}_i} w_{i:\mathbf{v}} g(\mathbf{r} + \mathbf{v})$$

and a finite set of the (quantified) outputs of the ith nonlinear filter with the parameters $(\mathbf{w}_i; \alpha_i, \beta_i)$, respectively. The image probability for the FOE model with the N filters $\mathbf{W} = \{(\mathbf{w}_i; \alpha_i, \beta_i) : i = 1, \ldots, N\}$ is

$$P(\mathbf{g}) = \frac{1}{Z} \exp\left(-\sum_{\mathbf{r} \in \mathbb{R}} \sum_{i=1}^{N} \zeta_i(v_i(\mathbf{r}); \alpha_i, \beta_i)\right)$$

$$= \frac{1}{Z} \exp\left(-|\mathbb{R}| \sum_{i=1}^{N} \sum_{u \in \mathbb{U}_i} V_i(u) F_i(u|\mathbf{g})\right)$$

where $V_i(u)$ and $F_i(u|\mathbf{g})$ denote, respectively, the potential values for and empirical marginals (relative frequencies) of the filter outputs $u = \zeta_i(\ldots)$ on the image $\mathbf{g}$. These marginals are the sufficient statistics of the FoE.

Both the N linear filters and the transformation parameters $\mathbf{W}$ are learned by gradient search for a local minimum of the relative energy $E_\mathbf{W}(\mathbf{g}^\circ) = \sum_{i=1}^{N} \sum_{u \in \mathbb{U}_i} V_i(u) F_i(u \mid \mathbf{g}^\circ)$ of a given training image, $\mathbf{g}^\circ$. To facilitate the learning, the chosen transformation function $\zeta_i(\ldots)$ is continuous and differentiable with respect to the variables α_i, β_i, and v, as well as yields a convex unimodal interaction energy. Moreover, it resembles typical heavy-tailed marginals of natural image statistics, e.g., has a strong kurtosis. The gradient search starts with the unit transformation parameters and orthogonal linear filters, which are obtained by the PCA and "whiten" (decorrelate) the training k^2-component vectors of training signals for all co-aligned $k \times k$ cliques.

4.3 Learning Second-Order Interaction Structures

Generic translation-invariant MGRF models in Section 4.2.3 describe each particular type of spatially homogeneous textures in terms of characteristic pixel/voxel coordinate offsets $\mathbb{N}$ and potentials $\mathbf{V} = [\mathbf{V}_\mathbf{v} : \mathbf{v} \in \mathbb{N}]$ that specify the geometric structure and quantitative strengths of interactions, respectively. Collecting the sufficient model statistics, i.e., the normalized histograms, or empirical probabilities of signal co-occurrences for each clique family for a given training sample, $\mathbf{g}°$, facilitates not only the approximate analytical MLE of the potentials, but also the search for the characteristic texture-dependent offsets $\mathbb{N}$.

Analytical approximations of the potentials allow for ordering a large set of clique families by their relative partial energies:

$$E_{\mathbf{v}}(\mathbf{g}°) = \rho_{\mathbf{v}} \sum_{(q,q')\in Q^2} \left(F_{\mathbf{v}}(q,q'\,|\,\mathbf{g}°) - P_{\mathrm{irf}}(q)P_{\mathrm{irf}}(q')\right) F_{\mathbf{v}}(q,q'\,|\,\mathbf{g}°) \qquad (4.22)$$

and select the most characteristic ones. The lower the relative partial energy, $E_{\mathbf{v}}(\mathbf{g}°) = \mathbf{V}_{\mathbf{v}}^{\mathsf{T}}\mathbf{f}_{\mathbf{v}}(\mathbf{g}°)$, the more relevant the clique family $\mathbb{C}_{\mathbf{v}}$ to the model.

Because all clique families share the same lattice sites, signal co-occurrences in the overlapping cliques are not statistically independent and the search for a characteristic structure depends on how strong are their dependencies. The simplest assumption that all clique families are (almost) independent outlines a class of "stochastic" textures determined by their basic interaction structures. In this case the characteristic set $\mathbb{N}$ can be learned by choosing the partial energies below an adaptive threshold τ derived from the empirical distribution of the energies $E_{\mathbf{v}}(\mathbf{g}°)$ for a large *search set* of the clique families $\mathbb{C} = \{\mathbb{C}_{\mathbf{v}} : \mathbf{v} \in \mathbb{N}_{\mathrm{search}}\}$. Translation-invariant stochastic textures, shown in Figure 4.10, have only close-range pixel neighborhoods of texture-dependent shape, whereas quasi-periodic textures have disjoint long- and close-range neighborhoods, which reflect dominant directions of periodicity. Many natural textures in medical images are of stochastic appearance, which simplifies their modeling. More "regular," e.g., quasi-periodic visual patterns, such as, e.g., mosaics in Figure 4.10, cannot be accurately modeled by only the basic structure. Both the guiding basic and minor fine repetitive details of these textures are visually important, although the partial energies for the families governing the fine

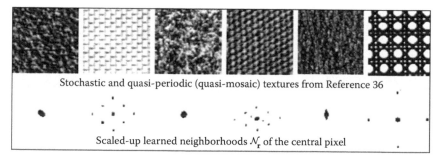

Stochastic and quasi-periodic (quasi-mosaic) textures from Reference 36

Scaled-up learned neighborhoods $\mathcal{N}_r$ of the central pixel

FIGURE 4.10
Learned multiple characteristic pairwise interactions.

interaction structure are usually much higher than for the basic structure, and hence cannot be recovered by simple thresholding.

An alternative assumption that the characteristic interactions should have little, if any, statistical dependence allows for separating the primary and secondary interactions in the search set, because only the primary ones are (almost) independent and hence characteristic for modeling a texture. The secondary interactions, which appear due to statistical interplay of the less energetic and almost independent primary ones, depend on the primary interactions and thus need not be considered characteristic. Under this more general and natural assumption, the guiding basic structure is reduced in size and the fine structure is recovered after eliminating the secondary interactions.

In the simplest case the superior low-energy outliers are separated from all other noncharacteristic clique families by placing the threshold θ at the $3 \ldots 4$ standard deviations below the mean energy for the search set. This threshold allows for modeling and simulating a number of stochastic textures, but often fails for other types of textures. A better threshold selection considers the empirical probability distribution of the partial (family-wise) energies for the search set as a mixture of a large noncharacteristic higher-energy "main-body" part and a considerably smaller characteristic lower-energy "tail": $P(E_\mathbf{v}) = wP_{\mathrm{lo}}(E_\mathbf{v}) + (1 - w)P_{\mathrm{hi}}(E_\mathbf{v})$. The marginal modeling framework detailed in Chapter 3 is then used to approximate both the mixture and its two parts with the LCDGs and find the threshold τ to separate the characteristic lower-energy clique families:

$$P_{\mathrm{lo}}(E_\mathbf{v}) \geq \frac{1-w}{w} P_{\mathrm{hi}}(E_\mathbf{v}) \quad \text{for } E_\mathbf{v} \leq \tau;$$
$$\mathbb{N}_\tau = \{\mathbf{v} : \mathbf{v} \in \mathbb{N}_{\mathrm{search}}; \ E_\mathbf{v}(\mathbf{g}^\circ) \leq \tau\}$$

(4.23)

Figures 4.11 and 4.12 illustrate the identification of a generic second-order MGRF, given a training image, provided that the interaction structure is learned by mixture modeling of the empirical distribution of the relative energies of Equation 4.22. In this example the search set consists of the 5100 candidate families: $\mathbb{N}_{\mathrm{search}} = \{\mathbf{v} = (\xi, \eta) : |\xi| \leq 50; \ 0 \leq \eta \leq 50\}$. The LCDG modeling accounts for the arbitrary shapes of the lower- and higher-energy parts of the energy distribution and accurately separates these parts with the threshold $\tau = 28$. The selected 168 characteristic families are shown in Figure 4.11 together with the gray-coded relative pixel-wise energies $E_\mathbf{r}(\mathbf{g}^\circ)$ over the template for the identified MGRF with zero potential values if the sites $\mathbf{r} \pm \mathbf{v}$ are outside the lattice:

$$E_\mathbf{r}(\mathbf{g}^\circ) = \sum_{\mathbf{v} \in \mathbb{N}} (V_\mathbf{v}(\mathbf{g}^\circ(\mathbf{r}), \mathbf{g}^\circ(\mathbf{r} + \mathbf{v})) + V_\mathbf{v}(\mathbf{g}^\circ(\mathbf{r} - \mathbf{v}), \mathbf{g}^\circ(\mathbf{r}))); \quad \mathbf{r} \in \mathbb{R}$$

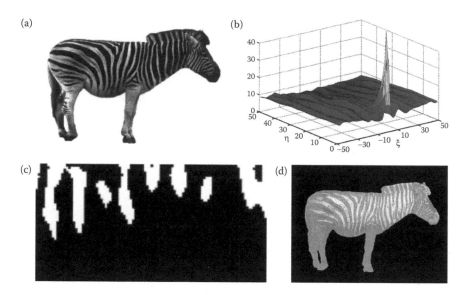

FIGURE 4.11

Zebra template (a); relative interaction negenergies $-E_{\xi,\eta}$ (b) for the search set $\mathbb{C}$ of the 5100 clique families; coordinate offsets $\mathbf{v} = (\xi, \eta)$ for the found 168 characteristic families (c), and the pixel-wise negenergies over the template for the identified MGRF (d).

Similar learning of the characteristic interaction structure for the second-order MGRF model of a starfish image, a kidney DCE-MRI, and a lung LDCT image is illustrated in Figures 4.13 through 4.15, respectively.

Because the assumed independence of the clique families does not hold due to statistical interplays between the interacting sites, the energy thresholding often produces more clique families than an accurate texture model actually should have. The interplay between two primary low-energy translation-invariant clique families $\mathbb{C}_i$ and $\mathbb{C}_j$ with the intra-clique offsets $\mathbf{v}_i$ and $\mathbf{v}_j$, respectively, produces the secondary one, $\mathbb{C}_k$ with the offset $\mathbf{v}_k = \mathbf{v}_i + \mathbf{v}_j$, having also a slightly higher, but still low interaction energy. Such families often do not belong to the basic structure, but due to their presence the simple thresholding cannot detect the families, which are responsible for minor, but visually important details of a texture in spite of their higher energy. Sequential learning, such that the already learned clique families are added one-by-one to the core model, can in principle recover both the basic and fine interaction structures, provided that the expected sufficient statistics to estimate the potentials can be closely approximated by their mean values for a collection of images generated by the MCMC sampling in accord with the core model.

Applications of stochastic modeling to medical image analysis including co-alignment, segmentation, and tracking objects of varying scale and appearance in video sequences (cine images) are exemplified in the subsequent chapters.

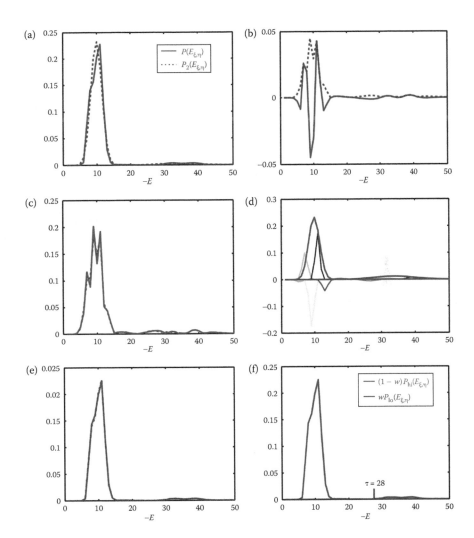

FIGURE 4.12
Empirical energy distribution $P(E_{\xi,\eta})$ and the estimated dominant mixture $P_2(E_{\xi,\eta})$ (a) of the lower- and higher-energy marginals; deviations $P(E_{\xi,\eta}) - P_2(E_{\xi,\eta})$ and absolute deviations $|P(E_{(\xi,\eta)}) - P_2(E_{(\xi,\eta)})|$ (b); mixture modeling of the scaled-up absolute deviation (c); final DGs (d) for the estimated LCDG model (e), and the conditional LCDG models (f) of the found lower- and higher-energy marginals yielding the threshold $\tau = 28$.

4.4 Bibliographic and Historical Notes

Classical second-order MGRF models of 2D/3D digital images and region maps, including auto-binomial and normal (Gaussian) random fields [24,134,157] and popular stochastic relaxation techniques to sample generative MGRFs: the heat-bath (Gibbs) and Metropolis-Hastings samplers

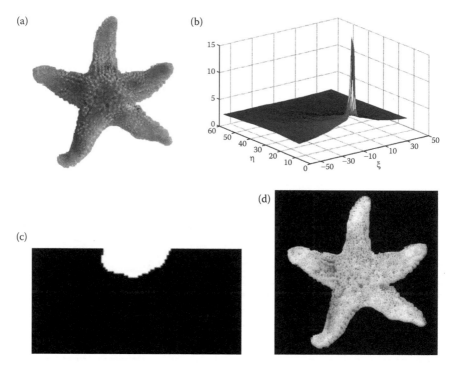

FIGURE 4.13
Starfish template (a); relative interaction negenergies $-E_{\xi,\eta}$ (b) for the search set $\mathbb{C}$ of the 5100 clique families; coordinate offsets $\nu = (\xi, \eta)$ for the found 61 characteristic families (c); and pixel-wise negenergies over the template for the identified MGRF (d).

[113,131,135]—came initially from statistical physics and measurement theory. The auto-binomial, or Potts random fields generalized physical Ising models of interacting two-state particles [17,246]. An early Gaussian model, called a simultaneous autoregressive (SAR), or GMRF, was often used to model homogeneous textures [129,157].

The auto-binomial MGRFs [246] were applied to modeling image textures from the early nineteen eighties [64,134]. The Potts models of arbitrary-shaped region maps with only the nearest (or, rarely, both the close- and long-range neighborhoods of lattice sites [120]) are used up to now as region priors to guide segmentation. The analytical MLE of the Potts potential in Section 4.2.1 is computed faster and is mostly more accurate, than the alternative least square (LS) [68]; coding [24], or MCMC and σ estimates [298].

All these initial MGRFs had mostly predefined potential functions, e.g., quadratic bivariate ones for the Gauss and Gauss-Markov models with several parameters to be learned, and accounted for either only the nearest 4- or 8-neighbor translation-, rotation-, and contrast/offset-invariant pairwise interactions, or all translation-invariant pairwise interactions within a fixed-size rectangular window centered at each pixel, or over the whole lattice. Generally, such models can allow for both close- and long-range interactions,

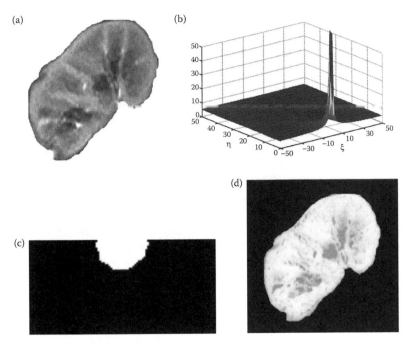

FIGURE 4.14
Kidney template (a); relative interaction negenergies $-E_{\xi,\eta}$ (b) for the search set $\mathbb{C}$ of the 5100 clique families; coordinate offsets $\mathbf{v} = (\xi, \eta)$ for the found 76 characteristic families (c), and pixel-wise negenergies over the template for the identified MGRF (d).

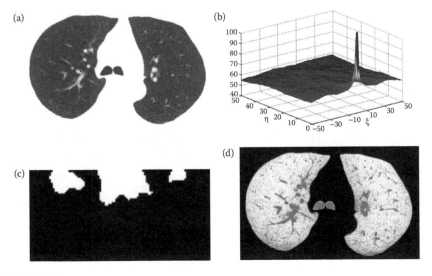

FIGURE 4.15
Lungs template (a); relative interaction negenergies $-E_{\xi,\eta}$ (b) for the search set $\mathbb{C}$ of the 5100 clique families; coordinate offsets $\mathbf{v} = (\xi, \eta)$ for the found 173 characteristic families (c), and pixel-wise negenergies over the template for the identified MGRF (d).

but in many cases only relatively close neighbors were accounted for image modeling [185].

The widespread development of MGRFs for modeling shapes and visual appearances of objects in images had begun after the seminal papers by Besag [24], Sklansky [134], Jain [64], and Geman and Geman [113] that had demonstrated sound advantages of stochastic modeling and probabilistic inference over earlier heuristic approaches to image analysis and simulation. Initially, homogeneous textures have been modeled in the nineteen eighties – early nineteen nineties with the second-order Potts or Gaussian models, especially, GMRF, such as SAR or more general SAR model with moving average (ARMA) models [52,68,129,157,179,242]. The general-case Gaussian random fields account for all pairwise interactions across the whole lattice and restrict the expected signal means, variances, and covariances. The traditional Potts models account for ordinal pairwise interactions of each lattice site with the nearest 4- or 8-neighbors. The GMRFs whiten the pairwise interactions in a fixed-size rectangular neighborhood of each pixel by a linear predictive filter. The prediction errors for all pixels form a spatially uniform IRF with zero mean and an unknown variance to be learned together with the fiter coefficients.

Although generally the GMRF and Potts models allow for arbitrary spatial structures of close- and long-range pairwise interactions, in a majority of practical cases only square local neighborhoods dominated initially in stochastic modeling of images and objects [185]. In medical applications, such models relied on anatomical facts that most of pixels or voxels belong just to the same objects as their close neighbors. Parameters of the predefined potentials for such spatially homogeneous models have been learned using the MLE or even the simplest LS estimates, despite their drawbacks and inaccuracies [68].

For the last two decades, the above simple models were followed by a host of much more versatile and powerful second- and higher-order MGRFs that have been developed specially for image processing and analysis. Among other applications, these MGRFs have been used successfully for image restoration and denoising [25,113,256], segmentation and surface reconstruction [112], edge detection [112], motion analysis [173], scene interpretation [212], texture analysis and synthesis [116,120,315,316], and so forth. At present, increasingly more complex new models continue to come to the forefront of attempts to better describe intricate natural images (e.g., [30,279,297]). Nonetheless, a reasonably large number of important practical problems of medical image analysis are still solved effectively even with the IRFs and simple second-order MGRFs, allowing for accurate learning (parameter estimation).

4.4.1 Image Filtering

Classical finite-difference approximations of the first- and second-order differential operators: the first-order 3×3 Sobel and Prewitt gradient filters and the second-order 2×2 Roberts and 3×3 Laplacian filters are often used as local edge detectors up to now. Modeling pre-attentive human visual perception of textures by an edge detector based on the difference of two offset Gaussians (the DOOG filter) worked well on both synthetic and natural images [199]. A comprehensive review [253] outlined most successful and popular early filtering in spatial and spectral (spatial frequency) domains, which is still of interest in image modeling.

4.4.2 Image Sampling

Statistical properties of the Gibbs and Metropolis-Hastings samplers were analyzed in depth in [113,131,177,307]. Generally, the image sampling calls for combinatorial numbers of macrosteps to closely approach the multivariate probability distribution specifying the univariate site-wise transitional probabilities [177]. Routing the stochastic relaxation across the lattice is called lattice coloring in Reference 24 and a visiting scheme in Reference 307.

In principle, the MCMC process of Algorithm 5 performing the pixel-wise stochastic relaxation generates a Markov chain of images, which are distributed in accord with a given MGRF [64,134,307]. Given a GPD, the MCMC-based *simulated annealing* (SA) performs in the parent population a stochastic coordinate-wise gradient search for the globally most probable image(s) [113]. An alternative stochastic approximation, called a controllable SA (CSA) in Reference 117, makes a set of sufficient statistics for the GPD, e.g., the empirical gray level co-occurrence marginals in a synthetic image, close to the like statistics in the training image. Although, generally, the MCMC-based search converges to the goal result after infinitely many steps and thus may not be very useful in practice, it is often employed for refining an image or region map in accord with its MGRF prior.

A fast-converging iterative conditional modes (ICM) algorithm by Besag [24] performs the like coordinate-wise, but deterministic gradient search for a local GPD maximum, which is the closest to the input image. The ICM follows Algorithm 5 with the Gibbs sampler, but places at each site $\mathbf{r}$ along the route the conditionally most probable signal $q' = \arg\max_{q \in \mathbb{Q}} P(g(\mathbf{r}) = q \mid \mathbf{g}^{\mathbf{r}})$.

4.4.3 Model Learning

Only learnable generic MGRFs can, at least, in principle, model realistic object shapes and appearances, which not necessarily should be spatially homogeneous [137,252]. However, learning a generic MGRF with an arbitrary system of high-order cliques and arbitrary potential functions of signal combinations on the cliques remains a challenging problem and eludes satisfactory solutions in the majority of cases [185,307].

Integral features of pairwise gray level co-occurrence histograms (GLCH) and gray level difference histograms (GLDH) or their normalized analogues: co-occurrence or difference marginals, respectively, have been used in image analysis over many decades [132]. Random field image models in Reference 242 also exploited specific characteristics of the GLCH matrices. Generic second-order MGRFs with multiple pairwise interactions, which have been introduced first in References 116 and 117, have such marginals (GLCHs or GLDHs) as sufficient statistics. Both nonparametric potentials and a characteristic interaction structure are learned from the training data using simple analytical approximations of the potential MLE. Simultaneous (parallel) analytical learning of the interaction structure by comparing interaction energies of the pairwise clique families in one or more training images, proposed in References 116 and 117, has been then extended in Reference 118 into a sequential empirical or approximate analytical process of selecting dominant interactions by excluding secondary ones, formed by statistical interplays of the dominant interactions.

The FRAME [315,316] and FoE (Field of Experts) [256] models are the most well-known high-order MGRFs. The maximum entropy property of exponential families is a common knowledge in the applied statistics for decades [15,37,231], but in image modeling this principle was applied first to derive the FRAME with its particular sufficient statistics–empirical marginals of quantified outputs of a bank of moving-window filters. The initial derivation did not refer to exponential families and introduced the "minimax" entropy principle [315] because the filtering can only decrease the entropy and the filters cannot be found by maximizing the model entropy. Actually, not only the FRAME, but also a vast majority of other MGRF image models, including the classical Gaussian random fields, auto-regressive GMRFs [157], and auto-binomial (Potts) models, as well as more recent generic second-order MGRFs with multiple arbitrary interactions [116,117,119], belong to the exponential families. All these models possess just the same maximum entropy property and differ only in the sufficient statistics, which are constrained to their training values, e.g., the mean image and the covariance matrix for the Gaussian field, or marginals of equal and nonequal adjacent signals for the Potts model, or marginals of multiple pairwise signal co-occurrences for the generic second-order MGRF.

Due to fast analytical learning, various joint MGRFs of spatially homogeneous images and region maps with multiple pairwise interactions were useful for accurate unsupervised segmentation of grayscale images with multimodal signal marginals [101] or remotely sensed higher-dimensional data [103]. As exemplified in the subsequent chapters, for segmenting a spatially inhomogeneous image, each region-of-interest is related to an individual dominant mode of the empirical marginal and texture homogeneity is restricted to only translational or translation-rotational invariance of selected signal statistics. Generally, the more accurate the identification of the models, the better the co-alignment and segmentation of many types of medical images.

5

Applications: Image Alignment

Image alignment, which is called also image registration, mapping or matching, superposes two or more images by establishing their pixel-to-pixel or voxel-to-voxel correspondences and bringing the corresponding pixels or voxels into coincidence. One of the most common goals is to closely superpose the same or similar objects-of-interest in two or more images taken, e.g., at different times, from different viewpoints, and/or with different modalities (sensors). The alignment is a crucial step in many applications of medical image analysis for clinical diagnostics, therapy planning, and more complete descriptions of anatomical objects that require an accurate fusion of different imaging modalities, like CT and MRI; detection of temporal changes in a sequence of images; integration of separate images, e.g., to form a 3D (volumetric) image from separate 2D slices, and so forth. Co-registered and fused MRI, CT, PET, SPECT, US, and other medical images not only provide more detailed information about a patient, but also ensure monitoring a disease, e.g., a tumor growth, verifying a treatment, and comparing patient's data to anatomical atlases or other patients.

In the most common scenarios, one or more *target* (moving, sensed, or source) images of the same or similar objects are co-aligned to a particular *reference*, or *prototype* image. Given a prototype, the targets are geometrically transformed to increase their mutual similarity. Generally, the targets differ from the prototype not only geometrically, but also perceptively, e.g., by global (spatially invariant) and/or local (spatially variant) contrast and offset deviations between the goal objects to be co-aligned. The object background may also vary substantially. In many cases the global perceptive deviations of an image can be excluded by normalizing the pixel/voxel-wise signals. In particular, image *equalization* provides invariance to arbitrary monotone transformations of signals. Spatially variant deviations could be partially taken into account by exploiting only ordinal relations (such as equal/unequal or greater/smaller) between the signals.

5.1 General Image Alignment Frameworks

Similarity criteria and techniques of image alignment depend on underlying models of images and their geometric and perceptive deviations.

The similarity is measured between either all the corresponding signals (intensities) in superposed areas/volumes or only local features (distinct spatial signal configurations). The latter include characteristic contours, corners, blob shapes, or other specific linear or areal objects, which can be identified and matched in the target and reference images. The feature-based and area/volume-based target-to-reference similarity criteria integrate quantitative measures of closeness between the corresponding feature descriptors or directly the pixel/voxel-wise signals, respectively.

Depending on admissible spatial and signal deviations between the reference and target images, the alignment can be rigid (global) and nonrigid (local or elastic). Affine, perspective (projective), and polynomial transformations of an image plane or volume are most frequent global geometric deviations. The affine transformations that translate, rotate, scale, and shear a target with respect to a reference are sufficient if the deformations of anatomical objects-of-interest are negligible comparing with required accuracies of the alignment. But typically these objects have considerable local deviations, so that the alignment has to involve also certain elastic transformations based, e.g., on radial basis functions or physical viscous fluid models, to warp a target to a reference.

Given a similarity criterion and a parametric model of the admissible deviations, the alignment is performed by a local or global search for the maximum target-to-reference similarity in the parameter space. The similarity criteria in medical image analysis are mostly multimodal in that space, and the local optimization converges to the closest to an initial target's position local maximum, resulting often in misalignment. Thus, proper initial positioning of the target with respect to the reference is very important. Common hybrid alignment frameworks combine both types of the similarity criteria in order to use image features at the initial stage and improve in this way the local maximization of the pixel-to-pixel or voxel-to-voxel signal similarity. The global optimization has no such drawbacks, but it is often computationally infeasible or too slow.

Due to considerable diversity of medical image modalities and anatomical structures, no generic framework for aligning medical images exists, and accurate alignment remains a challenging problem. Actual highly nonrigid deviations between the target and reference objects are often difficult to model, and one-to-one image correspondences may not exist due to missing or only partial measurements. That each imaging modality provides different information about the same anatomical structure complicates measuring signal- or feature-based similarity between the images (in particular, basic properties, e.g., intensities of the same tissues, bones, fluids, or lesions may vary considerably in multiple images). Moreover, aligning medical images of different resolution and with nonisotropic pixel/voxel dimensions may lead to intolerably excessive distortions. Intrapatient, inter-patient, and atlas-to-patient alignments have their own difficulties, too. Fast, robust, and efficient medical image alignment remains still a challenge, in spite of a number of existing efficient solutions, based in many cases on various stochastic models of reference and target images.

Generally, the image alignment framework establishes correspondence between a reference image, $\mathbf{g}_r$, and a target, $\mathbf{g}_t$, by a parametric geometric and perceptive transformation, $\mathbf{g}_{t:\theta} = \mathbf{T}(\mathbf{g}_t; \theta)$, depending on parameters θ from a certain set Θ. The transformation parameters for aligning the target and reference maximize a similarity criterion $\mathcal{C}(\mathbf{g}_{ref}, \mathbf{g}_\theta)$, specifying the alignment accuracy:

$$\theta^* = \arg\max_{\theta \subset \Theta} \{\mathcal{C}(\mathbf{g}_r, \mathbf{g}_{t:\theta} = \mathbf{T}(\mathbf{g}_t; \theta))\} \tag{5.1}$$

and are mostly found by numerical optimization. Starting from a certain initial alignment, θ_0, it converges iteratively to the local or global similarity maximum at θ^*.

5.2 Global Alignment by Learning an Appearance Prior

Let visual appearance of an object to be co-aligned with a prototype be a translation invariant texture, subject to arbitrary 2D affine geometric transformations and monotone perceptive transformations with respect to the prototype. Under this assumption, the monotone deviations are suppressed by equalizing all the images and the appearance can be modeled with an outline in Chapter 4 MGRF with multiple pairwise interactions. The characteristic interaction structure and Gibbs potentials of the model are learned from the prototype as detailed in Section 4.2.3. Then the dissimilarity between an equalized image and the prototype is measured by the interaction energy of the image: the lower the energy, the higher the similarity, and the alignment is performed by searching for the minimum-energy affine transformation of the image.

Because the interaction energy is mostly multimodal in the space of the affine parameters, an initial alignment, e.g., by exhausting only translations of the image with respect to the prototype, is performed. The latter initialization is justified by typical Gibbs energy distributions over the coordinate offsets, specifying the relative translations, such as shown in Figure 5.1. The energy-based alignment of complex textured objects is in many cases more robust and accurate than more conventional techniques employing, e.g., matching of the corresponding local features found by the scale-invariant feature transform (SIFT) or maximizing the mutual information (MI) of the image and prototype. Low variations between the objects, which are co-aligned with the prototype by minimizing the interaction energy, lead to building probabilistic shape priors for image segmentation by averaging the objects or collecting the pixel/voxel-wise "object-background" marginal probabilities.

(a)   (b)

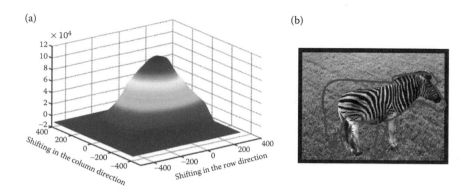

FIGURE 5.1
Gibbs energies (a) for relative target translations with respect to the reference and the initial
target position (b) with respect to the reference (template) in Figure 4.11.

Digital zebra photos, DCE-MRI of human kidney, and low dose CT (LDCT)
images of human lungs are commonly perceived as difficult for the conventional area- and feature-based alignment. Outlined below experiments
with such images, as well as similar results for other complex objects, e.g.,
starfish photos or brain images, show that the energy-based alignment can
outperform more commonly used image registration techniques, including
the area-based alignment by maximizing the MI or normalized MI (NMI) of
the object and prototype, as well as the feature-based alignment by establishing correspondences between the local features found with the SIFT. Some
alignment results for the zebra images with the learned MGRF model of the
prototype in Figure 4.11 are shown in Figure 5.2.

Plots of the MI/NMI and Gibbs energy values for the affine parameters
found at successive steps of the gradient search for the minimum energy in
Figure 5.3 explain one of the reasons behind the lower accuracy of the MI-
or NMI-based alignment. Both the MI and NMI have many local minima
that potentially hinder the search for the goal affine transformation, whereas
the energy curve is practically close to unimodal in these experiments.
The SIFT-based alignment in these experiments fails because of inaccurate
correspondences between the similar zebra stripes.

Figure 5.4 shows more diverse zebra objects and their final energy- and MI-
based alignment with the prototype. The prototype's contour, being back-
projected onto the objects, validates better performance of the energy-based
alignment. To quantitatively evaluate the accuracy, manually drawn masks
of the co-aligned objects are averaged in Figure 5.5. The common matching
area is notably larger for the energy-based alignment (91.6%) than for the
MI-based one (70.3%).

Similar results for the kidney and lung images with the learned MGRF
models of the prototypes in Figures 4.14 and 4.15, respectively, are

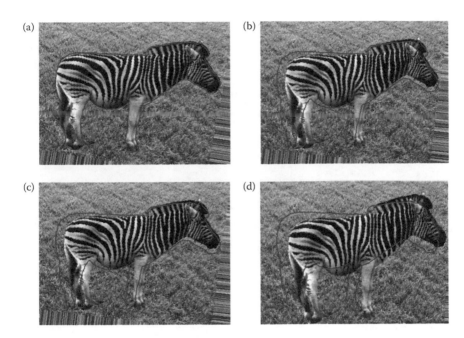

FIGURE 5.2
Final energy- (a), MI- (b), NMI- (c), and SIFT-based (d) alignment.

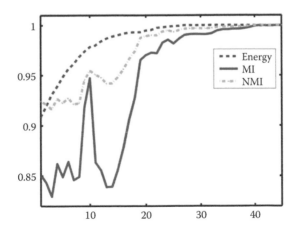

FIGURE 5.3
Energy, NMI, and MI at successive gradient search steps.

presented in Figures 5.6 through 5.11. The resulting common matching areas of the co-aligned object masks are in these cases 90.2% vs. 62.6% for the kidney DCE-MRI and 96.8% vs. 54.2% for the lung LDCT images.

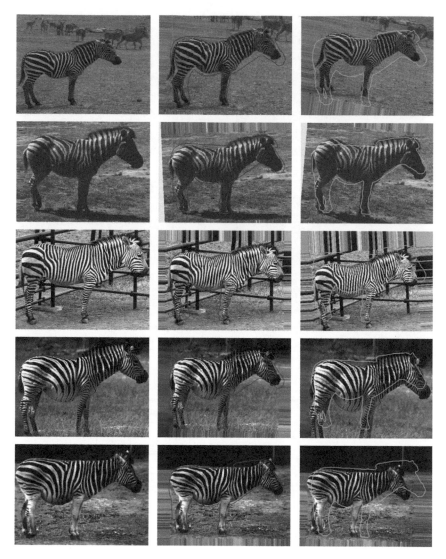

FIGURE 5.4
Original zebras (left) co-aligned using the Gibbs energy (middle) and MI (right) to measure the target-to-reference similarity.

5.3 Bibliographic and Historical Notes

Generally, the Gibbs energy is only one of a menagerie of image dissimilarity measures that quantify sparse feature-to-feature or dense pixel/voxel-wise signal-to-signal correspondences between the target and reference images

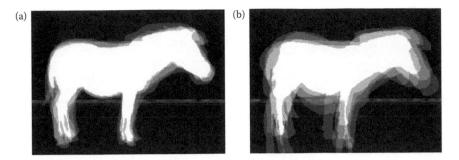

FIGURE 5.5
Relative overlap between the masks of objects for the energy-based (a; 91.6%) and MI-based alignment (b; 70.3%).

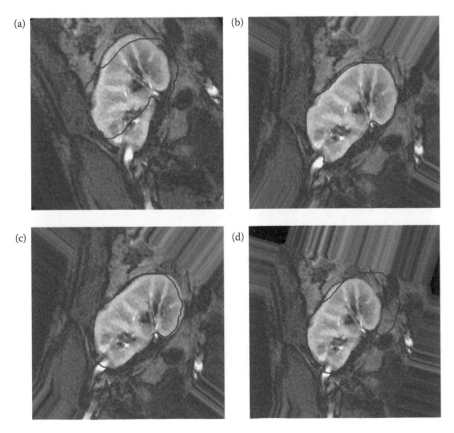

FIGURE 5.6
Initial (a) and final energy- (b), MI- (c), and SIFT-based (d) kidney alignment.

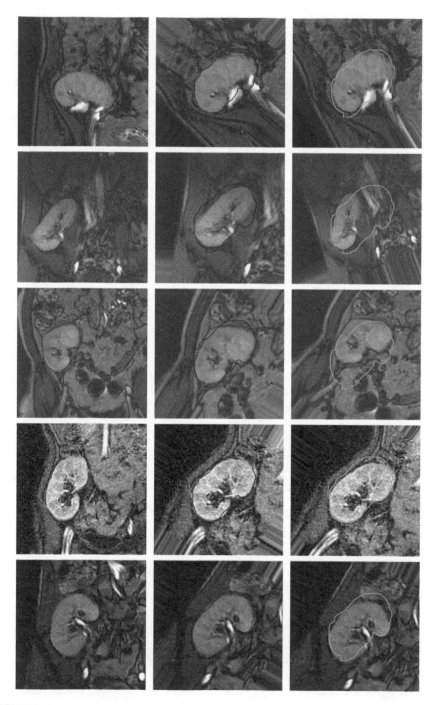

FIGURE 5.7
Original kidneys (left) co-aligned using the Gibbs energy (middle) and MI (right) to measure the target-to-reference similarity.

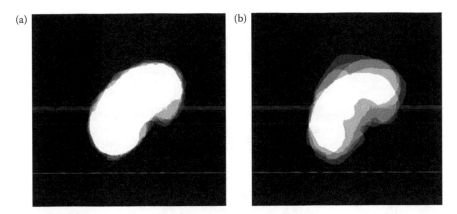

FIGURE 5.8
Relative overlap between the kidney masks for the energy-based (a; 90.2%) and MI-based alignment (b; 62.6%).

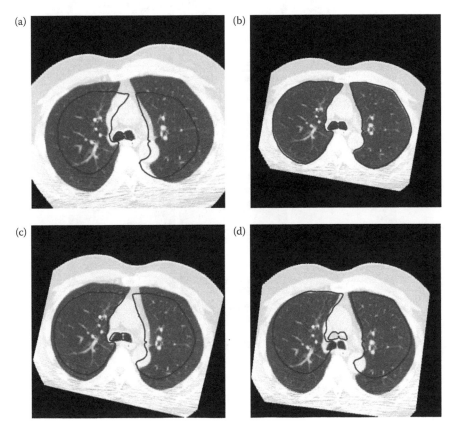

FIGURE 5.9
Initial (a) and final energy- (b), MI- (c), and SIFT-based (d) lungs alignment.

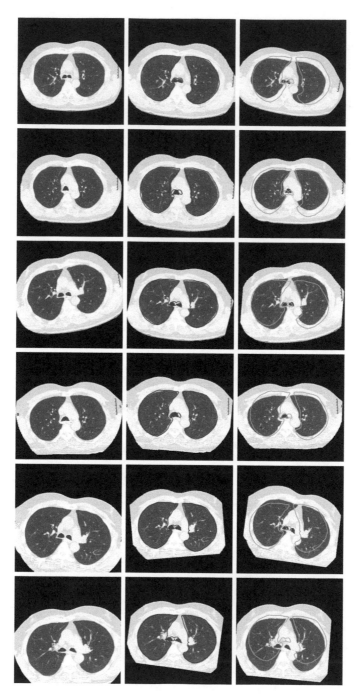

FIGURE 5.10
Original lungs (left) co-aligned using the Gibbs energy (middle) and the MI (right) to measure the object-to-prototype similarity.

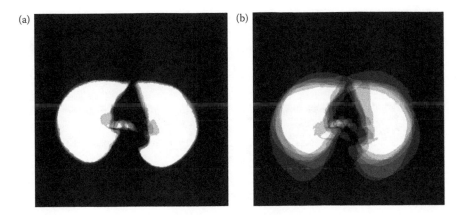

FIGURE 5.11
Relative overlap between the lung masks for the energy-based (a; 96.8%) and MI-based alignment (b; 54.2%).

and guide the alignment. Detailed surveys of feature- and area-based criteria of similarity between image features or visual appearances of objects can be found in References 167 and 317.

The feature-based alignment (registration) establishes one-to-one correspondences between distinctive local signal patterns, or features, such as contours, blobs, line intersections, and shapes or surfaces of specific points, lines, and areas in both the reference and target images, which are characteristic for objects-of-interest. The features are usually characteristic points, e.g., gravity centers or line endings, and the alignment quality depends on the accuracy of their correspondences. The most popular at present scale invariant feature transform (SIFT) by Lowe [188] reliably determines multiple reliable point-to-point correspondences between two images. The correspondences are described by local features, which may differ geometrically (by affine transformation) and perceptibly (by local contrast and offset signal deviations). The features present relative arrangements of the local maxima and minima produced by pyramidal scale-space linear filtering using the difference of Gaussians (DOG) filters. However, the SIFT-based registration works only if there exist distinctive and nonrepetitive local image features. Figures 5.12 and 5.13 illustrate pros and cons of the SIFT-based image alignment, which depends heavily on specificity and reliability of the features found.

To avoid feature extraction, the area-based registration matches directly image signals, mostly by maximizing either the classical least-square cross correlation, or unnormalized or normalized *mutual information* (MI) between the images [294,295]. The direct signal matching became recently most popular in the medical image alignment due to no data losses from feature detection, efficient alignment of images of the same or different modality or dimensionality under both rigid and elastic geometric deformations, and

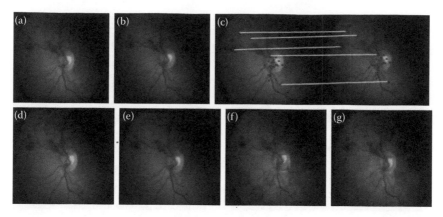

FIGURE 5.12
SIFT-based alignment of retinal images: the reference (a,d) and target (b,e); the candidate pixels (c) for aligning the (a) and (b) images, and checkerboard visualizations of the superposed (d) and (e) images before (f) and after (g) the alignment.

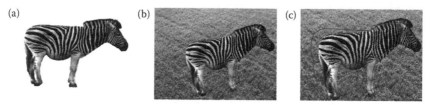

FIGURE 5.13
SIFT-based alignment of zebra images: the reference (a) and target (b) with candidate pixels for alignment, and the aligned target (c).

sub-pixel or voxel accuracy [239]. In most cases, such alignment needs no user interaction and allows for assessing the alignment accuracy both qualitatively and quantitatively. The signal dissimilarity measures are derived usually from a stochastic model of target and reference images that accounts for nonessential transformations of whole images or their parts (windows) and leads to statistically optimal estimates of transformational parameters.

Measuring similarity by correlation assumes that both objects are identical up to spatially uniform perceptive deviations. Hence, it is too sensitive to spatially variant and interdependent deviations between the corresponding signals due to different imaging modalities, sensor noise, and/or illumination variations. Alternative phase correlation and spectral-domain methods, based, e.g., on the Fourier-Mellin transform [7,53,107,250], are more robust to the correlated and frequency dependent noise, as well as to nonuniform time-varying illumination. Unfortunately, these methods typically allow for only very limited mutual geometric transformations between the images.

More powerful data similarity measures: MI [147,294] and normalized MI (NMI) [282]—account for general signal transformations that keep one-to-one dependency between two sets of signal values, i.e., preserve statistical dependencies between the signals. The MI compares a joint empirical probability distribution of corresponding signal pairs in two images to the joint distribution of pairs of independent signals, the marginals being estimated using either Parzen windows or discrete signal histograms [282].

The MI-based registration suits multi-modal images the best [294] and thus is widely used in the applied medical image analysis. The main advantage of the MI is its insensitivity to arbitrary one-to-one transformations of the target and reference signals that preserve their joint and marginal empirical probabilities. However, apart from these transformations, the objects should have almost identical shapes (up to their unessential affine geometrical transformations). The MI allows for both monotone and nonmonotone one-to-one transformations of the sets of signal values, although the nonmonotone ones may affect visual appearance too much and hinder thus the registration accuracy. Figure 5.14 exemplifies aligning the inter-subject kidney CT images by maximizing their MI [294,295].

The feature-based registration is effective only in the presence of distinctive and detectable features. Because medical images do not contain many such features, the signal matching is a widespread alternative in spite of its higher computational complexity and more frequent local minima traps during the optimization search. The aforementioned mutual information (MI) [294,295], and normalized mutual information (NMI) [282] are most well-known similarity measures suitable for multiple image modalities and nonrigid alignment. Both the reference and target images are considered each a sample from an IRF, and the MI and NMI evaluate the amount of information in the reference about the target (and vice versa) from pairwise statistical dependencies between the corresponding signals. Because the signals are independent, the MI and NMI are invariant to both arbitrary permutations of the corresponding lattice sites in the images and arbitrary one-to-one mappings of their signal sets.

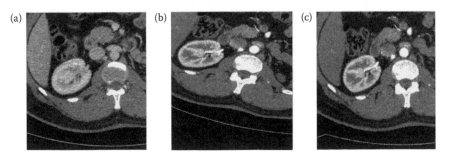

FIGURE 5.14
MI-based alignment of kidney CT images: the reference (a), target (b), and aligned (c) target.

Let $P_t(q_t)$, $P_r(q_r)$, and $P_{tr}(q_t, q_r)$ be (empirical) marginals of an individual target signal $g_t(\mathbf{r}) = q_t \in \mathbf{Q}_t$, an individual reference signal $g_r(\mathbf{r}) = q_r \in \mathbf{Q}_r$, and the corresponding pair (q_t, q_r) at the same lattice sites $\mathbf{r} \in \mathbb{R}$, respectively. Then the MI and NMI are defined as

$$MI(\mathbf{g}_r, \mathbf{g}_t) = H(\mathbf{g}_r) - H(\mathbf{g}_r \mid \mathbf{g}_t)$$

$$\equiv H(\mathbf{g}_t) - H(\mathbf{g}_t \mid \mathbf{g}_r) = \sum_{q_t \in \mathbf{Q}_t} \sum_{q_r \in \mathbf{Q}_r} P_{tr}(q_t, q_r) \log \left(\frac{P_{tr}(q_t, q_r)}{P_t(q_t) P_r(q_r)} \right)$$

$$NMI(\mathbf{g}_r, \mathbf{g}_t) = \frac{H(\mathbf{g}_r) + H(\mathbf{g}_t)}{H(\mathbf{g}_r, \mathbf{g}_t)} = 1 + \frac{MI(\mathbf{g}_r, \mathbf{g}_t)}{H(\mathbf{g}_r, \mathbf{g}_t)}$$

where $H(\ldots)$, $H(\ldots, \ldots)$, and $H(\ldots \mid \ldots)$ denote the Shannon's entropy, joint entropy, and conditional entropy of the signals, respectively:

$$H(\mathbf{g}_t) = - \sum_{q_t \in \mathbf{Q}_t} P_t(q_t) \log P_t(q_t);$$

$$H(\mathbf{g}_r) = - \sum_{q_r \in \mathbf{Q}_r} P_r(q_r) \log P_r(q_r);$$

$$H(\mathbf{g}_r, \mathbf{g}_t) = - \sum_{q_t \in \mathbf{Q}_t} \sum_{q_r \in \mathbf{Q}_r} P_{tr}(q_t, q_r) \log P_{tr}(q_t, q_r);$$

$$H(\mathbf{g}_r \mid \mathbf{g}_t) = - \sum_{q_t \in \mathbf{Q}_t} \sum_{q_r \in \mathbf{Q}_r} P_{tr}(q_t, q_r) \log \frac{P_{tr}(q_t, q_r)}{P_t(q_t)}$$

The following obvious properties hold for these entropies:

$$H(\mathbf{g}_r) \geq H(\mathbf{g}_r \mid \mathbf{g}_t) \geq 0;$$

$$H(\mathbf{g}_r, \mathbf{g}_t) = H(\mathbf{g}_t) + H(\mathbf{g}_r \mid \mathbf{g}_t) = H(\mathbf{g}_r) + H(\mathbf{g}_t \mid \mathbf{g}_r)$$

The NMI depends less than the MI on the overlap between the images [282] and both the MI and NMI call for an accurate estimation of the individual and joint marginals. These similarity measures are widely used for analyzing and aligning medical images. But taking no account of spatial relationships between the lattice sites, small numbers of distinct signal values in the target or the reference due to lossy rather than one-to-one signal mappings, and excessive image noise may heavily influence the alignment accuracy.

6

Segmenting Multimodal Images

Let a grayscale image be called "multimodal" if each region-of-interest in it is associated with a single dominant mode of the empirical marginal probability distribution of gray levels. One of the most common scenarios of unsupervised segmentation of these images considers each pair of an image and its region map a sample from a joint MGRF of conditionally independent pixel/voxel-wise image signals, given the region map, and interdependent region labels. To recover the goal region map for a given image, the MGRF model is identified first by precise approximation of the empirical marginal with the LCDG as shown in Chapter 3 and separated into the conditional LCDG models of each object. Under the same number of components, the LCDG approximates the empirical data better than a conventional Gaussian mixture with only positive components. The obtained conditional LCDG models of objects allow for initial segmentation that relates the pixel/voxel-wise image signals to the most probable modes. The initial region map is then iteratively refined using the MGRF of region labels with analytically estimated potentials. Comparative experiments showed that various complex multimodal medical images are segmented in this case more accurately than by several other known segmentation algorithms.

In contrast to a number of alternative solutions, the above scenario focuses on computationally simple, fast, and accurate identification of both the low-level models (conditional IRFs of image signals) and the high-level one (a Potts MGRF of region labels). This scenario circumvents difficulties encountered by more conventional unsupervised segmentation techniques in detecting practically meaningful borders between different objects. Correct borders are essential for object interpretation, but simultaneously present the main challenge. It holds even if all the dominant modes of the empirical marginal are clearly separated, because the borders are mostly specified by intersecting "tails" of the conditional object-wise marginals. Therefore, not only the main body of the conditional marginal for each object in the close vicinity of its dominant mode, but also its tails toward other modes have to be precisely approximated by the same LCDG to within the signal range.

6.1 Joint MGRF of Images and Region Maps

Let $P(\mathbf{g}, \mathbf{m})$; $(\mathbf{g}, \mathbf{m}) \in \mathbb{G} \times \mathbb{M}$; $\sum_{(\mathbf{g},\mathbf{m}) \in \mathbb{G} \times \mathbb{M}} P(\mathbf{g}, \mathbf{m}) = 1$, be a joint probability model of the L-modal images, $\mathbf{g}$, and their region maps, $\mathbf{m}$ in Equation 2.3, supported by the same lattice $\mathbb{R}$:

$$P(\mathbf{g}, \mathbf{m}) = P_u(\mathbf{m}) P_c(\mathbf{g} \,|\, \mathbf{m})$$

where $P_u(\mathbf{m})$; $\mathbf{m} \in \mathbb{M}$; $\sum_{\mathbf{m} \in \mathbb{M}} P_u(\mathbf{m}) = 1$, is an unconditional probability distribution of the maps; $P_c(\mathbf{g} \,|\, \mathbf{m})$; $\mathbf{g} \in \mathbb{G}$; $\sum_{\mathbf{g} \in \mathbb{G}} P_c(\mathbf{g} \,|\, \mathbf{m}) = 1$ for each $\mathbf{m} \in \mathbb{M}$, is a conditional probability distribution of images, given the map, and $\mathbb{G}$ and $\mathbb{M}$ are the parent populations of the images and region maps, respectively.

The Bayesian MAP estimate of the map $\mathbf{m}$, given an observed image $\mathbf{g}_{\text{obs}}$ (see Section 2.1.4):

$$\mathbf{m}^* = \arg \max_{\mathbf{m} \in \mathbb{M}} \ell(\mathbf{m} \,|\, \mathbf{g}_{\text{obs}})$$

maximizes the relative log-likelihood:

$$\ell(\mathbf{m} \,|\, \mathbf{g}_{\text{obs}}) = \frac{1}{|\mathbb{R}|} \left(\log P_c(\mathbf{m} \,|\, \mathbf{g}_{\text{obs}}) + \log P_u(\mathbf{m}) \right) \qquad (6.1)$$

To find this estimate, the chosen stochastic models $\mathbf{P}_u$ and $\mathbf{P}_c$ should be identified.

The conditional model $\mathbf{P}_c$ is an IRF of pixel/voxel-wise gray levels, or intensities with different marginals:

$$\mathbf{P}_\lambda = \left(p(q \,|\, \lambda) : q \in \mathbb{Q}; \sum_{q \in \mathbb{Q}} p(q \,|\, \lambda) = 1 \right)$$

for each object $\lambda \in \mathbb{L}$. The joint conditional distribution $P_c(\mathbf{g} \,|\, \mathbf{m})$ of the image signals for a given region map is then as follows:

$$P_c(\mathbf{g} \,|\, \mathbf{m}) = \prod_{\mathbf{r} \in \mathbf{R}} p(g(\mathbf{r}) \,|\, m(\mathbf{r})) \equiv \prod_{\lambda \in \mathbb{L}} \prod_{q \in \mathbb{Q}} [p(q \,|\, \lambda)]^{\nu_{\mathbf{m},\mathbf{g}}(q,\lambda)}$$

where

$$\nu_{\mathbf{m},\mathbf{g}}(q, \lambda) = |\{\mathbf{r} : \mathbf{r} \in \mathbb{R}; m(\mathbf{r}) = \lambda; g(\mathbf{r}) = q\}| \equiv f_{\mathbf{m}}(\lambda) f_{\mathbf{m},\mathbf{g}}(q \,|\, \lambda) |\mathbb{R}|$$

is the number of lattice sites supporting the signal q in the region λ; $f_{\mathbf{m}}(\lambda)$ denotes the empirical marginal probability of the label λ in the region map $\mathbf{m}$, and $f_{\mathbf{m},\mathbf{g}}(q \,|\, \lambda)$ is the empirical marginal probability of the site-wise signal

q in the region λ of the image $\mathbf{g}$. The conditional marginals $\mathbf{P}_\lambda$; $\lambda \in \mathbb{L}$, are the model parameters to be learned. The first term $\frac{1}{|R|} \log P_c(\mathbf{g} \mid \mathbf{m})$ of the log-likelihood in Equation 6.1 can be rewritten as

$$\sum_{\lambda \in \mathbb{L}} f_{\mathbf{m}}(\lambda) \left(\sum_{q \in \mathbb{Q}} f_{\mathbf{m},\mathbf{g}}(q \mid \lambda) \log p(q \mid \lambda) \right) \tag{6.2}$$

To accurately identify the conditional model, the marginal in each region is approximated with an LCDG as detailed in Chapter 3.

The unconditional model is the nearest-neighbor MGRF of region labels, such as in Section 4.2.1. For the 2D images, the nearest 8-neighborhood is taken into account, so that each pixel interacts with the closest horizontal, vertical, and left-right-diagonal neighbors. By symmetry considerations, the Gibbs potentials are assumed independent of relative orientation of pixel pairs, are the same for all regions, and depend only on equality or inequality of the pair of labels:

$$V(\lambda, \kappa) = \begin{cases} -\gamma & \text{if } \lambda = \kappa \\ \gamma & \text{if } \lambda \neq \kappa \end{cases}; \; \lambda, \kappa \in \mathbb{L}$$

Under these assumptions, it is the simplest, but widely employed up to now auto-binomial, or Potts model with the nearest neighborhood specified with the inter-pixel coordinate offsets $\mathbf{N}$, e.g., $\mathbf{N} = \{(1,0), (0,1), (-1,1), (1,1)\}$ for the 2D images:

$$P(\mathbf{m}) = \frac{1}{Z_{\mathbf{N}}} \exp \left(-\sum_{\mathbf{r} \in \mathbb{R}} \sum_{\mathbf{v} \in \mathbf{N}} V(m(\mathbf{r}), m(\mathbf{r}+\mathbf{v})) \right)$$
$$= \frac{1}{Z_{\mathbf{N}}} \exp \left(\gamma |\mathbf{C}_{\mathbf{N}}| (2f_{\mathrm{eq}}(\mathbf{m}) - 1) \right) \tag{6.3}$$

where $Z_{\mathbf{N}}$ denotes the normalizer (the partition function); $\mathbf{C}_{\mathbf{N}}$ is the family of neighboring pairs of the lattice sites, or the second-order cliques, supporting the Gibbs potentials:

$$\mathbb{C}_{\mathbf{N}} = \{(\mathbf{r}, \mathbf{r}+\mathbf{v}) : \mathbf{r} \in \mathbb{R}; \mathbf{r}+\mathbf{v}) \in \mathbb{R}; \mathbf{v} \in \mathbf{N}\};$$

$|\mathbf{C}_{\mathbf{N}}|$ denotes the cardinality of this clique family, and $f_{\mathrm{eq}}(\mathbf{m})$ is the empirical probability of equal labels in the cliques:

$$f_{\mathrm{eq}}(\mathbf{m}) = \frac{1}{|\mathbf{C}_{\mathbf{N}}|} \sum_{(\mathbf{r},\mathbf{r}') \in \mathbf{C}_{\mathbf{N}}} \delta(m(\mathbf{r}) - m(\mathbf{r}')) \tag{6.4}$$

Here, $\delta(z)$ is the Kronecker delta function. To identify this model, the potential value γ is approximated analytically, as in Equation 4.10.

To compute the second term, $\frac{1}{|\mathbb{R}|} \log P_{\mathrm{u}}(\mathbf{m})$, in the log-likelihood of Equation 6.1 for the region map $\mathbf{m}$, the unknown partition function $Z_{\mathbf{N}}$ can be approximated as

$$Z_{\mathbf{N}} \approx \exp\left(-\sum_{\mathbf{r}\in\mathbb{R}}\sum_{\mathbf{v}\in\mathbf{N}}\sum_{\lambda\in\mathbb{L}} V(\lambda, m(\mathbf{r}+\mathbf{v}))\right)$$

$$= \exp\left(-|\mathbb{C}_{\mathbf{N}}|\sum_{\lambda\in\mathbb{L}}(\gamma f_{\lambda}(\mathbf{m}) - \gamma(1 - f_{\lambda}(\mathbf{m})))\right)$$

$$= \exp\left(\gamma|\mathbb{C}_{\mathbf{N}}|(L - 2)\right)$$

This approximate partition function results in the following term $\frac{1}{|\mathbb{R}|} \log P_{\mathrm{u}}(\mathbf{m})$ in Equation 6.1:

$$\rho\gamma(2f_{\mathrm{eq}}(\mathbf{X}) + L - 3) \approx 4\gamma(2f_{\mathrm{eq}}(\mathbf{X}) + L - 3) \tag{6.5}$$

where $\rho = \frac{|\mathbb{C}_{\mathbf{N}}|}{|\mathbb{R}|} \approx |\mathbf{N}| = 4$.

At the first stage of maximizing the approximate log-likelihood of Equation 6.1, an initial region map $\mathbf{m}^{\circ}$ is obtained by precise unsupervised estimation of the conditional marginals P_{λ} for each object $\lambda \in \mathbb{L}$ using the LCDG modeling outlined in Chapter 3 and the Bayesian pixel/voxel-wise MAP classification. For simplicity, the total number of objects, L, is specified in this case manually and is not changed during the whole segmentation process. At the second stage, the initial map is refined by searching iteratively for a local log-likelihood maximum in the vicinity of the initial state. Each iteration involves three steps:

1. Update the current MGRF model $\mathbf{P}_{\mathrm{u}}$ of region maps by estimating the potential value γ from the current map using Equation 4.10: $\gamma^{\circ} = \frac{L}{2(L-1)}\left(Lf_{\mathrm{eq}}(\mathbf{m}^{\circ}) - 1\right)$.

2. Use the updated region map model, together with the conditional image-map model, $\mathbf{P}_{\mathrm{c}}$, to refine the current map by the MCMC stochastic relaxation.

3. Update the current conditional image-map model by collecting the empirical marginals, $\mathbf{P}_{\lambda}$; $\lambda = 1, \ldots, L$, for the objects and approximating them with the LCDGs.

Because at each step the approximate log-likelihood of Equations 6.1, 6.2, and 6.5:

$$\ell(\mathbf{m} \mid \mathbf{g}_{\mathrm{obs}}) \approx \sum_{\lambda\in\mathbb{L}} f_{\mathbf{m}}(\lambda)\left(\sum_{q\in\mathbf{Q}} f_{\mathbf{m,g}}(q \mid \lambda) \log p(q \mid \lambda)\right) + 4\gamma\left(2f_{\mathrm{eq}}(\mathbf{X}) + L - 3\right)$$

$$\tag{6.6}$$

Algorithm 6 Iterative Image Segmentation

---

1. Find the empirical marginal $\mathbf{P}_{emp}$ for a given image $\mathbf{g}$.

2. Estimate the initial LCDG model of L objects using Algorithm 3 of Section 3.4.1.

3. Refine the estimated LCDG model using Algorithm 4 of Section 3.4.2.

4. Partition the refined LCDG model into the L conditional object pseudo-marginals by minimizing the classification error in line with Section 3.4.3.

5. Form the current region map $\mathbf{m}^\circ$ by the pixel/voxel-wise Bayesian classification using the obtained conditional object models.

6. Estimate the potential value (γ°) for the Potts model using Equation 4.10 and the current region map: $\gamma^\circ = \frac{L}{2(L-1)} \left(L f_{eq}(\mathbf{m}^\circ) - 1 \right)$.

7. Refine the region map $\mathbf{m}^\circ$ using the pixel/voxel-wise MCMC stochastic relaxation, e.g., the Metropolis sampler, and the estimated Potts model of the maps.

8. Compute the approximate log-likelihood of Equation 6.6 for the refined map.

9. Collect the conditional empirical marginals using the refined region map $\mathbf{m}^*$ and build the updated LCDG models of objects.

10. Repeat Steps 5–9 iteratively until the log-likelihood remains almost the same for the two successive iterations; then output the final region map $\mathbf{m}^*$.

---

either increases, or at least does not decrease, the above iterations converge to a local log-likelihood maximum. The process terminates when the successive log-likelihood values remain equal to within a prescribed accuracy threshold. Algorithm 6 details the basic segmentation steps. Typical changes of this approximate log-likelihood at successive iterations are illustrated in Figure 6.1.

6.2 Experimental Validation

Robustness and feasibility of Algorithm 6 have been tested and validated on the same synthetic data and five types of medical images as in Section 3.5 where the unsupervised learning of the conditional LCDGs, or pseudo-marginals for these images were detailed.

6.2.1 Synthetic Data

The initial and refined conditional pseudo-marginals learned for the synthetic checkerboard image in Figure 3.5 were shown in Section 3.5.1;

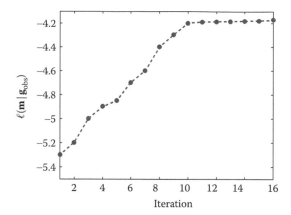

FIGURE 6.1
Convergence of iterative refinement of the region map built by Algorithm 6 for the chest LDCT image in Figure 3.11.

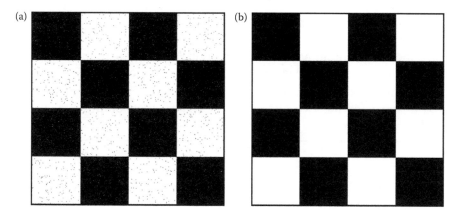

FIGURE 6.2
The initial (a) and final (b) region maps (the final error of 0.005%).

Figures 3.9 and 3.10. The initial region map obtained using the conditional LCDGs in Figure 3.10 is further iteratively refined by Algorithm 6 (Figure 6.2). Changes in the approximate likelihood $\ell(\mathbf{m}, \mathbf{g})$ become negligible after just four iterations, as shown in Figure 6.3. The initial and final estimated potential values for the map model are $\gamma = 1.9$ and $\gamma = 2.1$, respectively.

Table 6.1 shows that the original parameter values for the dominant and subordinate components of the conditional LCDGs are close to their final estimates. The segmentation error for the final region map in Figure 6.2. i.e., its difference from the ground truth in Figure 3.5 is only 0.005%.

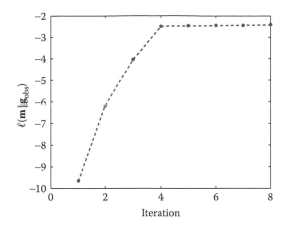

FIGURE 6.3

Convergence of Algorithm 6 segmenting the synthetic image.

TABLE 6.1

Original Parameters and Their Initial and Final Estimates for the Dominant ($i = 1, 2$) and Subordinate (3−10) Components of the LCDG Model for the Synthetic Data

Comp.		Weight w_i			Mean μ_i			Variance σ_i^2		
i	$\pm$	Original	Initial	Final	Original	Initial	Final	Original	Initial	Final
1	+	0.50	0.53	0.51	65	64	65	600	719	581
2	+	0.50	0.47	0.49	190	189	190	600	780	581
3	+	0.020	0.022	0.019	20	17	21	50	60	59
4	−	0.020	0.019	0.020	60	55	59	50	65	61
5	−	0.020	0.021	0.020	90	82	92	50	40	45
6	+	0.020	0.023	0.021	116	120	119	50	39	42
7	+	0.020	0.017	0.020	150	155	149	50	55	54
8	−	0.020	0.018	0.019	180	169	182	50	53	53
9	−	0.020	0.021	0.021	210	206	207	50	62	57
10	+	0.020	0.017	0.020	240	245	244	50	69	56

For comparison, the best multiple resolution segmentation (MRS) of the same synthetic image, which was obtained for the potential values of 0.3 and three levels of resolution had a notably larger error of 0.46%. The best segmentation with the iterative conditional modes (ICM) algorithm using the same potential values of 0.3 was even less accurate: the error of 0.77%. Although all the three region maps look good, Algorithm 6 is the best and produces more accurate borders between the two objects. This is quite expectable because the Gaussian autoregressive model of the MRS is less general than the joint MGRF model of Algorithm 6.

6.2.2 Lung LDCT Images

The segmentation has to separate lung tissues from their background in such a way that the lung borders closely approach the borders outlined by a radiologist. Spatial dependencies between the region labels are taken into account to preserve shapes and borders of the regions because intensities of individual lung tissues, such as arteries, veins, bronchi, and bronchioles, are similar to intensities of the chest tissues.

The initial region map is obtained by the pixel-wise classification using the conditional LCDGs in Figure 3.15 and then is further refined iteratively in accord with Algorithm 6. The log-likelihood changes become negligible after 12 iterations, as shown in Figure 6.1. The initial and final potential estimates for the region map model are $\gamma = 1.01$ and 1.30, respectively, and Table 6.2 presents also the initial and final parameter estimates of the dominant components for the conditional pseudo-marginals.

The final region map refined with the estimated MGRF parameters is shown in Figure 6.4 in comparison with the "ground truth" outlined by a radiologist; the initial region map; the final map refined with a heuristically selected potential, and the maps obtained by the multiple-resolution segmentation (MRS), iterated conditional mode (ICM) segmentation, and segmentation with a version of Algorithm 6, which models empirical marginals with conventional mixtures of only positive Gaussians. Large errors of the initial region map for the latter algorithm cannot be substantially reduced because the final refinement using the joint image-map MGRF model yields only minor accuracy improvements.

To highlight advantages of Algorithm 6 over the segmentation with deformable models (DM), the CT image in Figure 3.11 was segmented with the greedy algorithms using the image gradients (DMG) and the gradient vector flow (GVF) as an external guiding force. In both the cases the DM was manually initialized within the lung regions. The resulting DM positions in Figure 6.5 show that Algorithm 6 notably outperforms both the DMG and GVF. The latter algorithms fail most probably because inhomogeneities of the lung tissues disrupt gradient-based attraction of the DMs towards the region boundaries. As shown in Figure 6.6, the segmentation with Algorithm 6 does not lose abnormal lung tissues as the iterative thresholding (IT) algorithm.

TABLE 6.2

Initial and Final Parameter Estimates for the Dominant LCDG Components

Parameter	w_1	μ_1	σ_1^2	w_2	μ_2	σ_2^2
Initial	0.26	41	243	0.74	171	296
Final	0.27	42	256	0.73	171	289

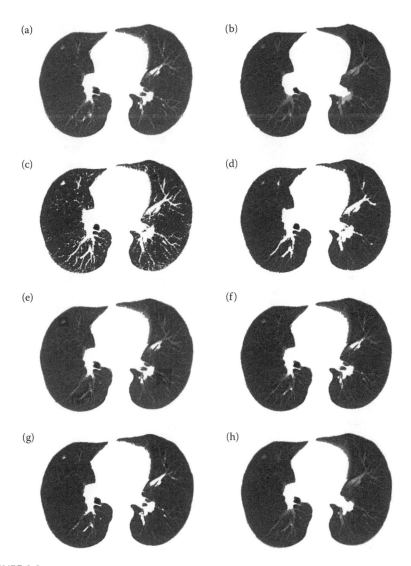

FIGURE 6.4
Initial (a;c) and final (b;d) segmentation by Algorithm 6 with the LCDG (a;c: the final error of 1.1% w.r.t. the ground truth) and a conventional Gaussian mixture model of the empirical marginal (the final error of 5.1%); the refined map (e) obtained from (a) with a heuristic MGRF potential (the final error of 1.8%); the best MRS (f: the error of 2.3% for the three-level resolution and potential value of 0.3; ICM g: the error of 2.9% for the potential value of 0.3) region maps; and the radiologist's ground truth (h).

In these and preceding experiments, the segmentation accuracy was evaluated with respect to the "ground truth" from an expert-radiologist, despite such a prototype may be incorrect due to unstable hand positioning during manual segmentation. A geometric phantom with the same regional

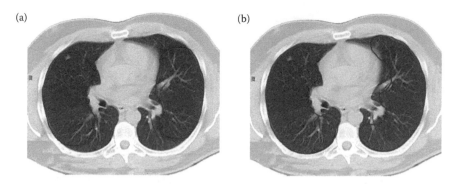

FIGURE 6.5
Lung regions found by DMG (a: the error of 35%) and GVF (b: the error of 15%) (the borders found are in red).

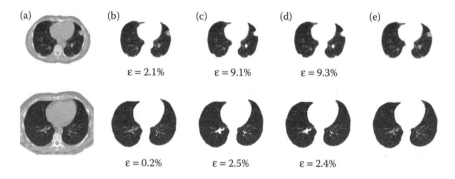

FIGURE 6.6
Original CT slices (a) and their region maps for Algorithm 6 (b), IT (c), and the version of Algorithm 6 using Gaussian mixture models of empirical marginals (d) with errors, ε, w.r.t. the radiologist's ground truth (e).

signal marginals as in the CT slices at hand allows for the alternative and more objective accuracy evaluations. The phantom, its ideal region map, and segmentation results for Algorithm 6 are shown in Figure 6.7. The error of 0.09% between the found regions and their ground truth confirms the high segmentation accuracy. For comparison, Figure 6.7 presents also the region maps for the IT, ICM, MRS, DMG, and GVF algorithms. More segmentation results for the 3D lungs are shown in Figure 6.8.

The above experiments, as well as the additional experiments with 120 different bimodal LDCT slices have shown that Algorithm 6 can outperform several more conventional algorithms. As indicated in Table 6.3, the most accurate among them MRS has the error range of 1.9%–9.8% and the mean error of 5.1% w.r.t. the ground truth, comparing with the notably smaller range of 0.1%–2.2% and the mean of only 0.32% for Algorithm 6.

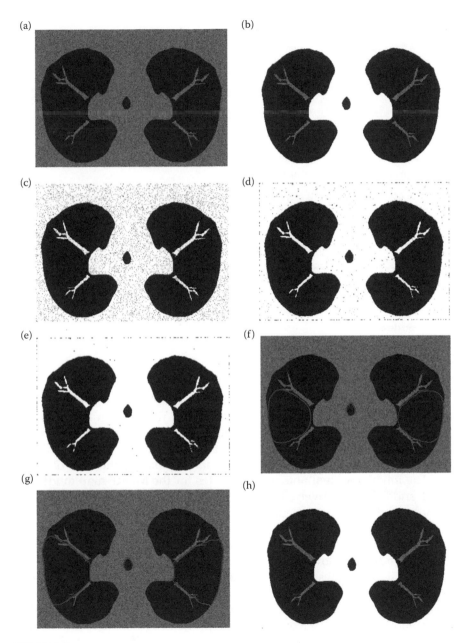

FIGURE 6.7
Synthetic phantom (a) and its regions for Algorithm 6 (b; the error of 0.09%); IT (c; the error of 6.0%), ICM (d; the least error of 2.9% with the potential value of 0.3); MRS (e; the least error of 2.0% with the potential value of 0.3 and three resolution levels); DMG (f; the error of 59%), and GVF (g; the error of 52%) w.r.t. the ground truth (h).

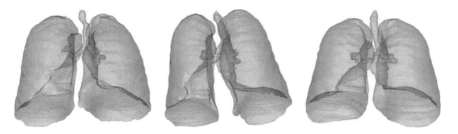

FIGURE 6.8
3D lung segmentation from LDCT images.

TABLE 6.3

Accuracy of Algorithm 6 (A6) w.r.t. IT, MRS, ICM, DMG, and GVF

Error, %	A6	IT	MRS	ICM	DMG	GVF
Min	0.1	2.8	1.9	2.0	10	4.1
Max	2.2	22	9.8	17	29	18
Mean	0.3	11	5.1	9.8	15	13
St. dev.	0.7	6.0	3.3	5.1	7.7	4.8

6.2.3 Blood Vessels in TOF-MRA Images

Precise segmentation of images with three dominant modes is obtained in a similar way. Figure 6.9 presents the initial and final region maps for the third object—the vessels—for Algorithm 6 and compares them with ICM, MRS, DMG, and GVF w.r.t. the expert's "ground truth." First eight refining iterations of Algorithm 6 converge to the final map having the error of about 0.5%. The initial and final potential estimates for the MGRF map model are $\gamma = 2.1$ and 2.6, respectively. The initial and final estimated parameters of the dominant LCDG components are shown in Table 6.4. The ICM and MRS have considerably higher errors, whereas DMG and GVF behave much better although still are less accurate than Algorithm 6, need manual initialization, and are considerably slower.

Figure 6.10 illustrates extracting the blood vessels using the Wilson-Noble's model (WN) of empirical marginals. The model estimation and segmentation quality are measured by the Levy distance between two distributions and the absolute error, respectively. The Levy distances of 0.11 and 0.00013 between the empirical distribution and its model and the absolute error of 0.12 and 0.0002, respectively, for the WN and Algorithm 6 indicate that the considerably worse approximation of the marginals strongly affects the accuracy of separating blood vessels from their background. Because of a typically higher separation threshold, e.g., $\tau_2 = 214$ versus our $\tau_2 = 188$ in this particular example, the WN-based segmentation misses some blood vessels, as shown in Figure 6.11.

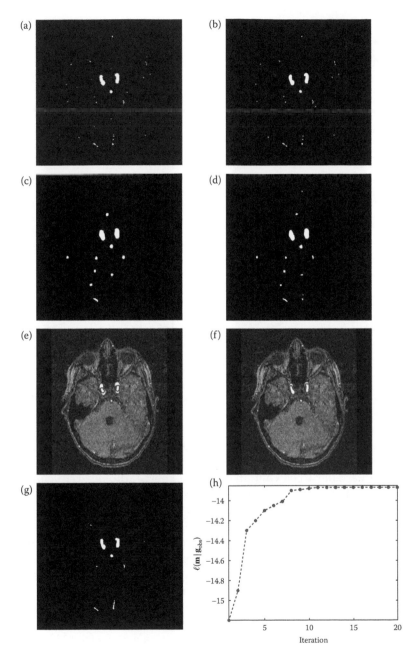

FIGURE 6.9
Initial (a) and final (b) maps of blood vessels from Algorithm 6 (the final error of 0.47%) vs. the maps from ICM (c: the least error of 20% with the potential values of 0.3); MRS (d: the least error of 9.1% with the potential values of 0.3 and three levels of resolution); DMG (e: the error of 0.95%), and GVF (f: the error of 0.53%) w.r.t. the radiologist's ground truth blood vessels) (g), and the convergence (h) of Algorithm 6 for the experiment in Figure 3.17a.

TABLE 6.4

Initial/Final Parameter Estimates of the Dominant LCDG
Components for the TOF-MRA Image

	Object i		
Parameter	1: Bones and Fat	2: Brain Tissues	3: Blood Vessels
Mean μ_i	23/23	103/102	208/204
Variance σ_i^2	116/109	335/349	256/261
Weight w_i	0.52/0.52	0.45/0.45	0.03/0.03

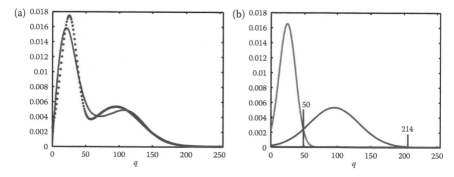

FIGURE 6.10

WN model (—) of the empirical marginal (—: a) and conditional models (b) of the three objects: bones/fat (—); brain tissues (—), and blood vessels (—), separated by the thresholds $\tau_1 = 50$ and $\tau_2 = 214$.

Experimental 3D results for the six subjects in Figures 6.11 and 6.12, as well as other experiments suggest that the WN model fails to detect large fractions of the brain vascular trees validated by an expert-radiologist, in contrast to Algorithm 6, which is more accurate in detailing these trees.

It is very difficult to get manually segmented complete and accurate vascular trees to validate segmentation algorithms. To quantitatively evaluate performance of Algorithm 6 in comparison with the WN one, three 3D phantoms in Figure 6.13 with known geometrical shapes similar to blood vessels have been created to act as the ground truth. The phantoms mimic bifurcations, as well as zero and high curvature existing in any vascular system, and their changing radii simulate both large and small blood vessels. To make marginal signal distributions for the phantoms similar to real MRA images, the empirical conditional marginals $\mathbf{P}_k = (p(q \mid k) : q \in \mathbb{Q})$; $k = 1, 2, 3$, were computed from image signals representing the CSF, brain tissues, and blood vessels in the MRA images segmented by a radiologist (in these experiments, 200 images were selected from a data set of more than 5000 images of 50 subjects). Then, the phantoms signals were generated using the inverse mapping. The resulting phantom's marginals are similar to those in Figure 3.20.

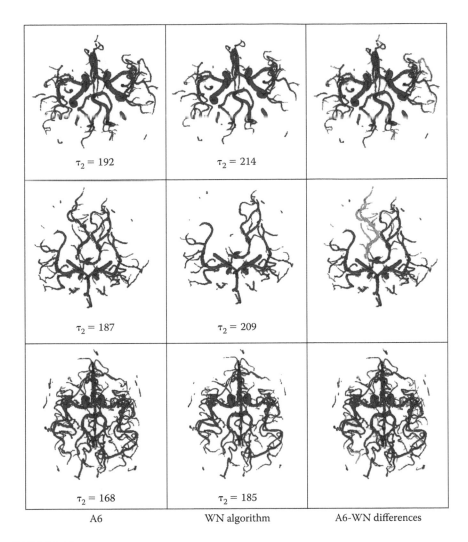

$\tau_2 = 192$ $\tau_2 = 214$

$\tau_2 = 187$ $\tau_2 = 209$

$\tau_2 = 168$ $\tau_2 = 185$

A6   WN algorithm   A6-WN differences

FIGURE 6.11
Each row relates to one patient; to highlight differences between the segmented vascular trees, voxels missed by the WN algorithm and detected by both the algorithms are colored in green and red, respectively.

The total segmentation error is a percentage of erroneous voxels with respect to the overall number of voxels in the ground truth (3D phantom). Figure 6.13 shows that on the average Algorithm 6 is an order of magnitude more accurate than the WN algorithm. The errors per each 2D slice for both the algorithms are plotted in Figure 6.14.

Results of segmenting 182 three-modal MRA images in Table 6.5 show that Algorithm 6 has the least error range (0.04%–1.2%), mean error (0.2%), and standard error deviation (0.4%), comparing to the six alternative algorithms.

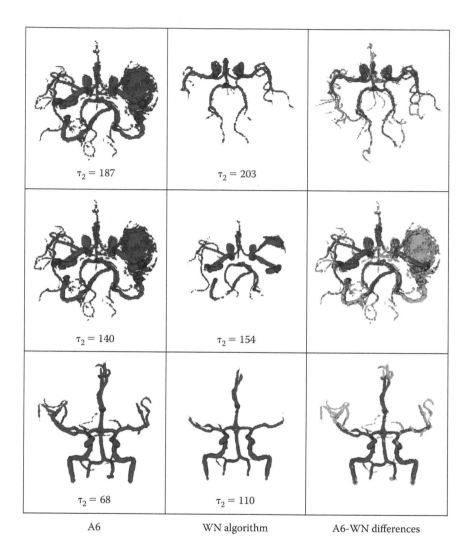

FIGURE 6.12
Each row relates to one patient; to highlight differences between the segmented vascular trees, voxels missed by the WN algorithm and detected by both the algorithms are colored in green and red, respectively.

The most accurate among them GVF has almost the same error range of 0.07%–1.2%, but the notably higher mean error of 0.5%.

6.2.4 Blood Vessels in PC-MRA Images

The like segmentation with three dominant modes (see also Section 3.5.5) is illustrated in Figure 6.15 by the initial and final region maps for the object 3 (blood vessels). The final map, obtained after the first five iterations

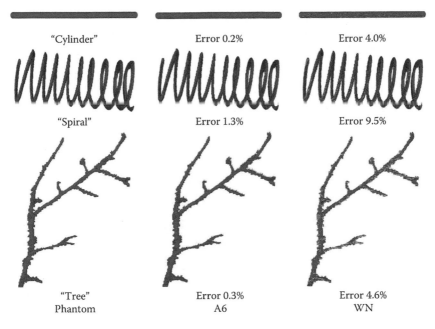

FIGURE 6.13
Segmenting 3D phantoms with Algorithm 6 and the WN algorithm (the same color coding as in Figure 6.11).

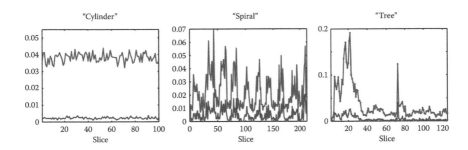

FIGURE 6.14
Total errors per slice for Algorithm 6 (—) and the WN algorithm (—).

of the refinement, has the error about 0.2% with respect to the expert's "ground truth." Figure 6.16 shows the dynamic changes in the log-likelihood $\ell(\mathbf{m} \mid \mathbf{g}_{obs})$. The initial and final potential estimates for the map model are $\gamma = 0.09$ and 0.12, respectively. The initial and final estimated parameters for the dominant LCDG components of are shown in Table 6.6.

Figures 6.17 and 6.18 illustrate the like segmentation using the Chang-Noble's model (CN) of the empirical marginal. The Levy distances

TABLE 6.5

Accuracy of Algorithm 6 w.r.t. WN, IT, MRS, ICM, DMG, and GVF

Error, %	A6	WN	IT	MRS	ICM	DMG	GVF
			Segmentation Algorithm				
Min	0.04	0.10	11	2.1	6.0	0.10	0.07
Max	1.2	12	29	11	21	1.9	1.2
Mean	0.2	6.2	16	8.3	13	0.9	0.5
St. dev.	0.4	7.4	5.9	3.1	4.7	0.5	0.5

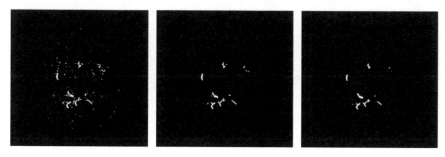

FIGURE 6.15
Initial (left) and final (middle) segmentation with Algorithm 6: the misclassification error of 0.2% w.r.t. the ground truth (right).

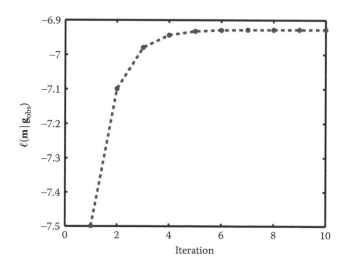

FIGURE 6.16
Convergence of Algorithm 6 at the map refining stage.

TABLE 6.6

Initial/Final Estimated Parameters of the Dominant LCDG
Components

Parameter	Object i in the PC-MRA Image		
	1: Bones and Fat	2: Brain Tissues	3: Blood Vessels
Mean μ_i	8.2/9.5	30/30	99/100
Variance σ_i^2	28/29	178/176	3010/2980
Weight w_i	0.25/0.25	0.73/0.71	0.02/0.04

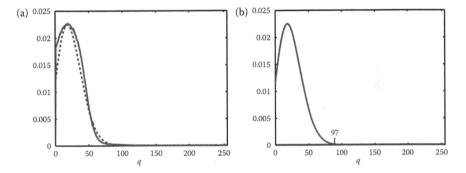

FIGURE 6.17
CN model (a: · · ·) of the marginal (–) and the conditional models (b) of the blood vessels (—) and other objects (—).

between the marginal and its model are 0.1 and 0.003 for the CN and Algorithm 6, respectively, despite their absolute deviations are about 0.09 in both the cases. The worse approximation of the marginal decreases the accuracy of separating the blood vessels from the background. In particular, the less accurate object separation threshold for the CN model comparing to Algorithm 6 results either in missing blood vessels or mixing them with surrounding tissues, as shown in Figure 6.18.

Just the same phantoms as for the TOF-MRA images validate the PC-MRA segmentation if the inverse signal mapping uses the marginal for the latter image. According to fractions of erroneous voxels w.r.t. the overall sizes of the "ground truth" 3D phantoms in Figure 6.19, Algorithm 6 is on the average an order of magnitude more accurate than the CN. The errors per each 2D slice for both the algorithms are plotted in Figure 6.20.

6.2.5 Aorta Blood Vessels in CTA Images

As mentioned in Section 3.5.6, the segmentation in this case assumes the four dominant modes in the empirical marginal, the third (light-gray) mode being associated with the goal blood vessels. Figure 6.21 presents their initial and

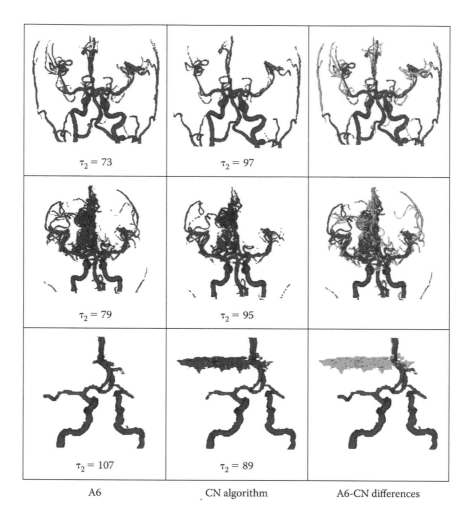

| A6 | CN algorithm | A6-CN differences |

FIGURE 6.18

Each row relates to one patient: to highlight differences between the segmented vascular trees, voxels missed by the CN algorithms and detected by both the algorithms are colored in green and red, respectively.

final region maps, the final map differing by about 0.6% from the expert's "ground truth." As shown in Figure 6.22, the map refinement converged after the first eight iterations. The initial and final potential estimates for the MGRF map model are $\gamma = 0.12$ and 0.17, respectively. The initial and final estimated parameters for the dominant components of the LCDGs model are shown in Table 6.7.

6.2.6 Brain MRI

The initial region map of the four dominant objects: dark bones and fat, gray matter, white matter, and CSF—is obtained by modeling the empirical

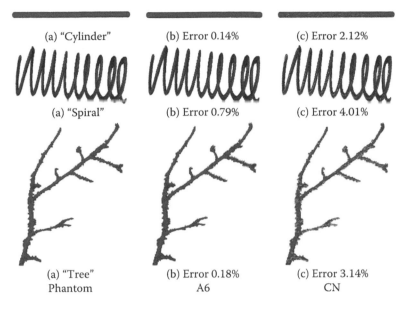

(a) "Cylinder"   (b) Error 0.14%   (c) Error 2.12%

(a) "Spiral"   (b) Error 0.79%   (c) Error 4.01%

(a) "Tree"   (b) Error 0.18%   (c) Error 3.14%
Phantom   A6   CN

FIGURE 6.19
Segmenting 3D phantoms (a) with Algorithm 6, (b) the CN algorithm, and (c) the same color coding as in Figure 6.18.

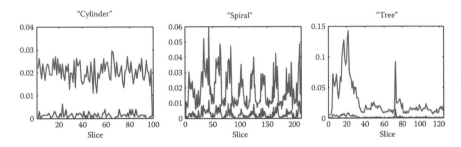

FIGURE 6.20
Total errors per slice for Algorithm 6 (—) and the CN algorithm (—).

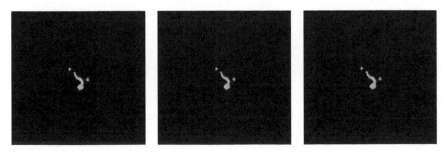

FIGURE 6.21
Initial (left) and final (middle) segmentation with Algorithm 6: the misclassification error of 0.6% w.r.t. the ground truth (right).

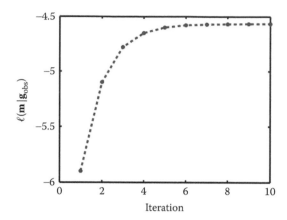

FIGURE 6.22
Convergence of Algorithm 6 at the map refining stage.

TABLE 6.7

Initial/Final Estimated Parameters of the Dominant LCDG Components for the CTA Image

Parameter	Object i			
	1: Background and Colon	2: Liver and Kidney	3: Blood Vessels	4: Bones
Mean, μ_i	24/23	102/103	214/217	248/250
Variance, σ_i^2	188/192	858/851	463/414	16/19
Weight, w_i	0.44/0.40	0.51/0.52	0.03/0.04	0.02/0.04

marginal with the LCDGs in Figure 3.25. The final map is obtained by refining the initial one, the refinement having converged in 15 iterations, as shown in Figure 6.23. The initial and final potential estimates are $\gamma = 2.0$ and 3.0, respectively, and Table 6.8 presents the estimated initial and final parameters of the dominant LCDG components. Figure 6.23 shows the initial and final region maps, having the final error of about 3% w.r.t. the expert's "ground truth." Comparisons in Figure 6.23 and Table 6.9 combining results for the 230 four-modal brain MRI demonstrate that the accuracy of the IT, ICM, MRS, DMG, and GVF segmentation algorithms is considerably lower than that of Algorithm 6. The latter algorithm has the smallest error range of 0.61%–2.9%; mean error of 0.79% and standard deviation of 0.60%, whereas the most accurate alternative algorithm (once again, the GVF) yielded the error range of 2.6%–14% with the mean error of 6.2%. The 3D results of segmenting the white matter from the MRI are shown in Figure 6.24.

The above experiments show that Algorithm 6 holds promise in segmenting images with multimodal marginals, such that their dominant modes

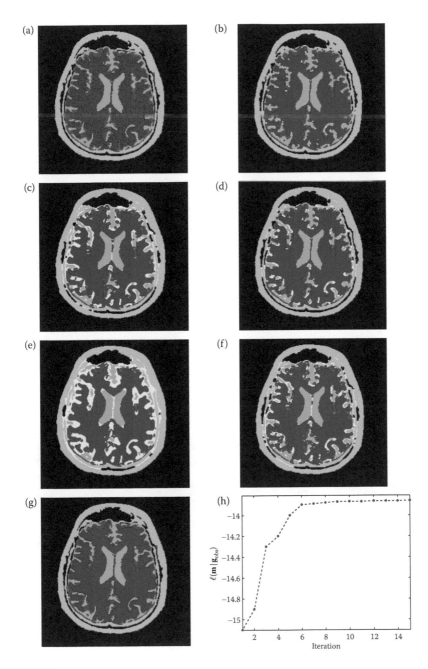

FIGURE 6.23
Initial (a) and final segmentation (b: the error of 2.2%) of brain tissues by Algorithm 6 vs. the ICM (c: the least error of 14% for the potential value of 0.3); MRS (d: the least error of 7.9% with the potential value of 0.3 and three levels of resolution); DMG (e: the error of 24%), and GVF (f: the error of 9.8%) w.r.t. the expert's ground truth (g), and the convergence (h) of Algorithm 6 for the experiment in Figure 3.22a. The errors are highlighted by yellow color.

TABLE 6.8

Initial/Final Estimated Parameters of the Dominant LCDG Components for the Brain MRI

Parameter	Object i			
	1: Bones and Fat	2: White Matter	3: Gray Matter	4: CSF
Mean, μ_i	23/22	85/86	127/126	207/210
Variance, σ_i^2	181/187	206/211	793/789	306/295
Weight, w_i	0.23/0.22	0.50/0.50	0.19/0.20	0.08/0.08

TABLE 6.9

Accuracy of Algorithm 6 (A6) in Comparison to the IT, MRS, ICM, DMG, and GVF Algorithms

Error, %	A6	IT	MRS	ICM	DMG	GVF
Minimum	0.69	4.9	5.9	16	10.3	2.6
Maximum	3.1	35	18	33	23	14
Mean	0.84	20	9.2	23	13	6.2
St. dev.	0.74	8.6	3.8	6.9	3.8	2.8

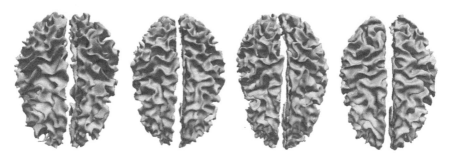

FIGURE 6.24
3D white matter segmentation from brain MRI.

relate to the goal objects-of-interest. The marginal is precisely approximated with the LCDG in order to separate the objects by simple signal threshold-ing, and the MGRF potential is analytically estimated in order to refine the obtained region map. The final maps are considerably closer to the ground truth than the like maps produced by several other image segmentation algorithms, including those based on deformable models.

6.3 Bibliographic and Historical Notes

A total number of classes for pixel- or voxel-wise classification or regions for segmenting medical images is often difficult to determine automatically [181], but usually is evident from the prior anatomical knowledge. Early segmentation techniques assumed spatially uniform intensities or textures [230], so that supervised classifiers could partition a feature space derived from the labeled training images [26,262].

The nonparametric nearest-neighbor (NN) classification needs no probabilistic assumptions about features and classes. A simple k-NN classifier relates each pixel or voxel to the class with the closest k training intensities, whereas a generalized k-NN classifier applies the majority vote tor these k intensities. The like vote is used for a nonparametric Parzen window based classification. Parametric classifiers, e.g., the ML or Bayesian ones, assume that the images or collections of their features are sampled independently from a particular stochastic model of an image with homogeneous regions, having certain visual appearances and, possibly, shape characteristics.

Today's medical image analysis employs a menagerie of classification and segmentation methods, which combine signal thresholding, clustering, region growing, and other techniques accounting for proximity between adjacent and distant signals both on the lattice and in the signal spaces. Such classifiers and segmentation tools include artificial neural networks and their combinations, trees and networks of classifiers, various DMs, and statistical decision algorithms based on MGRF image and region map models. A few such algorithms are detailed in this and subsequent chapters.

The approximate partition function of the Potts model in Section 6.1 was introduced in [24]. The log-likelihood of Equation 6.1 is a complex multi-modal function of the region map $\mathbf{m}$. To closely approximate the Bayesian MAP estimate, $\mathbf{m}^*$, of the region map, Section 6.1 employs conventional two-stage segmentation [34,278], but with more accurate model identification.

Table 6.10 lists the two algorithms (CN and WN) for segmenting blood vessels and five more general segmentation algorithms, including the classical DMG and GVF DMs (see Section 2.4), compared with Algorithm 6. The CN's mixture model of the PC-MRA signal extends the WN model, applicable to both the TOF and PC-MRA. To segment the brain blood vessels, the WN approximates the empirical marginal with a bi-modal mixture of three conditional components: two Gaussians and a uniform distribution, – using the EM algorithm:

$$P(q) = w_0 \frac{1}{Q} + w_1 \varphi(q \mid \mu_1, \sigma_1) + w_2 \varphi(q \mid \mu_2, \sigma_2); \quad q \in \mathbb{Q} = \{0, 1, \ldots, Q-1\};$$

$$w_0 + w_1 + w_2 = 1$$

TABLE 6.10

Conventional Segmentation Algorithms for Experimental Comparisons

	Algorithm	Author(s)	References
CN	Chang-Noble model based segmentation	A. Chung and J. Noble	[59]
DMG	Gradient-based deformable model (DM)	M. Kass e.a.	[158]
GVF	Gradient vector flow based DM	C. Xu and J. Prince	[309]
ICM	Iterative conditional modes	J. Besag	[25]
IT	Iterative thresholding based segmentation	S. Hu and E. Hoffman	[145]
MRS	Multiple resolution segmentation	C. Bowman and B. Liu	[32]
WN	Wilson-Noble model based segmentation	D. Wilson and J. Noble	[305]

The CSF and background outside the head have lower signal magnitudes, whereas the higher magnitudes represent the brain tissues, eyes, skin, and bones. The blood vessels correspond to the upper tail of the higher magnitude mode and are segmented by comparing the Gaussian components of the mixture to the uniform component associated with the background noise [305]: the lattice site $\mathbf{r}$ is labeled "blood vessel" if

$$g(\mathbf{r}) > \max_{k=1,2} \left\{ \mu_k + \sigma_k \sqrt{2 \ln \left(\frac{w_k Q}{\sigma_k w_0 \sqrt{2\pi}} \right)} \right\}$$

The CN algorithm employs the mixture of the two (vessels and background) components and models the background with the Rician probability distribution, i.e., the distribution of the square root of the sum of the six squared Gaussian random variables, which have different means and the same variance.

The IT algorithm separates a bimodal marginal $\mathbf{P}_{\text{emp}}(\mathbf{g}) = (P_{\text{emp}}(q \mid \mathbf{g}) : q \in \mathbb{Q})$ for a chest CT image by K-means clustering with $K = 2$ (Algorithm 7).

Algorithm 7 Iterative Thresholding of the Bi-Modal Empirical Marginal

---

Initialization: Selecting an initial threshold, τ_0, by comparing the voxel-wise CT signals for the pure air and the chest wall.

Iteration i: Compute a new threshold, $\tau_i = \left\lfloor \frac{1}{2} \left(\mu_{\text{lo}:i-1} + \mu_{\text{hi}:i-1} \right) \right\rfloor$, where

$$\mu_{\text{lo}:i-1} = \frac{\sum\limits_{q=0}^{\tau_{i-1}} q P_{\text{emp}}(q \mid \mathbf{g})}{\sum\limits_{q=0}^{\tau_{i-1}} P_{\text{emp}}(q \mid \mathbf{g})}; \quad \mu_{\text{hi}:i-1} = \frac{\sum\limits_{q=\tau_{i-1}+1}^{Q-1} q P_{\text{emp}}(q \mid \mathbf{g})}{\sum\limits_{q=\tau_{i-1}}^{Q-1} P_{\text{emp}}(q \mid \mathbf{g})}$$

Terminate if $\tau_i = \tau_{i-1}$ and output the lung/nonlung threshold $\tau = \tau_i$.

After the candidate lung voxels are extracted by comparing the signals to the found threshold, τ, the 3D connected components are analyzed to identify the lungs and discard their background, including too small components occupying each less that 1% of the total lung volume, which is measured with the number of the extracted lung voxels. The resulting lung regions (the two largest labeled connected components) are filled in and their interior cavities are eliminated by topological analysis. After large airways are identified and segmented, a three-region map is built to separate the lungs, the trachea together with the left and right mainstream bronchi, and all other voxels. The left and right lungs are identified at every CT slice. If a slice contains only a single large connected lung component, an area of its possible separation into two parts is formed by morphological erosion/dilation, and dynamic programming is applied to search for the best separating path through this area. The morphological closing, erosion, and dilation are used then also to smooth the lung boundaries, in particular, exclude some shape imperfections caused by pulmonary blood vessels and bronchi.

The multiple resolution segmentation (MRS) uses the modified AIC to estimate the number of image textures to be separated in a given image. Each individual texture is described with a nonhomogeneous Gaussian autoregressive model. The segmentation begins at the coarser resolution level of the quadtree representation, and the region map obtained at a current resolution level is an initial condition at the next level.

6.4 Performance Evaluation and Validation

Let $\mathcal{R}_s$, $\mathcal{R}_{gt}$, $\mathcal{R}_s^c$, and $\mathcal{R}_{gt}^c$ denote a segmented region, $\mathcal{R}_s \subseteq \mathbb{R}$; its ground truth, $\mathcal{R}_{gt} \subset \mathbb{R}$; and their complements on the lattice $\mathbb{R}$, respectively: $\mathcal{R}_s \cup \mathcal{R}_s^c = \mathbb{R}$ and $\mathcal{R}_{gt} \cup \mathcal{R}_{gt}^c = \mathbb{R}$. Then the true positive (TP), false positive (FP), true negative (TN), and false negative (FN) results are defined as follows (Figure 6.25):

TP $= |\mathcal{R}_s \cap \mathcal{R}_{gt}|$ is the overlap, or intersection area, i.e., the number of the common sites (pixels or voxels) in $\mathcal{R}_s$ and $\mathcal{R}_{gt}$.

FP $= |\mathcal{R}_s \cap \mathcal{R}_{gt}^c| = |\mathcal{R}_s| - TP$ is the number of the sites in $\mathcal{R}_s$, which are absent in the ground truth $\mathcal{R}_{gt}$, i.e., the difference between the segmented area and the TP.

TN $= |\mathcal{R}_s^c \cap \mathcal{R}_{gt}^c| = |\mathbb{R} - \mathcal{R}_s \cap \mathcal{R}_{gt}|$ is the number of the sites, which do not belong to both the segmented region and ground truth.

FN $= |\mathcal{R}_{gt} \cap \mathcal{R}_s^c| = |\mathcal{R}_{gt}| - TP$ is the number of the sites in the ground truth which are absent in the segmented region:

$$TP + FP + TN + FN = |\mathbb{R}|; \; TP + FP + FN = |\mathcal{R}_s \cap \mathcal{R}_{gt}|.$$

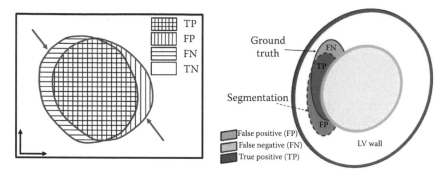

FIGURE 6.25
Agreement between the ground truth $\mathcal{R}_{gt}$ and segmented $\mathcal{R}_s$ regions.

The *Dice similarity coefficient* (DSC) characterizes an agreement between the segmented and ground truth regions [71]:

$$\text{DSC} = \frac{2 \cdot \text{TP}}{2 \cdot \text{TP} + \text{FP} + \text{FN}} \tag{6.7}$$

The closer the DSC to "1," the better the agreement between the regions. The ground truth in medical image segmentation is usually provided by one or more experts-radiologists delineated the goal objects in the images.

The DSC is used sometimes together with the relative total *absolute difference* (AD) between the segmented and ground truth regions with respect to the ground truth: $\text{AD} = \frac{FN+FP}{FN+TP} \times 100\%$. The closer the DSC and AD to one and zero, respectively, the more accurate the segmentation.

Distances between the borders of the segmented region and its ground truth are also used to measure the segmentation accuracy [249]. The *Hausdorff distance* (HD) from the region $\mathcal{R}_s$ to the region $\mathcal{R}_{gt}$ is the maximum Cartesian distance from the sites in $\mathcal{R}_s$ to their nearest sites in $\mathcal{R}_{gt}$ (Figure 6.26):

$$\text{HD}(\mathcal{R}_s, \mathcal{R}_{gt}) = \max_{\mathbf{r} \in \mathcal{R}_s} \left\{ \min_{\mathbf{s} \in \mathcal{R}_{gt}} D(\mathbf{r}, \mathbf{s}) \right\}$$

where $D(\mathbf{r}, \mathbf{s})$ is the Cartesian distance between the sites $\mathbf{r}$ and $\mathbf{s}$. The bidirectional HD is defined as $\text{HD}_{bi}(\mathcal{R}_s, \mathcal{R}_{gt}) = \max \left\{ \text{HD}(\mathcal{R}_s, \mathcal{R}_{gt}), \text{HD}(\mathcal{R}_{gt}, \mathcal{R}_s) \right\}$.

To comparing the region boundaries, other statistics of the distances $\min_{\mathbf{s} \in \mathcal{R}_{gt}} D(\mathbf{r}, \mathbf{s})$ and $\min_{\mathbf{r} \in \mathcal{R}_s} D(\mathbf{r}, \mathbf{s})$ from the boundary sites of one region to the closest sites of another region are often used instead of the maximal values in the HD or its bidirectional version. Such statistics, in particular, the average distance together with the standard deviation of the distances, or a particular percentile, e.g., the 95th percentile of the distances, etc, are often called the *modified HD* (MHD).

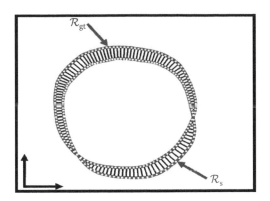

FIGURE 6.26
Measuring distances (black lines) between the ground truth and segmented boundaries.

Receiver operating characteristic (ROC) plots [104] allow to compare segmentation or classification algorithms by their performance and test sensitivity of segmentation to a certain operating parameter, e.g., a chosen threshold. The ROC is plotted in a unit square on the plane of the TP (y-axis) and FP (x-axis) rates (abbreviated below TPR and FPR, respectively):

$$\text{TPR} = \frac{\text{TP}}{\text{TP} + \text{FN}}; \ 0 \leq \text{TPR} \leq 1, \quad \text{and} \quad \text{FPR} = \frac{\text{FP}}{\text{TN} + \text{FP}}; \ 0 \leq \text{FPR} \leq 1$$

The ideal (errorless) segmentation relates to the ROC point $(0, 1)$, and the steeper the line $(0,0) - (\text{TPR}, \text{FPR})$ for an algorithm w.r.t. the main diagonal $(0,0) - (1,1)$, the better its performance. The TPR and FPR are also called *recall* (or *sensitivity*) and *false alarm rate*, respectively. The performance of an algorithm is also evaluated by its *accuracy*, $\frac{\text{TP}+\text{TN}}{\text{TP}+\text{FN}+\text{FP}+\text{TN}}$; *precision*, $\frac{\text{TP}}{\text{TP}+\text{FP}}$, and *specificity*, $\frac{\text{TN}}{\text{FP}+\text{TP}} \equiv 1 - \text{FPR}$.

An *area under the ROC curve* (AUC) is often used to compare and rank two or more algorithms: the closer the AUC to 1.0, the higher the performance.

7

Segmenting with Deformable Models

Deformable models (DM), or active contours and surfaces, which are power-ful tools of image segmentation, may incorporate various stochastic models of visual appearances and shapes of goal objects. Parametric or nonparametric (geometric) DMs are evolving towards intricate object boundaries under the external and internal forces outlined in brief in Chapter 2 (Section 2.4). If external forces depend on joint probabilities of image signals and region labels in individual points within and outside the object, such an active boundary could be called a *stochastic DM*.

Often the guiding joint probabilities are derived from a simple stochastic model combining an unconditional MGRF of hidden region labels and a conditional IRF of pixel/voxel-wise observed signals, as, e.g., in Chapters 5 and 6. The conditional signal marginals for each region are recovered from a mixed empirical marginal for the entire image by the LCDG modeling (Chapter 3), and the Gibbs potentials to refine the region map are estimated analytically as in Chapter 4.

External forces depending only on joint "signal–region label" probabilities in individual points are suitable for segmenting piecewise homogenous or only slightly inhomogeneous images. But considerable signal inhomogeneities or strong noise call for adding a shape-related energy term. One of the common shape descriptors is a *distance map* of Equation 2.32 presenting the signed Cartesian distances of lattice sites from a current boundary. A generalized shape can be learned from the distance maps for a set of co-aligned training objects.

Comparative experiments have shown that stochastic DMs outline various objects of interest more accurately than their deterministic counterparts. Advantages of the probabilistic external forces include an automated initialization, low sensitivity to the initialization, and abilities to represent complex shapes with concavities.

7.1 Appearance-Based Segmentation

The appearance is modeled with a conditional IRF of image signals with arbitrary marginals, being the same for the lattice sites of one region. By assumption, each individual region is associated with one of the dominant modes of the mixed multi-modal image-wide marginal, and the IRF is identified using the LCDG approximation of the empirical marginal in accord with Chapter 3. The unconditional Potts MGRF of region maps accounts for only pairwise dependencies between the region labels in the nearest 8- or 26-neighborhood of each pixel or voxel, respectively. By symmetry considerations, the second-order Gibbs potentials are the same for all the pixel/voxel pairs and regions and have only two values: $-\gamma$ and γ; $\gamma \geq 0$, for the equal or unequal labels, respectively. As shown in Chapters 2 and 4, the analytic approximate MLE of the potential is $\gamma = \frac{L^2}{(L-1)} \left(p_{eq}(\mathbf{m}) - \frac{1}{L} \right)$ where L is the number of the dominant modes in the identified LCDG, i.e., the number of regions to be found in the image $\mathbf{g}$, and $p_{eq}(\mathbf{m})$ is the empirical frequency of the equal region labels for the nearest neighbors in the map $\mathbf{m}$, which was obtained by classifying every signal $g(\mathbf{r})$ in the lattice sites $\mathbf{r} \in \mathbb{R}$.

After identifying both the models, the active contour evolves by greedy searching for a closest local minimum of the total energy. A stochastic external force for each control point $\mathbf{b}_k = \mathbf{b}(u_k)$ of a current deformable contour $\mathcal{B} = \{\mathbf{b}(u) : u \in [0,1]\}$ evolving within a region λ is defined as

$$\zeta_{ext}(\mathbf{b}_k) = \begin{cases} -p_c \left(g(\mathbf{b}_k) \mid m(\mathbf{b}_k)\right) p_u \left(m(\mathbf{b}_k)\right) & \text{if } m(\mathbf{b}_k) = \lambda \\ p_c \left(g(\mathbf{b}_k) \mid m(\mathbf{b}_k)\right) p_u \left(m(\mathbf{b}_k)\right) & \text{if } m(\mathbf{b}_k) \neq \lambda \end{cases} \qquad (7.1)$$

At every greedy search step, the nearest neighborhood of each control point $\mathbf{b}_i \equiv \mathbf{b}(u_i)$ is analyzed, and the neighbor ensuring the smallest total energy becomes the new position for that control point, as illustrated in Figure 7.1. The evolution continues until the whole active contour, i.e., all its current control points, do not move anymore. Algorithm 8 details the above greedy evolution.

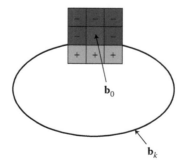

$\mathbf{b}_0$

$\mathbf{b}_k$

FIGURE 7.1
Greedy propagation of an active contour: interior (green) and exterior (red) nearest neighbors of the control point $\mathbf{b}_0$.

Algorithm 8 Segmenting a Region λ in a 2D Image **g** by Greedy Propagation of a Deformable Contour $\mathcal{B}_\lambda$

---

1. Apply Algorithm 6 to the image **g** partially, i.e., identify the conditional LCDG models of the L objects and the unconditional probabilities of region labels in Equation 4.10.

2. Form an initial L-region map **m** for **g** with a site-wise Bayesian classifier.

3. Find the site $\mathbf{r} \in \mathbb{R}$ with the maximum joint probability $p(g(\mathbf{r}), m(\mathbf{r}) = \lambda)$ to automatically initialize the deformable contour.

4. **For each** control point $\mathbf{b}_k; k = 0, \dots, n-1$, on the current deformable contour $\mathcal{B}_\lambda$, indicate exterior (the negative sign, "$-$") and interior (the positive sign, "$+$") positions w.r.t. the contour of each of the eight nearest neighbors, as shown in Figure 7.1.

5. **If** the control point is assigned to the region λ, i.e., $m(\mathbf{b}_k) = \lambda$, **AND** some of its exterior neighbors are also assigned to the region λ, **then** expand the contour by moving the control point to the exterior position giving the minimum total energy; **otherwise**, keep the current position of this point.

6. **If** the control point is not assigned to the region λ, i.e., $m(\mathbf{b}_k) \neq \lambda$, **then** contract the contour by moving this point to the interior position giving the minimum total energy.

7. Mark each site visited by the deformable contour.

8. **If** the current control point moves to an already visited site, **then** find the edge formed by the already visited sites and use the edge points as the new control points of the active contour.

9. **If** the iteration adds new control points, **then** use the cubic spline interpolation of the whole contour and smooth all its control points with a low pass filter.

10. Repeat Steps 4–9 **until** all the control points remain steady (no positional changes).

7.1.1 Experimental Validation

Robustness and computational performance of Algorithm 8 are tested below on different real-world and biomedical objects of intricate shapes and appearances, such as star fish, hand, bones etc.

7.1.1.1 Starfish

Each such image exemplified in Figure 7.2 contains two dominant objects: the darker background and the brighter starfish. Figure 7.3 shows both

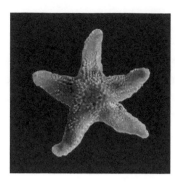

FIGURE 7.2
Starfish image.

the empirical marginal for this image and steps of identifying its pseudo-marginal, or LCDG model with the two dominant and six subordinate DGs in accord with Chapter 3.

The modeling produces two conditional LCDG models of the objects. After the first six refining iterations increase the model log-likelihood from -6.9 to -2.2, the refinement terminates since the log-likelihood begins to decrease. The minimum classification error of 0.02% between the starfish and background for the final LCDGs is obtained for the separating threshold $\tau = 82$, which relates the first and the last three subordinate DGs the starfish and background LCDGs, respectively. The site-wise Bayesian classifier uses the latter conditional pseudo-marginals to produce an initial region map of the observed image in Figure 7.2. The resulting potential estimate for the Potts model is $\gamma = 2.2$.

Figure 7.4 shows two initial active contours: (1) a circle with the radius of 20 sites centered at the site with the maximum joint probability of the image signal and starfish label for the estimated conditional object models and unconditional region map model and (2) a circle with the larger radius (120 sites) including some parts of the background. That in both the cases the active contour evolved to the same final starfish boundary indicates that Algorithm 8 is relatively insensitive to its initialization.

7.1.1.2 Hand

The active contour based on Algorithm 8 preserves topological properties of various goal shapes better than other geometrical deformable models, such as, e.g., a geodesic active contour (GAC). Figure 7.5 compares the GAC with the parametric deformable model of Algorithm 8 on segmenting a human hand on a relatively low-resolution image (540×640 pixels). Because two middle fingers are very close to each other, the initial GAC changes its topology and splits into two separate curves. The final GAC consists of a larger outer curve and a disjoint inner curve shown in Figure 7.5. That the two

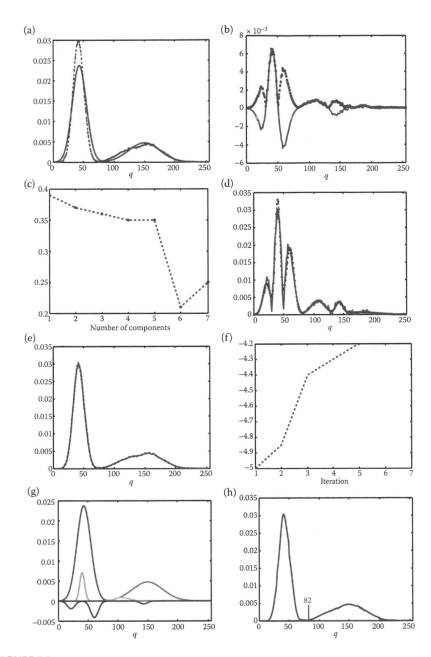

FIGURE 7.3

Empirical marginal $\mathbf{P}_{emp}(\mathbf{g})$ (–) for the image in Figure 7.2, approximated with a mixture $\mathbf{P}_2$ (–) of two dominant DGs (a); the deviation and absolute deviation between $\mathbf{P}_{emp}(\mathbf{g})$ and $\mathbf{P}_2$ (b), estimating the number of subordinate DGs (c); the mixture modeling of the absolute deviation (d); the final bimodal pseudo-marginal LCDG model of the empirical marginal $\mathbf{P}_{emp}(\mathbf{g})$ (e); the log-likelihood changes during the model refinement (f); all the DG components of the final LCDG (g), and the conditional LCDGs for each object (h).

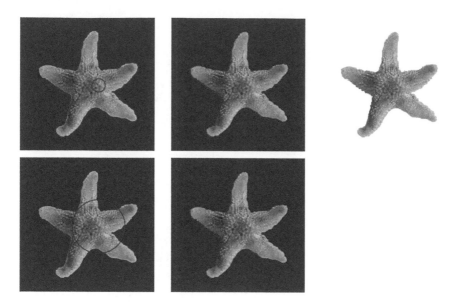

FIGURE 7.4
Initialized active contour (left column) and its final position for Algorithm 8 (middle column) giving the same error of 0.004% w.r.t. the ground truth (right column) in both the cases.

middle fingers became a "single wide finger with a hole" in the final segmentation is obviously undesirable. The corresponding results of Algorithm 8 in Figure 7.5 show that the boundaries of each finger are kept separate, and the final contour reflects the correct shape of the hand.

7.1.1.3 Bones

Figure 7.6 compares the GAC with the parametric deformable model of Algorithm 8 on two adjacent bones in a CT image of 872×440 pixels. Because these bones are very close to each other, two separate GACs merge at a weak gap between the two bone cells and the resulting single final GAC encloses both the bones. Again, Algorithm 8 keeps the curves separated throughout the evolution and correctly finds the boundary of each cell.

7.1.1.4 Various Other Objects

Figure 7.7 and Table 7.1 show advantages of guiding the active contour with the external force of Equation 7.1 in Algorithm 8 w.r.t. the conventional greedy algorithms DMG and GVF, relating the external forces to image gradients and a gradient vector flow, respectively. By speed and accuracy, Algorithm 8 outperforms the DMG and GVF. More objects segmented accurately with Algorithm 8 are shown in Figures 7.8 through 7.11.

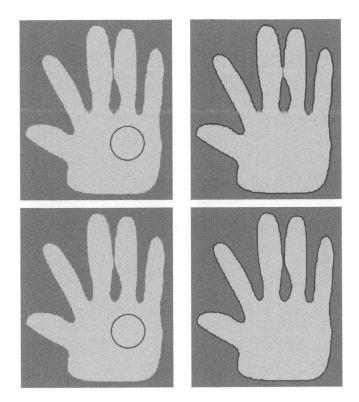

FIGURE 7.5
Hand segmentation with the GAC (top) and Algorithm 8 (bottom): The initial (left column) and final (right column) boundaries.

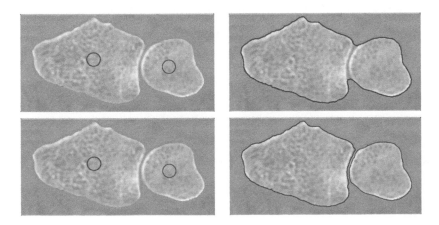

FIGURE 7.6
Segmenting carpal bones on a CT image with the GAC (top) and Algorithm 8 (bottom): the initial (left column) and final (right column) boundaries.

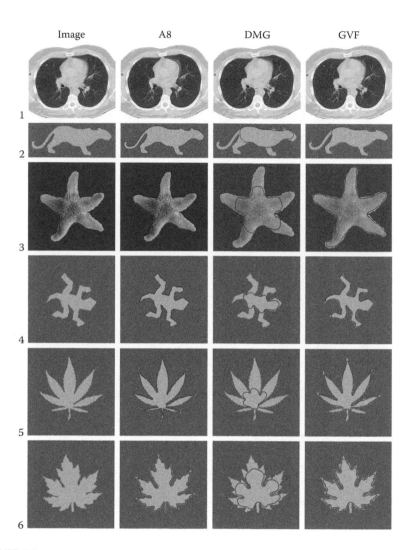

FIGURE 7.7
Segmenting objects of various shapes with Algorithm 8 (A8) and more conventional DMG and GVF greedy algorithms. The final boundaries are shown in red.

TABLE 7.1

Segmentation Time, s/Error, % for Algorithms and Images in Figure 7.7

	1	2	3	4	5	6
Image, Pixels	512×512	300×800	512×512	900×900	1000×1000	1100×1100
A8	140/1.2	120/0.002	150/0.001	150/0.004	200/0.003	210/0.002
DMG	420/35	410/32	490/32	580/41	610/67	650/19
GVF	280/15	260/8.0	300/8.6	290/13	360/13	390/5.9

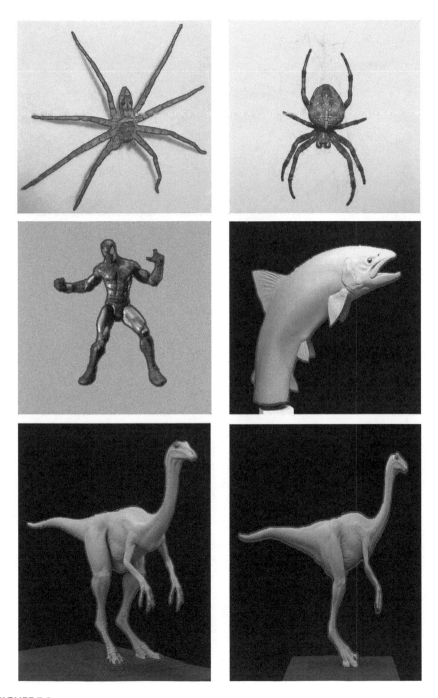

FIGURE 7.8
Segmentation with Algorithm 8.

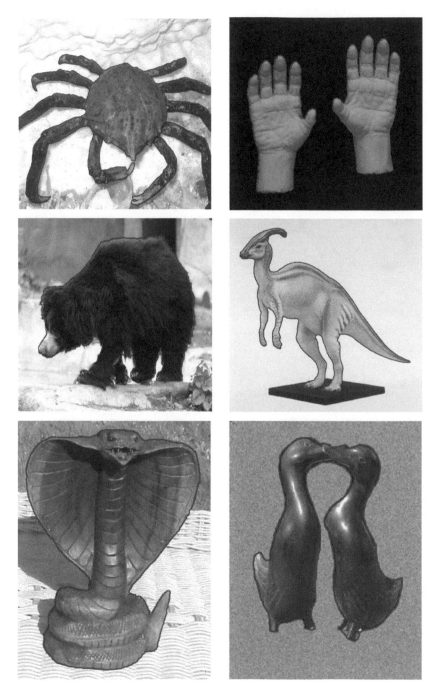

FIGURE 7.9
Segmentation with Algorithm 8.

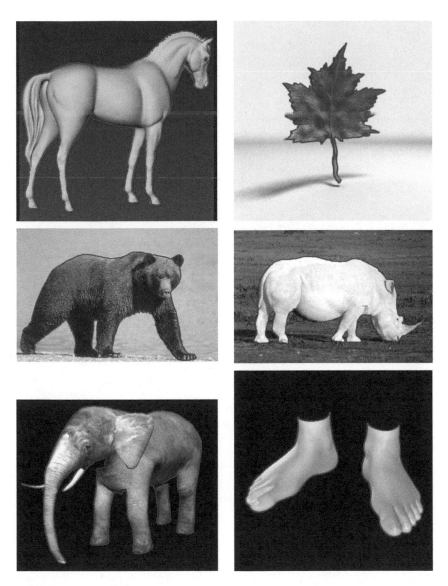

FIGURE 7.10
Segmentation with Algorithm 8.

7.2 Shape and Appearance-Based Segmentation

The validation in Section 7.1.1 confirmed that the parametric active boundary of Algorithm 8 is a powerful tool for segmenting images of intricate objects. Nonetheless, it might fail in the presence of high signal noise, under poor

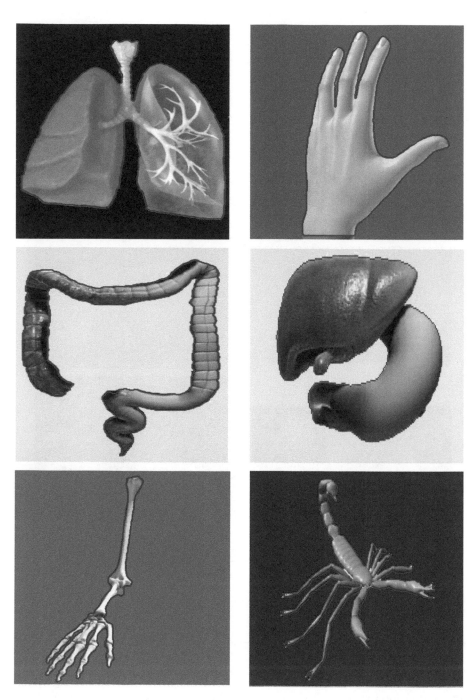

FIGURE 7.11
Segmentation with Algorithm 8.

image resolution, and for diffused or partially occluded object boundaries. One of the possible reasons of such failures is that no prior information about the objects' shapes is used, although in many applications, especially, in medical image analysis, most of the goal objects (i.e., anatomical organs) have well constrained shapes. The segmentation can obviously benefit from using shape constraints to complement the appearance descriptors of the objects.

Comparing to Section 7.1, let the external force of Equation 7.1 be modified by combining the conditional object models and the unconditional region map model, estimated for a given image, with a probabilistic shape model, learned from a set of training shapes. The conditional models of signals describe visual appearance of the objects; the MGRF of region maps controls continuity of the regions occupied by the objects, and the shape model takes account of signed distance maps for the training shapes. The modified external force is

$$
\zeta_{\text{ext}}(\mathbf{b}_k) = \begin{cases} -p_c(g(\mathbf{b}_k) \mid m(\mathbf{b}_k))p_u(m(\mathbf{b}_k))p_s(d(\mathbf{b}_k) \mid m(\mathbf{b}_k)) & \text{if } m(\mathbf{b}_k) = \lambda \\ p_c(g(\mathbf{b}_k) \mid m(\mathbf{b}_k))p_u(m(\mathbf{b}_k))p_s(d(\mathbf{b}_k) \mid m(\mathbf{b}_k)) & \text{otherwise} \end{cases}
$$
(7.2)

where $d(\mathbf{b}_k)$ is the signed distance in the position $\mathbf{b}_k$ and the conditional probability distributions $\mathbf{P}_s = (p_s(d \mid \lambda)) : d \in \{-d_{\max}, -d_{\max} + 1, \ldots, 0, 1, \ldots, d_{\max}; \lambda \in \{1, \ldots, L\})$ describe the signed distance map inside and outside each object λ. Specifically, examples below, in Section 7.2.2, assume only two-object images ($L = 2$); e.g., a kidney vs. all other tissues.

7.2.1 Learning a Shape Model

Algorithm 9 builds an average shape model for a given training set of images in order to find the above conditional distributions $\mathbf{P}_s$ of the signed distances. Figures 7.12 through 7.14 illustrate basic steps of this algorithm. Figure 7.15 evaluates the accuracy of the affine co-alignment of the N training images by averaging their region maps before and after the alignment. Obviously, the shapes coincide more significantly after the alignment, i.e., the alignment does decrease their variability.

7.2.2 Experimental Validation

The performance of the shape and appearance based segmentation is illustrated below in application to various 2D star fish and kidney images.

7.2.2.1 Starfish

Just as in Section 7.1.1, the segmentation assumes that each image has only two dominant objects ($L = 2$): the darker background and the brighter

---

Algorithm 9 Shape Modeling for the Modified External Force of Equation 7.2

---

1. Manually segment objects of interest on N images from a training database, as shown in Figure 7.12a and b.

2. Co-align the N training images using 2D rigid registration outlined in Chapters 2 (Section 2.1.5) and 5, as shown in Figure 7.12c.

3. Convert the co-aligned images into binary region maps shown in Figure 7.12d.

4. Calculate the 2D object boundaries $\mathcal{B}_{[n]}$ for all the manually segmented N biregional maps obtained in Step 3.

5. For each of the training N shapes calculated at Step 3, form the signed distance map, i.e, the map of the signed distances from each lattice site r inside and outside the object to the object boundary:

$$d_n(\mathbf{r}) = \begin{cases} 0 & \text{if } \mathbf{r} \in \mathcal{B}_{[n]} \\ D(\mathbf{r}; \mathcal{B}_{[n]}) & \text{if } \mathbf{r} \text{ is inside the object's boundary } \mathcal{B}_{[n]} \\ -D(\mathbf{r}; \mathcal{B}_{[n]}) & \text{otherwise} \end{cases}$$

(7.3)

where $D(\mathbf{r}; \mathcal{B}_{[n]})$ denotes the minimum Cartesian distance between the lattice site $\mathbf{r}$ and the boundary $\mathcal{B}_{[n]}$. Such distance maps (Figure 7.12e and f are constructed only once for subsequent segmentation of various images of the same object.

6. Compute the empirical conditional distributions $\mathbf{P_s}$ for the co-aligned shapes as shown in Figure 7.12g.

7. Calculate the average signed distance map of each object:

$$d(\mathbf{r}) = \frac{1}{N} \sum_{n=1}^{N} d_n(\mathbf{r}); \quad \mathbf{r} \in \mathbb{R}$$

(7.4)

Figure 7.13 shows an average signed distance map of Equation 7.4 for the kidney and the average shape obtained by thresholding the average map at zero level. The average empirical conditional distributions in Figure 7.14 are formed in the similar way, by averaging the empirical distributions obtained at Step 6 (Figure 7.12).

---

starfish. Figure 7.16 illustrates the affine registration of an arbitrary starfish image to an already co-aligned training database.

Figure 7.17 shows the empirical marginal for the image in Figure 7.16c and basic steps of identifying its pseudo-marginal (LCDG) model with two dominant and six subordinate DGs and producing two conditional LCDG

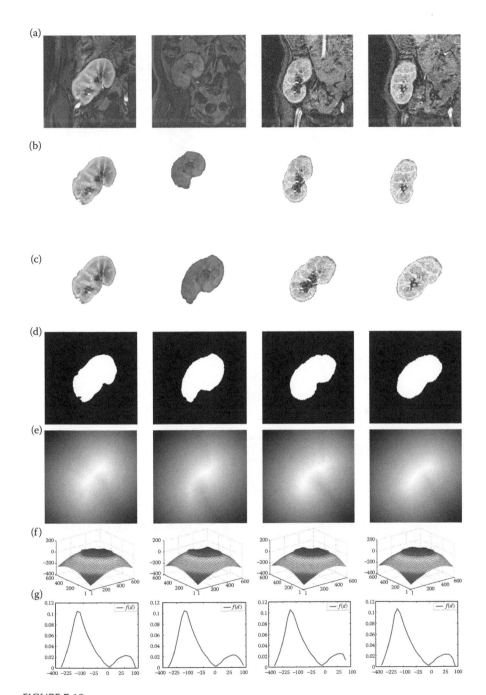

FIGURE 7.12
Basic shape modeling steps of Algorithm 9.

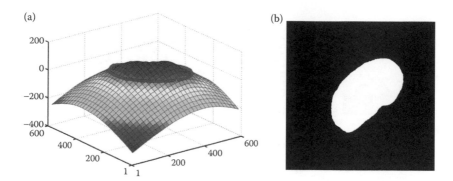

FIGURE 7.13
The average signed distance map (a) and shape (b) of the kidney.

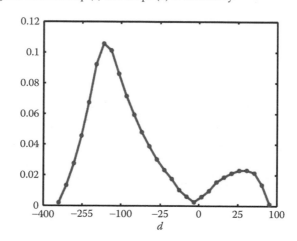

FIGURE 7.14
Averaging conditional distributions shown in Figure 7.12g.

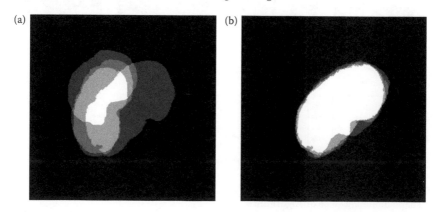

FIGURE 7.15
Overlaps of the training shapes before (a) and after (b) the image alignment.

(a)   (b)   (c)

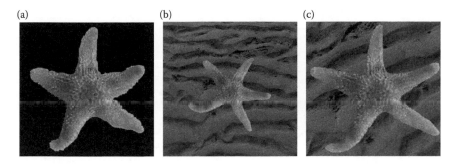

FIGURE 7.16
Image (a) from a co-aligned starfish database; a nonaligned starfish (b), and its affine registration (c) to the image (a).

models of the objects in accord with Chapter 3. Comparing to the like starfish image modeling in Section 7.1.1, only the model refinement differs in the number of iterations (10) increasing the model log-likelihood from -4 to -2.9. The threshold ($\tau = 82$) separating the starfish and background signals; the corresponding minimum classification error (0.0002), and the resulting allocation of the three subordinate DGs to each dominant DG are the same or closely similar.

Figure 7.18 shows the average signed distances for all the co-aligned starfish maps. The LCDG modeling of the empirical marginal distribution of the signed distances results in more accurately separated conditional distributions of the average signed distances inside and outside the learned starfish shape.

Figure 7.19 illustrates the shape and appearance based segmentation using the active contour. In this case the segmentation had the error of 0.4% w.r.t. the ground truth. Additional results for real starfish images are given in Figure 7.20. Robustness of such segmentation is tested in Figure 7.21 for the case when the same starfish is placed to the uniform background and the whole image is distorted by the uniform independent random noise. When the signal-to-noise ratio (SNR) changes from 20 dB to -1.5 dB, the segmentation error increases from 0.0001% to only 2.9%.

7.2.2.2 Kidney

Similar results for the kidney DMRI are shown in Figures 7.22 through 7.25.

These and other experiments have validated abilities of the external force of Equation 7.2 to guide an evolving active contour towards complex boundaries with concavities. Comparing with the active contours in Section 7.1, which are mostly suitable for objects of homogeneous appearance, adding the shape model, learned with Algorithm 9, increases the segmentation accuracy and robustness for inhomogeneous appearances.

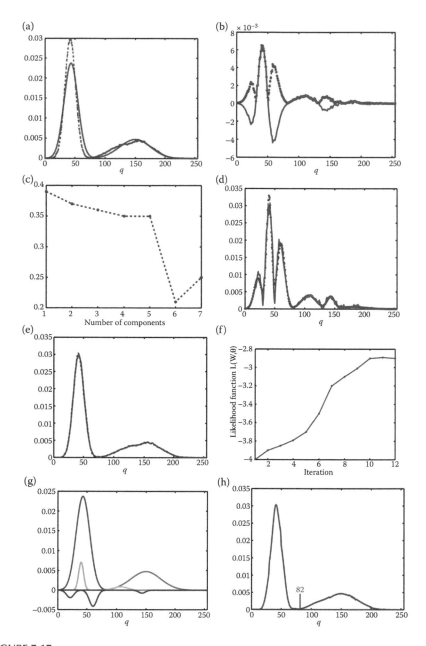

FIGURE 7.17
Empirical marginal $\mathbf{P}_{emp}(\mathbf{g})$ (–) for the image in Figure 7.16c, approximated with a mixture $\mathbf{P}_2$ (–) of two dominant DGs (a); the deviation and absolute deviation between $\mathbf{P}_{emp}(\mathbf{g})$ and $\mathbf{P}_2$ (b); estimating the number of subordinate DGs (c); the mixture modeling of the absolute deviation (d); the final bimodal pseudo-marginal LCDG model of the empirical marginal $\mathbf{P}_{emp}(\mathbf{g})$ (e); the log-likelihood changes during the model refinement (f); all the DG components of the final LCDG (g), and the conditional LCDGs for each object (h).

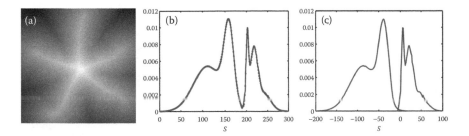

FIGURE 7.18
Average signed distances (a) for the aligned starfish images; the empirical marginal (b) of the average signed distances, modeled with the LCDG (–) and separated into the starfish and background pseudo-marginals (c).

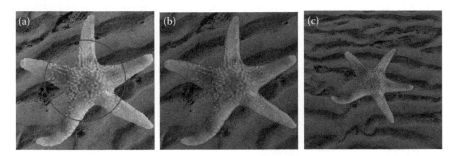

FIGURE 7.19
Initial active contour (a) for the aligned starfish in Figure 7.16c; the segmented aligned image (b), and the final starfish boundary (c) with the error of 0.4% w.r.t. the ground truth. This boundary was reduced to the original nonaligned image by inverting the affine transformation used for the alignment.

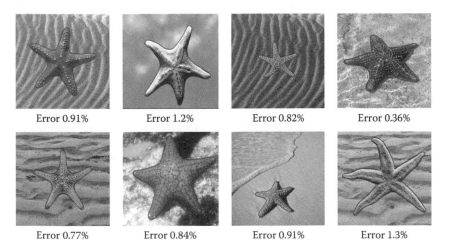

| Error 0.91% | Error 1.2% | Error 0.82% | Error 0.36% |
| Error 0.77% | Error 0.84% | Error 0.91% | Error 1.3% |

FIGURE 7.20
Segmentation under shape deformations and appearance variations.

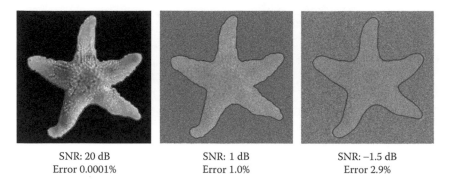

| SNR: 20 dB | SNR: 1 dB | SNR: −1.5 dB |
| Error 0.0001% | Error 1.0% | Error 2.9% |

FIGURE 7.21
Segmentation errors vs. the signal-to-noise ratio (SNR): The boundaries found are in red.

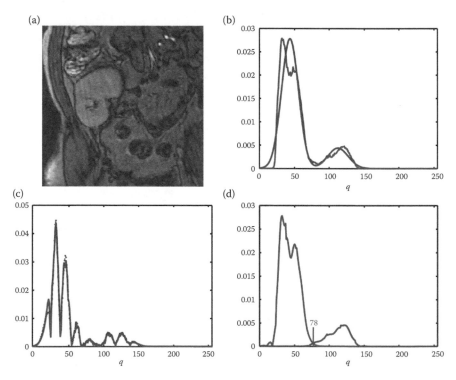

FIGURE 7.22
DMRI slice (a); its empirical marginal $\mathbf{P}_{emp}(\mathbf{g})$ (b) approximated with the bimodal mixture $\mathbf{P}_2$ of the dominant DGs (–); the scaled-up absolute deviation between $\mathbf{P}_{emp}(\mathbf{g})$ and $\mathbf{P}_2$ (c) approximated with the mixture of eight subordinate DGs, and the conditional LCDG models of each object (d) for the best separating threshold $\tau = 78$.

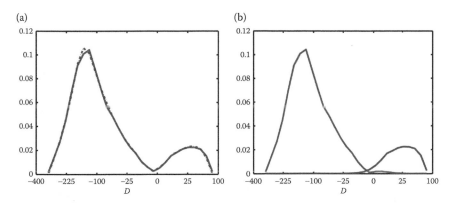

FIGURE 7.23
Signed distances from the lattice sites inside and outside the kidney to the kidney boundary: (a) the empirical marginal and its LCDG model and (b) the conditional LCDGs for both types of the distances.

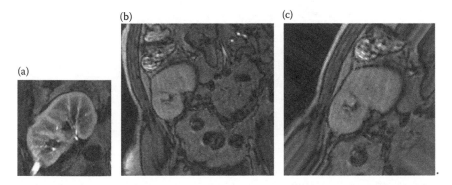

FIGURE 7.24
Kidney from the co-aligned training set (a); a nonaligned kidney (b) to be segmented; and its affine alignment to (a) by maximizing mutual information (c).

Aligning each new image to the training database excludes translations, rotations, and scalings of the goal objects. However, the segmentation could be inaccurate under large non-affine global and local geometric deformations of the goal object. The shape and appearance priors, discussed in Chapter 8, help in handling these problems.

7.3 Bibliographic and Historical Notes

Typical external forces of Equation 2.31 lead an active contour toward step edges in a grayscale image **g**. But both these and other traditional forces,

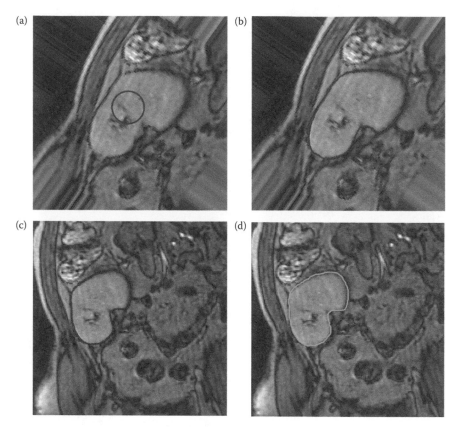

FIGURE 7.25
Initial active contour (a) for the co-aligned kidney; the segmented aligned image (b); the final kidney boundary (c) with the error of 0.23% w.r.t. the ground truth, or the radiologist's segmentation (d). The boundary was reduced to the original nonaligned image by inverting the affine transformation used for the alignment.

such as, e.g., based on lines, edges (gradients), or gradient vector flow (GVF) cannot closely approach intricate boundaries with concavities, being often met in medical objects. Moreover, high computational complexity makes the deformable models with most of such external forces too slow comparing with alternative segmentation techniques.

The total energy of an evolving contour is minimized most frequently using a greedy strategy [303]. The first and still most well-known greedy guidance of a deformable model by image gradients (DMG) was proposed in [158]. More flexible active contours, relating the external force to GVF, were proposed in [309], and geodesic active contours (GAC) were explored in [48,123]. The conventional speed functions, accounting for image intensities, object edges (e.g., [195]), or GVF (e.g., [310]), usually fail on noisy images with low object-background intensity gradients.

The level-set-based active contours, which evolve in a discrete time-space domain in accord with zero level of a level-set function [226], such as a map of the signed distances of Equation 2.32, are most popular in the today's medical image analysis due to flexibility and easy parameterization. The level-set-based segmentation improves after employing shape priors, such as e.g. in [244,289]. However, it still may remain erroneous under the large image noise and other inhomogeneities. Embedding stochastic forces into a level-set-based geometric deformable model to account for shape and appearance priors increases the segmentation accuracy, as exemplified in Chapter 8.

8

Segmenting with Shape and Appearance Priors

The priors to control a parametric deformable boundary are learned from the same co-aligned training images of objects as in Section 7.2. The shape prior follows from approximating an evolving boundary with a linear combination of distance vectors for a set of training boundaries, provided that the boundary is described with a vector of distances between a set of successively ordered boundary points and their common centroid. The visual appearance prior is built by using an MGRF with multiple spatially homogeneous pairwise interactions to model the training images and estimating the interaction geometry and Gibbs potentials analytically, as in Chapter 4. To more accurately separate a goal object from an arbitrary background, the empirical signal marginals inside and outside the deformable boundary at every evolution step are modeled with the LCDGs in the same way as in Sections 7.1 and 7.2.

Segmentation that involves the analytical shape and appearance priors together with the object/background LCDG models is faster than with many other geometric and parametric deformable boundaries. Experiments with various images confirmed robustness, accuracy, and high speed of the deformable boundaries guided by the shape and appearance priors.

8.1 Learning a Shape Prior

Boundaries of many medical objects in 2D images can be closely approximated with piecewise-linear curves. Such a curve $\mathcal{B}$ is specified by K control points $\mathcal{B} = (\mathbf{b}_k : k = 1, \ldots, K)$, defining linear segments and taking up intersections of the boundary with a polar system of K° equiangular rays (i.e., with the same angular pitch $2\pi/K^\circ$). The rays are emitted from the common center $\mathbf{b}_0$, being a centroid, $\mathbf{b}_0 = \frac{1}{K} \sum_{k=1}^{K} \mathbf{b}_k$, of the control points. Generally, there may be rays with no or more than one intersection of a certain boundary, so that the number of the control points K may differ from the number of the rays K°. For simplicity, $K = K^\circ$ below, although both the parametric

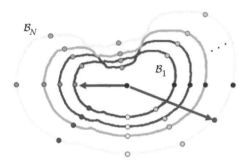

FIGURE 8.1
Mutually aligned training boundaries.

deformable model defined and its learning framework hold for the general case, too.

For the definiteness, the control points be enumerated clockwise, with zero angle for the first position $\mathbf{b}_1$ of each boundary $\mathcal{B}$, and the boundary is described with a vector $\mathbf{d} = [d_k : k = 1, \ldots, K]$ of the squared Cartesian distances $d_k = |\mathbf{b}_k - \mathbf{b}_0|^2$ from the center to the circularly ordered control points.

To build the shape prior, the N training images are mutually aligned to ensure the same centroid, $\mathbf{b}_0$, of all boundaries of the goal objects and unify their poses (orientations and scales) w.r.t. the system of the equiangular rays, as exemplified in Figure 8.1.

The shape prior $\mathcal{B}_{\mathrm{pr}}$ combines the co-aligned boundaries $\mathcal{B}_n = [\mathbf{b}_{n:1}, \ldots, \mathbf{b}_{n:K}]$; $n = 1, \ldots, N$, in such a way that their common center is always preserved and the control points remain at the corresponding rays:

$$\mathcal{B}_{\mathrm{pr}} = \left[\mathbf{b}_{\mathrm{pr}:k} = \mathbf{b}_0 + \sum_{n=1}^{N} w_n \left(\mathbf{b}_{n:k} - \mathbf{b}_0 \right); \ k = 1, \ldots, K \right] \qquad (8.1)$$

where w_n; $n = 1, \ldots, N$, are weights of the training boundaries. Any collection $\{w_1, \ldots, w_N\}$ of the weights produces a unique boundary, which shares the same centroid and is described by a linear combination of the training descriptors: $\mathbf{d}_{\mathrm{pr}} = \sum_{n=1}^{N} w_n \mathbf{d}_n$ with the same weights. An evolving boundary can be analytically approximated with the closest shape prior, and the evolution has to decrease the approximation errors.

Therefore, the space of the distance vectors describing the parametric deformable boundaries is closed w.r.t. linear operations, in contrast to the space of descriptors for the most popular level set-based ones. The latter deformable models evolve as zero level of a 2D map of the signed shortest distances from each lattice site to the boundary, being positive or negative inside or outside the boundary, respectively. The geometric shape prior is a linear combination of the signed distance maps for the co-aligned training images. However, the space of the distance maps is not closed w.r.t. linear operations because a linear combination of the signed distance maps may not necessarily be a valid map of distances to the same boundary and its zero level may significantly deviate from the training boundaries or even cannot be interpreted as a valid boundary.

Large sizes, $|\mathbb{R}|$, of the signed distance maps hinder their principal component analysis (PCA) to simplify the geometric shape prior. The distance vectors are much smaller ($K \ll |\mathbb{R}|$) and thus can be easily simplified by the PCA. Moreover, because their space is closed w.r.t. linear operations, the parametric shape prior has no singularities.

Let $\mathbf{d}_{\text{ave}} = \frac{1}{N} \sum_{n=1}^{N} \mathbf{d}_n$; $\mathbf{D} = [\mathbf{d}_n - \mathbf{d}_{\text{ave}} : n = 1, \ldots, N]$; and $\mathbf{U} = \mathbf{D}\mathbf{D}^{\mathsf{T}}$ denote the "average" shape descriptor; the $K \times N$ data matrix with the centered training distance vectors as its columns, and the symmetric $K \times K$ Gram matrix of sums of squares and pairwise products of the vector components, respectively. The PCA of the matrix $\mathbf{U}$ produces K eigenvectors $[\mathbf{e}_k : k = 1, \ldots, K]$ sorted by their eigenvalues $\lambda_1 \geq \lambda_2 \geq \ldots \geq \lambda_K \geq 0$. Due to mostly almost identical or very similar training shapes, many bottom-rank eigenvalues are close to zero, so that the relevant eigenvectors can be discarded. The characteristic top-rank eigenvectors ($\mathbf{e}_k : k = 1, \ldots, K^\circ$); $K^\circ < K$, are often selected by prescribing or choosing empirically a fraction α of the variance of the training shapes w.r.t. their average shape that should be preserved in the prior: $\sum_{k=1}^{K^\circ} \lambda_k \approx \alpha \sum_{k=1}^{K} \lambda_k$, e.g., with $\alpha = 0.8 \ldots 0.9$.

Let an arbitrary deformable boundary $\mathcal{B}$ on a given image aligned with the training set be described with the distance vector $\mathbf{d}$. Then the descriptor of the shape prior $\mathcal{B}_{\text{pr}}$, being the closest to this boundary in the least square sense, is a linear combination of the characteristic training eigenvectors $\mathbf{d}_{\text{pr}} = \mathbf{d}_{\text{ave}} + \sum_{k=1}^{K^\circ} w_k \mathbf{e}_k$ where $w_k = \mathbf{e}_k^{\mathsf{T}}(\mathbf{d}_{\text{obs}} - \mathbf{d}_{\text{ave}})$. Each sign-alternate difference $\Delta_k = d_{\text{pr}:k} - d_k$ between the squared distances to the control points along the same ray k determines the direction and force to move the current boundary $\mathcal{B}$ toward the closest shape prior $\mathcal{B}_{\text{pr}}^*$ with the descriptor $\mathbf{d}_{\text{pr}}^*$.

Just as with the level-set based deformable boundary using the geometric shape prior, segmentation results with the above parametric deformable model depend essentially on how accurately similar shapes were mutually aligned at both the training and segmentation stages (see, e.g., Chapter 5). To initialize a deformable boundary at the latter stage, an image $\mathbf{g}$ to be segmented is aligned with one of the training images, selected arbitrarily as a prototype.

8.2 Evolving a Deformable Boundary

In addition to the learned shape prior, the evolution is guided by a simple object appearance prior and even simpler appearance models of the object and background on each current image to be segmented. To specify and learn the appearance prior, the mutually co-aligned training objects are considered samples of a spatially homogeneous MGRF with multiple pairwise pixel interactions. its interaction structure and Gibbs potentials are analytically estimated, as detailed in Chapter 4. To account for the current image appearance, the LCDG model of the empirical marginal of image signals is built and separated into the conditional pseudo-marginals of the goal object and its background, as detailed in Chapter 3.

The evolution $\mathcal{B}_t \to \mathcal{B}_{t+1}$ of the deformable boundary in discrete time, $t = 0, 1, \ldots, T$, is specified by the system of difference equations

$$\mathbf{b}_{k:t+1} = \mathbf{b}_{k:t} + \Xi(\mathbf{b}_{k:t})\mathbf{u}_k; \ k = 1, \ldots, K \tag{8.2}$$

where $\Xi(\mathbf{b}_{k:t})$ is a speed of the k-th control point $\mathbf{b}_{k:t}$ at step t and $\mathbf{u}_k = \frac{\mathbf{b}_{k:t} - \mathbf{b}_0}{|\mathbf{b}_{k:t} - \mathbf{b}_0|}$ is the unit vector along the k-th ray. The boundary speed in the experiments below depends on the shape prior, MGRF-based appearance prior, and LCDG models of the current object and background appearances:

$$\Xi(\mathbf{b}_{k:t}) = \begin{cases} \exp(-\beta\Delta_{k:t})P_{\text{lcdg:ob}}(g(\mathbf{b}_{k:t}))p_{\text{mgrf:}\mathbf{b}_{k:t}}(g(\mathbf{b}_{k:t})) & \text{if } \Delta_{k:t} \geq 0 \\ -\exp(-\beta\Delta_{k:t})P_{\text{lcdg:bg}}(g(\mathbf{b}_{k:t}))p_{\text{mgrf:}\mathbf{b}_{k:t}}(g(\mathbf{b}_{k:t})) & \text{if } \Delta_{k:t} < 0 \end{cases}$$

$$\tag{8.3}$$

where $g(\mathbf{b}_{k:t})$ is the image signal for the k-th point $\mathbf{b}_{k:t}$ of the evolving contour at step t; $\Delta_{k:t} = d_{\text{pr:}k:t} - d_{k:t}$ is the difference between the squared distances for this point and the corresponding point of the closest shape prior ($d_{k:t} = |\mathbf{b}_{k:t} - \mathbf{b}_0|^2$ and $d_{\text{pr:}k:t} = |\mathbf{b}_{\text{pr:}k:t} - \mathbf{b}_0|^2$); the constant β controls the evolution speed ($0 < \beta < 1$ for smooth propagation); $P_{\text{lcdg:ob}}(q)$ and $P_{\text{lcdg:bg}}(q)$; $q \in \mathbf{Q}$, are the estimated object and background pseudo-marginals, respectively, and $p_{\text{mgrf:}\mathbf{r}}(q)$; $q \in \mathbf{Q}$, is the conditional signal probability for the site $\mathbf{r}$, given the learned MGRF and fixed image signals in its characteristic neighbors of $\mathbf{r}$:

$$p_{\text{mgrf:}\mathbf{r}}(q) = \frac{\exp(-E_{\text{mgrf:}\mathbf{r}}(q)))}{\sum\limits_{s \in \mathbf{Q}} \exp(-E_{\text{mgrf:}\mathbf{r}}(s))}$$

Here, $E_{\text{mgrf:}\mathbf{r}}(q)$ is the conditional Gibbs energy of the signal q in the site $\mathbf{r}$ for the learned MGRF appearance prior, provided that the image $\mathbf{g}$ is fixed

---

Algorithm 10 Guiding the Deformable Boundary with the Learned Shape/Appearance Priors and Current Object/Background Appearances

---

Initialization: $t = 0$:

1. Align a given image **g** to a selected prototype $\mathbf{g}_1$ by finding the closest affine transformation (Chapter 5).
2. Initialize the deformable boundary with the training boundary $\mathcal{B}_1$ for the prototype $\mathbf{g}_1$.
3. Find the conditional LCDG models of the current object and background appearances.

Evolution: $t \leftarrow t + 1$:

1. Evolve the deformable boundary in accord with Equation 8.3.
2. **If** the overall absolute movement of the deformable boundary, $\sum_{k=1}^{K} |d_{k:t+1} - d_{k:t}| \leq \tau$ (a small predefined threshold), **then** terminate the evolution; **otherwise** repeat Evolution Step 1.

Segmentation: Transfer the final boundary to the initial (nonaligned) image **g** by the inverse affine transformation.

---

in all other lattice sites. For the learned set **A** of the characteristic clique families $a \in \mathbf{A}$, specified each with the intraclique coordinate offset, $\mathbf{v}_a$, and the Gibbs potential, $[V_a(q, s) : (q, s) \in \mathbf{Q}^2]$, this energy, as outlined in Chapter 4, is obtained by summing the potentials for all cliques containing the site **r**, e.g.,

$$E_\mathbf{r}(q) = \sum_{a \in \mathbf{A}} (V_a(g(\mathbf{r} - \mathbf{v}_a), q) + V_a(q, g(\mathbf{r} + \mathbf{v}_a)))$$

if $\mathbf{r} \pm \mathbf{v}_a \in \mathbb{R}$ for all $a \in \mathbf{A}$. Algorithm 10 summarizes the above segmentation.

8.3 Experimental Validation

Algorithm 10 is evaluated below on intricate real-world starfish and zebra images with visually obvious ground truth (the actual object boundaries) and dynamic contrast-enhanced MRI (DCE–MRI) of human kidneys. The latter are usually noisy and have continuously changing and low contrast. Their ground truth was presented by an expert-radiologist. About one third of all images of each type were used to learn the priors.

Basic segmentation steps of Algorithm 10 are shown in Figures 8.2, 8.3, and 8.4. These and additional examples in Figures 8.5, 8.6 and 8.7, as well as comparisons in Table 8.1 for 130 starfish, 200 zebra, and 50 kidney DCE-MR images confirm the accuracy and robustness of the described parametric deformable boundary. Guided by the shape/appearance priors and simple appearance models of the goal object and its background, this deformable boundary notably outperforms, by both the accuracy and processing time, one of the best level set-based geometric deformable models (GLS) outlined briefly in Section 8.4. One of the possible reasons is that linear combinations of the level-set distance maps specifying the geometric shape priors may unpredictably distort the produced zero-level shape comparing to the training ones. Also, Algorithm 10 is faster due to mostly analytical computations.

Experiments with these and other natural images confirmed promising performance of guiding the parametric deformable model with the learned shape and appearance priors. However, in this case the boundaries of the training and test objects should be reasonably similar, up to an arbitrary affine transformation, and the goal objects have to be accurately aligned to their prototypes in spite of their different backgrounds on the basis of the learned object appearance prior. These requirements restrict applicability

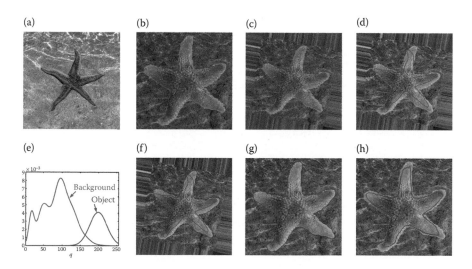

FIGURE 8.2
Training starfish prototype (a); an image to segment (b); its alignment to the prototype (c); the initial deformable boundary (d: in blue); the estimated object and background pseudo-marginals $\mathbf{P}_{lcdg:ob}$ and $\mathbf{P}_{lcdg:bg}$ (e); the initial (blue) and final (red) segmentation (f) of the image (c) with Algorithm 10, the final segmentation (g) after its inverse affine transformation to the initial image (b) (the total error of 0.74% w.r.t. the ground truth), and the final segmentation (h) with the GLS (the total error of 12%).

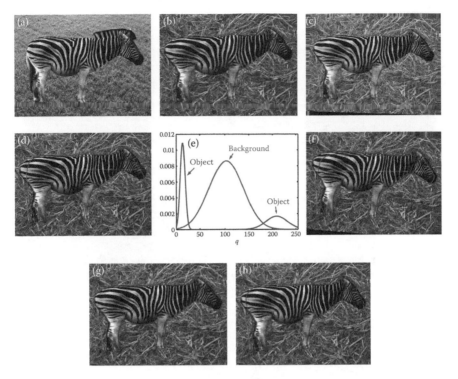

FIGURE 8.3
Training zebra prototype (a); an image (b) to segment; its alignment (c) to the prototype; the initial deformable boundary (d: in blue); the estimated object and background pseudo-marginals $\mathbf{P}_{\mathrm{lcdg:ob}}$ and $\mathbf{P}_{\mathrm{lcdg:bg}}$ (e); the initial (blue) and final (red) segmentation (f) of the image (c) with Algorithm 10; the final segmentation (g) after inverse affine transformation to the initial image (b) (the total error of 0.26% w.r.t. the ground truth), and the final segmentation (h) with the GLS (the total error of 9.1%).

of this parametric deformable boundary comparing to other parametric and geometric deformable models, although many of these latter also rely on the accurate mutual image alignment and may notably decrease their performance on low-contrast images.

8.4 Bibliographic and Historical Notes

One of the most efficient level-set based geometric DMs with a shape prior (abbreviated *GLS* here and in the subsequent chapters) was introduced

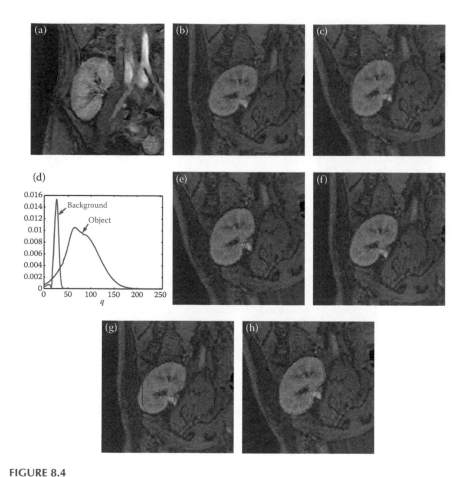

FIGURE 8.4
Training kidney prototype (a); an image (b) to segment; its alignment (c) to the prototype with the initial deformable boundary (in blue); the estimated object and background pseudo-marginals $\mathbf{P}_{\text{lcdg:ob}}$ and $\mathbf{P}_{\text{lcdg:bg}}$ (d); the final (red) segmentation (e) of the image (c) with Algorithm 10; the final segmentation (f) after the inverse affine transformation to the initial image (b) (the total error of 0.63% w.r.t. the ground truth (h)), and the final segmentation (g) with the GLS (the total error of 4.9% w.r.t. the ground truth (h)).

in [289] and used, in particular, for segmenting the inner left ventricle (LV) wall border of the heart. The shape prior is represented with a linear combination of characteristic signed distance maps, which are learned from co-aligned training heart cavity images in accord with Algorithm 11.

To efficiently evolve the DM and account simultaneously for the goal shape, the closest prior to each ongoing distance map is taken into account. The gradient and coordinate-wise descent methods are used to search for the prior $(\alpha_1, \ldots, \alpha_k)$ and affine transformation parameters that minimize

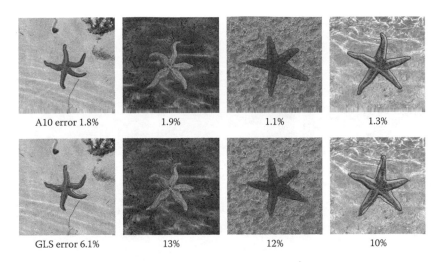

| A10 error 1.8% | 1.9% | 1.1% | 1.3% |
| GLS error 6.1% | 13% | 12% | 10% |

FIGURE 8.5
Final starfish boundaries and errors for Algorithm 10 (A10) and the GLS.

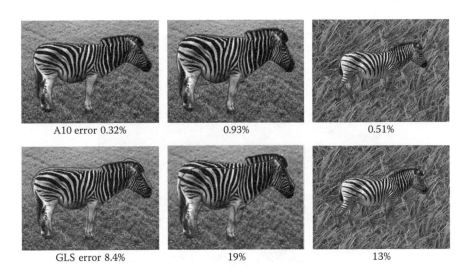

| A10 error 0.32% | 0.93% | 0.51% |
| GLS error 8.4% | 19% | 13% |

FIGURE 8.6
Final zebra boundaries and errors for Algorithm 10 (A10) and the GLS.

signal dissimilarities in each region and deviations between the prior and goal shapes. But because the space of the signed distance maps is not closed with respect to linear operations, zero level of the linear combination may produce a boundary of a wrong shape or even a physically invalid boundary.

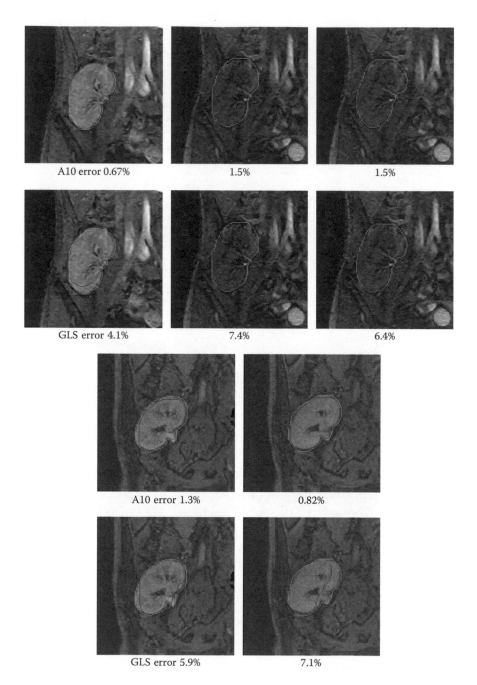

FIGURE 8.7
Final kidney boundaries (red) on DCE-MRI for Algorithm 10 and the GLS w.r.t. the ground truth (green).

TABLE 8.1

Segmentation Accuracy and Time for Algorithm 10 (A10) and the Level-Set Based GLS[a]

	A10	GLS	A10	GLS	A10	GLS
Images (number)	**Starfish (130)**		**Zebra (200)**		**Kidney (50)**	
Minimum error, %	0.15	5.2	0.21	7.3	0.25	3.9
Maximum error, %	2.0	15	1.1	19	1.5	8.3
Mean error, %	1.0	10	0.54	10	0.83	5.8
Standard deviation, %	0.67	3.1	0.31	3.3	0.45	1.5
Average time, s	50	550	60	790	23	250

[a] One-third of the images (43, 67, and 17 starfish, zebra, and kidney images, respectively) were used as the training sets.

Algorithm 11 Learning the Shape Prior

---

1. Manually outline an object-of-interest on given n training 2D/3D images and choose one of the obtained region maps $\mathbf{m}_i; i = 1, \ldots, n$, specifying the outlined shapes as a reference.

2. Co-align all the other training shapes by gradient minimization of the total mismatch energy $e(\mathcal{T}_1, \ldots, \mathcal{T}_n)$ for all pairs of the maps under their constrained affine transformations $\mathcal{T}$.

   a. The transformation $\mathcal{T}_i$ of each map includes translation, rotation, and uniform scaling.

   b. The reference shape is not transformed (zero translation and rotation; unit scale).

   c. The mismatch energy e_{ij} for each pair of the maps is the total squared difference between these maps relative to their total squared sum:

$$e_{ij}(\mathcal{T}_i, \mathcal{T}_j) = \frac{\sum_{\mathbf{r} \in \mathbb{R}} (m_i(\mathbf{r}) - m_j(\mathbf{r}))^2}{\sum_{\mathbf{r} \in \mathbb{R}} (m_i(\mathbf{r}) + m_j(\mathbf{r}))^2};$$

$$e(\mathcal{T}_1, \ldots, \mathcal{T}_n) = \sum_{i=1}^{n} \sum_{j \neq i; j=1}^{n} e_{ij}(\mathcal{T}_i, \mathcal{T}_j)$$

1. Form the signed distance maps of Equation 2.32, $\mathbf{W}_i = [W(\mathbf{r} : \mathbf{r} \in \mathbb{R}]^{\mathsf{T}}$ for the aligned shapes.

2. Find the mean distance map $\overline{\mathbf{W}} = \frac{1}{n} \sum_{i=1}^{n} \mathbf{W}_i$ and the shape deviation maps $\widetilde{\mathbf{W}}_i = \mathbf{W} - \overline{\mathbf{W}}; i = 1, \ldots, n$.

---

3. Use the PCA to find k; $k \leq n$, most significant eigenshapes Ω_j; $j = 1, \ldots, k$, representing all the training set.

   a. Form the shape variability matrix $\mathcal{W} = \left[\widetilde{\mathbf{W}}_1 \ldots \widetilde{\mathbf{W}}_n\right]$ from the column-vector representations $\widetilde{\mathbf{W}}_i$ of the deviation maps.

   b. Form the $n \times n$ symmetric matrix $\frac{1}{n}\mathcal{W}^\mathsf{T}\mathcal{W}$ and find its eigenvectors ω_j and eigenvalues λ_j; $j = 1, \ldots, n$; $\lambda_1 \geq \lambda_2 \geq \ldots \leq \lambda_n$.

   c. Select the top k; $k \leq n$, characteristic eigenvectors by thresholding the eigenvalues and form the corresponding characteristic eigenshapes $\Omega_j = \mathcal{W}\omega_j$; $j = 1, \ldots, k$.

4. Form the parametric shape prior (the signed distance map) as a linear combination

$$\mathbf{W}_{\mathrm{pr}:\boldsymbol{\alpha}:\mathcal{T}} = \overline{\mathbf{W}}_\mathcal{T} + \sum_{j=1}^{k} \alpha_j \Omega_{j:\mathcal{T}}; \quad \boldsymbol{\alpha} = (\alpha_1, \ldots, \alpha_k)$$

where $\alpha_1, \ldots, \alpha_k$ are the mixing weights of the shape prior and $\mathcal{T}$ denotes the affine transformation of the prior:

$$W_{\mathrm{pr}:\boldsymbol{\alpha}:\mathcal{T}}(\mathbf{r}) = \overline{W}(\mathcal{T}(\mathbf{r})) + \sum_{j=1}^{k} \alpha_j \Omega_j(\mathcal{T}(\mathbf{r})).$$

9

Cine Cardiac MRI Analysis

Noncontrast cine cardiac magnetic resonance images (CMRIs) are widely used at present for examining and evaluating global cardiac function. However, its regional quantification is established less well. To analyze wall thickness and thickening function on such images, two major data processing steps are performed: (1) segmenting inner and outer borders of the left ventricle (LV) from surrounding tissues and (2) estimating the wall thickness.

Integrating the accurate LV wall segmentation and the wall thickness measurenent and analysis is an extensive research area. However, most of the existing frameworks for analyzing the CMRI have serious limitations. Some of them require considerable user input and interaction, i.e., are prone to inter-observer variability. The LV wall segmentation using deformable models (DMs) with inadequate LV appearance and shape priors often fails under excessive image noise, poor resolution, diffused boundaries, or occluded shapes. The segmentation based only on the shape prior still results in large errors caused by discontinuities in boundaries, large image noise, and other inhomogeneities. Parametric shape-based segmentation is unsuitable for discontinuous cardiac objects due to a very small number of distinct landmarks. Wall thickness measurements, which are often based on the wall centerline, are typically too sensitive to imperfect contours and image noise, as well as require reliable point-to-point correspondences between the outer and inner borders.

An efficient and robust automated framework for analyzing the cine CMRI, outlined in Figure 9.1, overcomes some of these limitations. Accurate LV wall segmentation from cine CMRI is a challenging problem due to considerable intensity and shape variations of the LV wall at different image slices and within the same slice over the cardiac cycle. To increase the segmentation accuracy under large image noise and other inhomogeneities, the LV wall borders are segmented from a cine CMRI using a powerful geometric level set-based DM guided by stochastic speed function. The latter depends on a shape and appearance model of the heart, integrating the shape prior with the first-order intensity and second-order spatial interaction model.

Accurate point-to-point correspondences between the myocardial borders are established via a potential field, formed by solving the Laplace partial differential equation (PDE) within the segmented wall. The correspondences are used to evaluate both global functional and local physiological indexes, such as global end diastolic (EDV) and systolic volumes (ESV), global

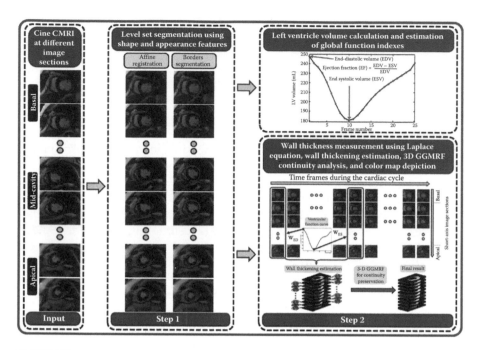

FIGURE 9.1
Cine CMRI analysis framework.

ejection fraction (EF), and local wall thickness and thickening. The cavity areas derived from the inner region are also used to estimate the global indexes, e.g., the EF.

9.1 Segmenting Myocardial Borders

The stochastic speed function for evolving the DM depends on a probabilistic shape prior, pixel/voxel-wise image intensities, and second-order pixel/voxel spatial interactions integrated into a joint bi-level object-background MGRF model (Figure 9.2) describing an aligned to the shape prior input image, $\mathbf{g}$, and its region map, $\mathbf{m}$:

$$P(\mathbf{g}, \mathbf{m}) = P(\mathbf{g} \mid \mathbf{m})P(\mathbf{m}) \tag{9.1}$$

Here, $P(\mathbf{g} \mid \mathbf{m})$ is a conditional distribution of the cine CMRI, given the map, and $P(\mathbf{m}) = P_{\text{sp}}(\mathbf{m})P_{\text{V}}(\mathbf{m})$ is an unconditional distribution of the maps, where $P_{\text{sp}}(\mathbf{m})$ is the shape prior and the GPD $P_{\text{V}}(\mathbf{m})$ with the potentials $\mathbf{V}$ specifies the MGRF of spatially homogeneous maps $\mathbf{m}$.

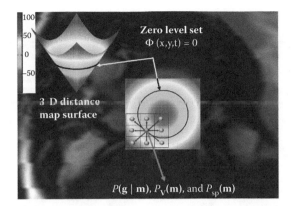

FIGURE 9.2
Combining (1) the first-order intensity model $P(\mathbf{g}\mid\mathbf{m})$, (2) the second-order MGRF model $P_V(\mathbf{m})$ of region maps, and (3) the shape prior $P_{\text{sp}}(\mathbf{m})$ to evolve the boundary (zero-level set).

To model visual appearance of the LV in each dataset to be segmented, an empirical marginal distribution of pixel/voxel-wise intensities is separated into two parts, associated with the dominant object and background modes, by using the precise LCDG approximation described in Chapter 3. To suppress noise impacts and ensure homogeneity of the segmented regions, spatial interactions of the region labels of a map $\mathbf{m}$ are taken into account by using the popular binary nearest-neighbor Potts MGRF described in Chapter 4.

In addition to the visual appearance characteristics, the level set evolution is constrained by probabilistic shape priors for the inner and outer borders of the LV wall. These priors were built from a set of training images collected for different subjects. To reduce variations of the training heart shapes and maximize their overlap for estimating the prior, the training images are mutually co-aligned by affine 2D transformations, which maximize their mutual information (MI). To construct the prior, a medical expert delineated the LV wall borders, specifying the region maps for the co-aligned training images. Then, the shape priors for the inner and outer contours are defined as spatially variant IRFs of region labels:

$$P_{\text{sp}}(\mathbf{m}) = \prod_{\mathbf{r}\in\mathbb{R}} p_{\text{sp}:\mathbf{r}}(m_{x,y}); \quad m(\mathbf{r}) \in \mathbb{L} = \{0,1\} \tag{9.2}$$

where 0 and 1 are the background and object labels, respectively, and $p_{\text{sp}:\mathbf{r}}(1)$ and $p_{\text{sp}:\mathbf{r}}(0) = 1 - p_{\text{sp}:\mathbf{r}}(1)$ denote the empirical pixel/voxel-wise object and background probabilities, estimated from the co-aligned training maps.

The framework exploits three shape priors, being built for the basal, mid-cavity, and apical levels at the learning stage after a medical expert divided the slices (cross sections) of each CMRI scan into basal, mid-cavity, and apical levels. During the segmentation, the first frame of each slice is

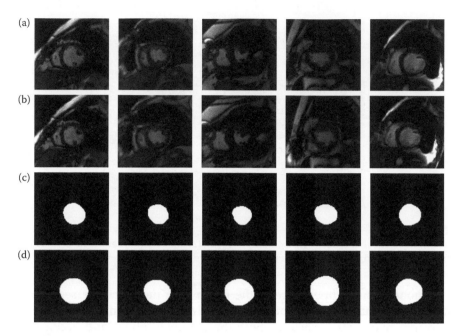

FIGURE 9.3
Forming the inner and outer shape priors: training samples (a) collected for different subjects, their affine co-alignment (b), and the manually segmented inner (c), and outer (d) borders.

automatically registered to the three shape priors and related to the basal, mid-cavity, or apical class by the maximum similarity to the prior. Figures 9.3 and 9.4 illustrate the process of building the shape priors for the mid-cavity level. The pixel-wise object probabilities, $p_{\text{sp}:\mathbf{r}}(1)$ are estimated for each lattice site from its empirical probability of being in the inner or outer LV area, which is manually segmented by the expert on the training images, co-aligned by maximizing their MI. The alignment enhances the overlap between the training maps and reduces variability of the prior shapes.

The learned shape prior, site-wise image intensities, and spatial interactions between the region labels contribute to the speed function, $\Xi(\mathbf{r})$, guiding the DM: $\Xi(\mathbf{r}) = \kappa \vartheta(\mathbf{r})$ where κ is the mean contour curvature and $\vartheta(\mathbf{r})$ specifies the contour evolution magnitude and direction:

$$
\vartheta(\mathbf{r}) = \begin{cases} -P_{1:\mathbf{r}} & \text{if } P_{1:\mathbf{r}} > P_{0:\mathbf{r}} \\ P_{0:\mathbf{r}} & \text{otherwise} \end{cases} \tag{9.3}
$$

where $P_{l:\mathbf{r}} = \frac{\Omega_{l:\mathbf{r}}}{\Omega_{1:\mathbf{r}}+\Omega_{0:\mathbf{r}}}$ and $\Omega_{l:\mathbf{r}} = p(q \mid l) p_{\mathbf{v}:\mathbf{r}}(l) p_{\text{sp}:\mathbf{r}}(l)$, assuming the heart and background label $l = 1$ or 0, respectively; $p(q \mid l)$ is a site-wise probability

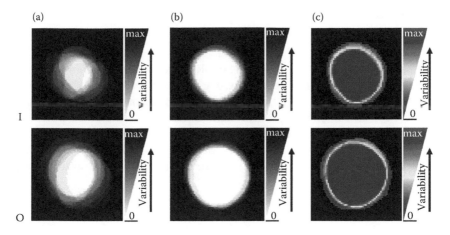

FIGURE 9.4
Gray-coded inner (I) and outer (O) shape priors before (a) and after (b) the affine MI-based alignment of the training database in Figure 9.3 with the color-coded visualization (c) of the prior (b).

Algorithm 12 Level Set-Based Segmentation of the LV Wall

Input: A grayscale image **g**.
Output: The segmented LV wall border.

1. Build the inner and outer shape priors from the co-aligned training images and their binary region maps.

2. **For each** input image **g**:

   a. Co-align **g** to one of the training images using the 2D affine transformation.

   b. Estimate the LCDG models of marginal intensity distributions with two dominant modes (Chapter 3).

   c. Form an initial region map **m** by the site-wise classification using the LCDG models.

   d. Estimate analytically the Gibbs potentials for the second-order Potts MGRF model of the map **m** (Chapter 4).

   e. Find the speed factor $\vartheta(\mathbf{r})$ of Equation 9.3.

   f. Segment **g** by evolving the zero-level set of the speed function found.

---

of the signal $q \in \mathbf{Q}$ for the LCDG appearance model of the current heart or background; and $p_{\mathbf{V}:\mathbf{r}}(l)$ is a label probability for the site **r** of the region map **m** in the MGRF model $P_{\mathbf{V}}(\mathbf{m})$ at the current evolution step: $p_{\mathbf{V}:\mathbf{r}}(0) = 1 - p_{\mathbf{V}:\mathbf{r}}(1)$. Algorithm 12 summarizes basic steps of the LV wall borders segmentation.

9.2 Wall Thickness Analysis

To assess and characterize the overall physiology of a patient in clinical and research applications, quantitative global or local (regional) indexes, such as wall thickening, are determined by heart ventriculometrics. Estimating thickness and thickening of the wall requires accurate correspondences (matches) between the inner and outer borders of the segmented LV wall. One of efficient ways to find the corresponding points is to place between the boundaries a potential field, $\gamma(\mathbf{r})$ where $\mathbf{r} = (x, y)$, being a solution of the planar Laplace PDE:

$$\nabla^2 \gamma(\mathbf{r}) \equiv \frac{\partial^2 \gamma(\mathbf{r})}{\partial x^2} + \frac{\partial^2 \gamma(\mathbf{r})}{\partial y^2} = 0$$

Let the inner and outer boundaries are equipotential and differ by their potentials. Then streamlines, which are orthogonal everywhere to all the intermediate equipotential surfaces of the field, establish natural point-to-point correspondences between two borders, e.g., $\mathbf{B}_a$ and $\mathbf{B}_b$ in Figure 9.5. Given the boundary potentials, all the potentials, $\gamma(\mathbf{r})$, can be found with the iterative numerical Jacobi method for the second-order central finite difference equations, being the finite-difference analogues of the Laplace PDE:

$$\gamma_{i+1}(x, y) = \frac{1}{4} \left(\gamma_i(x + \xi, y) + \gamma_i(x - \xi, y) + \gamma_i(x, y + \eta) + \gamma_i(x, y - \eta) \right)$$

$$(9.4)$$

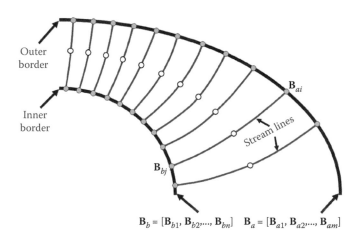

$$\mathbf{B}_b = [\mathbf{B}_{b1}, \mathbf{B}_{b2}, ..., \mathbf{B}_{bn}] \quad \mathbf{B}_a = [\mathbf{B}_{a1}, \mathbf{B}_{a2}, ..., \mathbf{B}_{am}]$$

FIGURE 9.5
Point-to-point correspondences between two boundaries via a potential field.

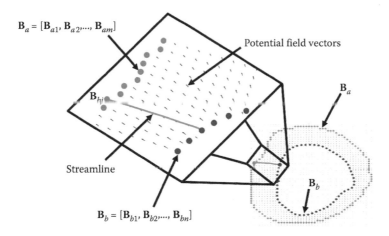

FIGURE 9.6
Point-to-point correspondences between the inner (red) and outer (cyan) LV wall borders (an enlarged section around the indicated streamline shows gradient vectors for the estimated potential field).

where i, ξ, and η denote the iteration and the lattice x- and y-resolution steps, respectively.

The *wall thickness* is measured by Euclidean distances between the corresponding inner and outer wall border points. Finding the correspondences between the LV wall borders from the solution of the Laplace PDE is exemplified in Figure 9.6. After the potential field between the borders is found by solving Equation 9.4, its gradient vectors induce the streamlines linking the corresponding border points. The *wall thickening* is evaluated for each image section by measuring changes between the end-systolic and end-diastolic wall thickness (Figure 9.7). For computing the thickening, the inner borders of all image frames at the same image section are re-sampled to the same number of points as at the end-diastolic phase (Figure 9.8). Then, the correspondences between the myocardial borders are found once again by solving the Laplace PDE and the site-wise changes across each MR scan are used to construct a 3D model of the LV (Figure 9.1, step #2).

9.2.1 GGMRF-Based Continuity Analysis

To preserve continuity and suppress (smooth) inconsistencies, deviations between the measured, $\delta = \{\delta_{\mathbf{r}} : \mathbf{r} \in \mathbb{R}\}$, and smoothed voxel-wise wall thickening values, $\widetilde{\delta} = \{\widetilde{\delta}_{\mathbf{r}} : \mathbf{r} \in \mathbb{R}\}$, are considered samples of a generalized 3D Gauss-Markov random field (GGMRF) prior with a diagonal covariance matrix. The smoothed thickening is also distributed in line with the GGMRF that accounts for interactions of each voxel $\mathbf{r}$ in its nearest

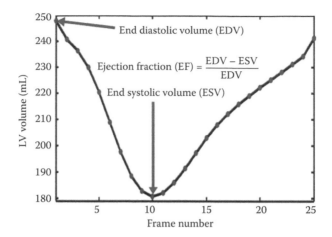

FIGURE 9.7
LV volume curve, integrating the cavity areas over the entire heart through the physiological cardiac cycle, with time points used to estimate wall thickening.

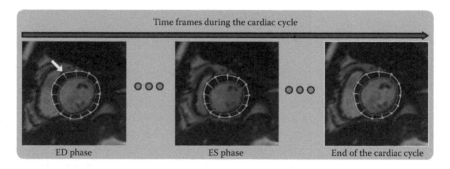

FIGURE 9.8
Re-sampling the inner borders at all image frames during the cardiac cycle to determine the wall thickening (the yellow arrow indicates an anatomical landmark to start the counter-clockwise re-sampling).

26-neighborhood, $\mathbb{N}_r$ (Figure 9.9). The measurements are replaced with their maximum *a posteriori* (MAP) estimates:

$$\hat{\boldsymbol{\delta}} = \arg\min_{\tilde{\boldsymbol{\delta}}} \left\{ \sum_{r \in \mathbb{R}} \left| \delta_r - \tilde{\delta}_r \right|^\alpha + \rho^\alpha \lambda^\beta \sum_{r \in \mathbb{R}} \sum_{s \in \mathbb{N}_r} b_{s,r} \left| \tilde{\delta}_s - \tilde{\delta}_r \right|^\beta \right\} \qquad (9.5)$$

obtained, due to the unimodal function to be minimized, by the computationally simple voxel-wise ICM.

The factors ρ and λ determine scales of the prior and smoothing GGMRF, respectively; the power $\beta \in [1.01, 2.0]$ controls the smoothing level ($\beta = 2$ for smooth and 1.01 for relatively abrupt edges); the power $\alpha \in \{1, 2\}$

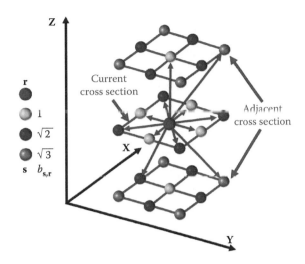

FIGURE 9.9
Pairwise voxel interactions with the nearest 26-neighbors at the current and two adjacent planar image sections.

determines either the Gaussian, $\alpha = 2$, or Laplace, $\alpha = 1$, prior for the estimates, and the coefficients $b_{r,s}$ quantify the second-order GGMRF interactions within the neighborhood. Experiments in Section 9.3 below were conducted with $\rho = 1$, $\lambda = 5$, $\beta = 1.01$, $\alpha = 2$, and $b_{s,r} \in \{1, \sqrt{2}, \sqrt{3}\}$ for all the adjacent voxel pairs $(r, s) : s \in \mathbb{N}_r$ (Figure 9.9).

For visual local assessment, the initial or estimated wall thickening can be displayed as a parametric map by relating these values over the entire LV volume to their maximum value in all image sections and mapping to the corresponding wall voxel. Basic steps of the wall thickening estimation are summarized in Algorithm 13.

9.3 Experimental Results

Performance evaluation metrics at each processing stage (the LV wall segmentation and the wall thickness/thickening estimation), including the ROC-analysis of combinations of the intensity, spatial interaction, and prior shape characteristics, were outlined in Section 6.4. The DSC and AD (absolute difference) metrics, which are instrumental in studying linear measurements, like wall thickening for all the test CMRI, are characterized below by their means and standard deviations (std). Although a per-sector wall thickening is considered in many cases, a myocardium dysfunction can be confined to a local heart wall territory.

Algorithm 13 Wall Thickening Estimation

Input: Segmented LV wall borders.
Output: Wall thickening values.
For each image section, repeat Steps 1 to 7:

 1. **Initial condition:** Set the maximum and minimum (zero) potentials $\gamma(\mathbf{r})$ at the inner and outer LV wall border, respectively.

 2. Estimate the potential field γ between these two iso-surfaces using the Jacobi technique (Equation 9.4) and the initial bounding conditions of Step 1.

 3. Iterate Step 2 until convergence (i.e., no change in the estimated field).

 4. Compute gradient x- and y-components for the final field at Step 3.

 5. Form streamlines using the gradient vectors of Step 4 and find correspondences between the iso-contours.

 6. Estimate the wall thickness by calculating the Euclidian distances for each pair of the corresponding points.

 7. Estimate the wall thickening from the thickness values at the ED and ES phases of the cardiac cycle.

Perform the continuity analysis on the estimated wall thickening using Equation 9.5.

9.3.1 LV Wall Correspondences

The accuracy of establishing correspondences between the inner and outer LV wall borders via the potential field was evaluated on simulated 2D images of two types: synthetic geometric phantoms with known point-to-point correspondences (e.g., concentric circles or more complex shapes with sharp corners and concavities), and realistic LV wall phantoms with outer borders obtained by deforming real inner ones. Figure 9.10 presents three synthetic concentric 2D phantoms that mimic enclosed areas between myocardial borders in a cine CMRI. Relative deviations of the corresponding points, which have been found for all inner contour points in each phantom via the potential field, from the true correspondences was about 1.0%.

The absolute deviation for each inner border point of the phantom is evaluated with the Euclidean distance, d_1 in Figure 9.11, between the corresponding point, chosen on the outer border via the potential field, and the true outer point. The point-wise relative error, $\varepsilon = 100 \left(\frac{d_1}{d_2} \right)$ %, is measured with respect to the true Euclidian distance between this inner point and its true correspondence: d_2 in Figure 9.11.

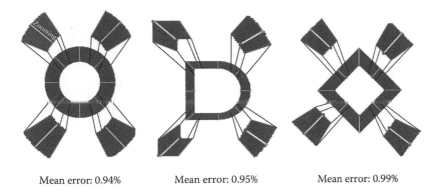

Mean error: 0.94%   Mean error: 0.95%   Mean error: 0.99%

FIGURE 9.10
True (red) vs. estimated (green) point-to-point correspondences.

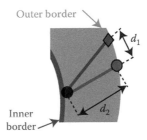

FIGURE 9.11
Measuring the relative correspondence error: ●—an inner point; ●—the true outer point; ■—the estimated corresponding point.

To mimic the real LV wall more realistically, the outer contours of a simulated LV wall are generated by deforming the actual inner contours of the cine images. The deformation inflates a closed equispaced contour (iso-contour), thus establishing their true point-to-point correspondences. Because the LV wall width, or thickness, varies from one to another patient, three deformation types: small, moderate, and large ones—were used to assess the relative correspondence errors. Their mean ± std percentages are shown in Figure 9.12.

9.3.2 LV Wall Segmentation

The entire framework was evaluated on 26 *in vivo* CMRI data sets collected from 11 patients having prior myocardial infarctions, by clinical indexes, and undergoing myoregeneration therapy. About ten image sections, typically, with 25 temporal image frames, were obtained for complete coverage of the LV for each patient. The breath-hold cine images were acquired using the 1.5 T Espree system (Siemens Medical Solutions Inc., USA) using segmented

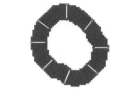 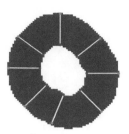

Errors: 1.0 ± 0.04%　　　　　　Errors: 1.0 ± 0.08%　　　　　　Errors: 1.0 ± 0.17%

FIGURE 9.12
True (red) vs. estimated (green) point-to-point correspondences between the manually segmented inner LV wall boundary and the outer border obtained by small (left), moderate
(middle), and large (right) deformations of the inner boundary (with the mean ± std relative
errors in establishing their correspondences).

TrueFISP contrast, with phased array wrap-around reception coils, and the
following typical parameters: TR – 4.16 ms; TE – 1.5 ms; 80° flip angle;
1 average; 12 k-space lines per segment; in-plane spatial resolution of
1.4 mm × 3.1 mm; and 8 mm slice thickness. All the patients took part in
approved by the Institutional Review Board investigations of a novel myoregeneration therapy, and had given informed consents before the imaging.

The segmentation accuracy is evaluated by applying to the segmented and
true contours the ROC, DSC, and AD metrics (Section 6.4). In these experiments one third of the data sets were selected for training and the remaining
sets were used for testing. For modeling the CMRI appearance, the marginals
have two dominant modes: (1) for the cavity and similar mid-gray tissues,
and (2) for the LV wall and darker tissues. Figure 9.13 illustrates the basic
steps of building the LCDG models of the two intensity classes associated
with these modes (Chapter 3).

Segmenting the LV wall borders on a time series data of one subject is
shown in Figure 9.14, and additional results on the test cine CMRI for different subjects and at different image sections are presented in Figure 9.15.
To evaluate the segmentation accuracy, both the DSC and AD statistics of the
agreement between the segmented and true borders on all the test CMRI
are summarized in Table 9.1. The ground truth was obtained by manual
contouring of the LV borders by an expert-radiologist.

Integrating the first-order LCDG intensity model (I), the second-order
MGRF model quantifying spatial interactions of the region labels (S), and the
probabilistic shape prior (P) allows for capturing main geometric features of
the heart. To show the advantages of combining all the three learned models (I+S+P), the test CMRI were also segmented using either only the I; or
I+S, or I+P models to guide just the same level-set-based deformable model.
Results for one subject in Figure 9.16 show that the accuracy of the I and I+S
algorithms decreases on low-contrast object-background edges, so that, e.g.,
the papillary muscles become a part of the LV wall. The shape prior (I+P)

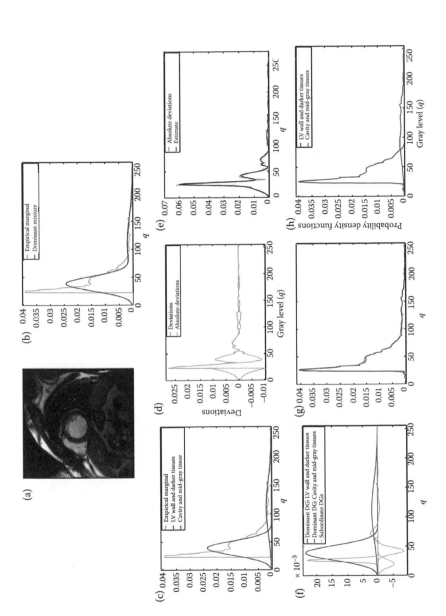

FIGURE 9.13

Typical cine CMRI (a); its empirical marginal with the dominant mixture model (b); the two dominant DGs (c); the sign-alternate and absolute deviations between the empirical and dominant marginals (d); the subordinate mixture model of the absolute deviation (e); the individual LCDG components (f); the final estimated LCDG model of the empirical marginal (g); and the final estimated LCDG models for each intensity class (h).

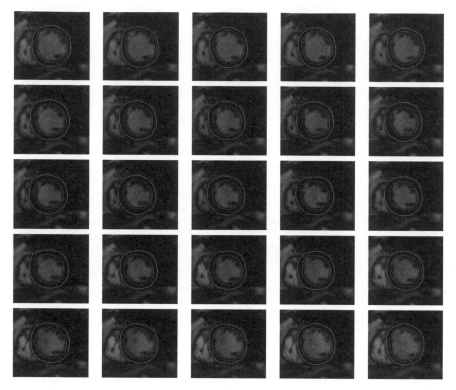

FIGURE 9.14
Inner (red) and outer (cyan) contours segmented on a complete time series reliably determine the actual LV wall borders.

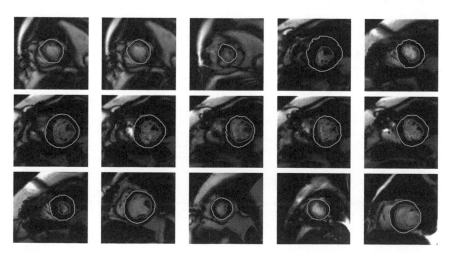

FIGURE 9.15
Segmentation of sine CMRI cross sections for different subjects.

TABLE 9.1

Accuracy of Segmenting the Inner (ILVB) and Outer (OLVB) LV Wall Borders of the Test Data Sets with the I+S+P, I+P, I+S, I, and GLS Algorithms

Algorithm	Dice Similarity (DSC)				Absolute Distance (AD), mm			
	ILVB	*p*-value	OLVB	*p*-value	ILVB	*p*-value	OLVB	*p*-value
I+S+P	0.91 ± 0.08		0.95 ± 0.03		1.4 ± 1.0		1.0 ± 0.5	
I+P	0.89 ± 0.13	$\leq 10^{-4}$	0.93 ± 0.09	$\leq 10^{-4}$	2.6 ± 0.7	$\leq 10^{-4}$	1.2 ± 0.4	$\leq 10^{-4}$
I+S	0.84 ± 0.07	$\leq 10^{-4}$	0.88 ± 0.12	$\leq 10^{-4}$	3.2 ± 1.6	$\leq 10^{-4}$	1.5 ± 0.5	$\leq 10^{-4}$
I	0.81 ± 0.08	$\leq 10^{-4}$	0.75 ± 0.13	$\leq 10^{-4}$	$4.1 + 1.0$	$\leq 10^{-4}$	7.7 ± 6.9	$< 10^{-4}$
GLS	0.78 ± 0.26	$\leq 10^{-4}$	0.85 ± 0.18	$\leq 10^{-4}$	4.4 ± 2.7	$\leq 10^{-4}$	3.9 ± 2.4	$\leq 10^{-4}$

Note: The mean $\pm$ std accuracy of segmenting $2,225$ 2D slices of the 3D images; small *p*-values indicate statistical significance of lower accuracies of other algorithms w.r.t. the I+S+P.

(a) (b) (c) (d) (e)

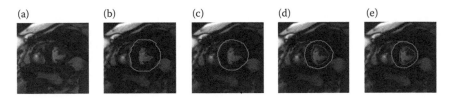

FIGURE 9.16
Image to segment (a) and its segmentation using the I (b), I+S (c), I+P (d), and I+S+P (e) algorithms.

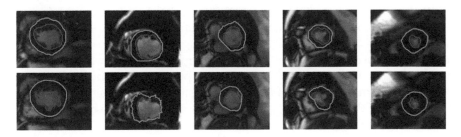

FIGURE 9.17
Comparative results for the inner (red) and outer (cyan) LV borders for the I+S+P (upper row) and shape-guided level-set deformable model (GLS: bottom row) for one image frame and two different sections for the five subjects.

helps to escape these errors, in particular, exclude the papillary muscles, but the accuracy is improved even further after combining all the three models (I+S+P). Figure 9.17, comparing qualitatively the segmentation accuracy on the five test data sets, highlights the I+S+P advantages over one of the most efficient shape-guided level-set based deformable model (GLS) referred to in Section 8.4.

Table 9.1 summarizes the DSC and AD statistics for all the test CMRI and compares the GLS, I, I+S, I+P, and I+S+P algorithms. According to

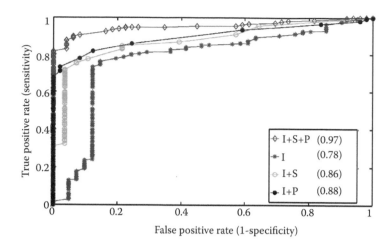

FIGURE 9.18
ROC curves for different combinations of the learned I, S, and P models for the level set guidance: the combined I+S+P (◇); I (∗); I+S (○); and I+P (●) models, the I+S+P resulting in the greatest AUC, 0.97.

its consistently higher DSC and lower AD values, the I+S+P framework performs notably better, than the other algorithms. Their statistically significant differences are confirmed by unpaired t-tests of the DSC and AD values for each algorithm, in particular, the GLS, evidenced by the less than 0.05 p-values. These comparisons highlight advantages of learning the shape prior in addition to the appearance and spatial interaction models.

Robustness of the I+S+P w.r.t. the five other algorithms is validated by its largest AUC in Figure 9.18. A "steep drop" phenomenon in some parts of these curves is due to a big number of true positive (TP) and small number of false positive (FP) points. One "difficult" FP point can affect a relatively large collection of the TP points. In other words, to eliminate a single "difficult" FP point, many TP points have to be eliminated, too, as can be seen in the steep drop in the TP fraction at a FP rate of approximately 0.125 in the red ROC curve.

The I+S+P guidance is not limited to the data collected under the aforementioned scanning protocol. To show this, the algorithm was tested on the cine CMRI data from the MICCAI 2009 Cardiac MR LV Segmentation Challenge against the most accurate in this challenge morphology-based algorithm (see Section 9.4). Comparisons for three subjects with the highest, moderate, and lowest accuracy of the morphological segmentation are presented in Table 9.2.

The segmentation provides clinically useful global LV parameters, such as the end-diastolic (EDV) and end-systolic (ESV) volumes, or the largest and smallest cavity sizes, respectively, and the related global indicator of

TABLE 9.2

Inner (ILVB) and Outer (OLVB) LV Wall Border Accuracy of the I+S+P
and Morphological Algorithms on Three MICCAI 2009 Cardiac MR
LV Segmentation Challenge Data Sets (the Mean ± Std Accuracy)

	DSC		AD, mm	
Algorithm	ILVB	OLVB	ILVB	OLVB
I+S+P	0.91 ± 0.07	0.96 ± 0.02	1.2 ± 1.3	0.9 ± 0.5
Morphological	0.88 ± 0.05	0.94 ± 0.04	2.0 ± 0.6	2.0 ± 1.2

the LV volume variation over time, called the ejection fraction (EF): $EF = \frac{EDV-ESV}{EDV} = 1 - \frac{ESV}{EDV}$. After delineating the cavity contour at each image slice at each time instant (image frame) of the cardiac cycle, a physiological curve showing temporal LV cavity volume changes over the cardiac cycle is constructed to estimate the EF. The total LV volume is produced by numerical integration, which sums contributions of the enclosed areas on the individual image slices using quadratic interpolation (the Simpson's rule). The EDV and ESV, and hence the EF are obtained from the total ventricular functional curve (Figure 9.7).

The Bland-Altman analysis (Section 9.4), which measures the agreement between the EDV, ESV, and EF obtained by the I+S+P segmentation and the ground truth in Figure 9.19, confirms the good accuracy of the estimated global functional indexes, although demonstrates that the ESV is slightly overestimated (the bias of 4.8), whereas the EDV has virtually no bias (-0.01). The systematic overestimation of the ESV might lead to the underestimated EF. Larger variations of the computed ESV vs. EDV relate to a limited accuracy of determining the end-systole time due to the temporal acquisition resolution.

9.3.3 Wall Thickening

After segmenting the inner and outer LV wall borders, their point-to-point correspondences are found via the Laplace-equation-based potential field in order to estimate the wall thickness and thickening. Figure 9.20 illustrates the estimation of the wall thickness from the point-to-point correspondences on the segmented cine images. To derive a pixel-wise color-coded map for visual assessment of the wall thickening (δ) functional parameter, each value δ is normalized by relating it to the maximum value measured in all image sections for the pre- or post-treatments of a given subject. The standard model of myocardial segments is used to assess the estimated (quantified) wall thickening values.

Figure 9.21 presents the δ-parametric maps over multiple image sections and mean wall thickening, $\bar{\delta}$, for each of the 17 heart segments corresponding to these maps in order to show to what extent the 3D GGMRF continuity

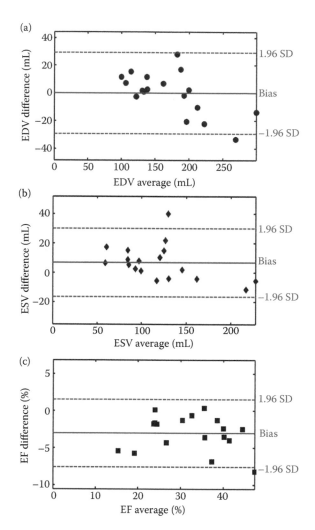

FIGURE 9.19
The Bland-Altman plots for global functional indexes showing the difference between the I+S+P segmentation and the ground truth (*y*-axis) vs. its average (*x*-axis). The 95% confidence intervals (the mean difference ±1.96 × standard deviation) are indicated for the EDV (a), ESV (b), and EF (c).

analysis for the pre- and post-therapy treatment of one test subject smoothes both regional and apex-to-base transitions between the δ-values.

The above efficient and robust cine CMRI analysis combines the accurate level-set-guided deformable model segmentation based on the learned intensity, spatial interactions, and shape prior models with the wall thickness estimation. The latter establishes accurate correspondences between the myocardial borders via a potential field solving the Laplace PDE within the

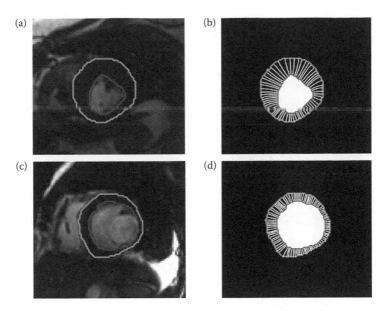

FIGURE 9.20
Inner (red) and outer (cyan) borders of typical cine CMRI at the end-systolic (a) and end-diastolic (c) phases of the cardiac cycle and streamlines of the potential fields for estimating the wall thickness at the end-systolic (b) and end-diastolic (d) phases.

segmented wall. The correspondences allow for estimating both the global and local functional indexes, such as the ESV, EDV, or EF, and the wall thickness changes, or wall thickening for patients undergoing a myoregenerative therapy after heart damage due to heart attacks. Incorporating all the three learned models: the shape prior, the first-order LCDG intensity descriptors, and the second-order spatial interaction descriptors, increases the segmentation accuracy and robustness in terms of various metrics (the ROC curves, DSC, and AD).

9.4 Bibliographic and Historical Notes

Accurate segmentation of the LV wall borders from either noncontrast cine cardiac MRI (CMRI), or contrast-enhanced cardiac MRI ones (CE-CMRI) is an important step toward reliable CAD systems, geometric modeling of the heart, and bio-mechanical modeling for surgical simulations [213]. It is also very useful for reliable assessment of myocardial viability and diagnostics of ischemic heart disease and LV dysfunction [175]. The wall mass, cavity volumes, and global performance indexes, e.g., stroke volume (SV), ESV, EDV, EF, as well as the local performance indexes, such as wall thickening

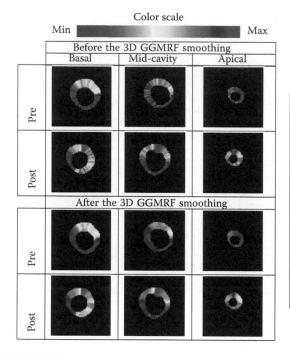

i	Pre	Post	Imp, %
1	5.4	7.1	32.0
2	3.3	4.2	27.0
3	1.4	1.9	29.0
4	2.8	5.9	112.0
5	5.0	5.3	6.0
6	4.6	6.9	50.0
7	4.8	5.6	15.0
8	2.2	2.4	11.0
9	2.2	2.3	4.7
10	1.6	1.7	5.5
11	3.0	3.7	21.0
12	5.8	7.2	24.0
13	3.0	3.9	30.0
14	2.8	3.2	16.0
15	1.7	2.9	65.0
16	3.4	4.5	32.0
17	0.0	0.0	0.0

FIGURE 9.21

Color-coded maps of wall thickness changes for pre- and post-treatment test data before and after the 3D GGMRF smoothing with $\sigma = 1$, $\lambda = 5$, $\beta = 1.01$, $\alpha = 2$, and $b_{s,r} = \sqrt{2}$. The red and blue color scale ends relate to the maximum and minimum thickness, respectively. Average wall thickening, $\bar{\delta}$ (mm), for the 17-segment model (see Section 9.4 is tabulated for the results shown (i: section; Imp,%: improvement).

and strain, are important indicators to quantify the status of cardiac physiology in both health and disease [19]. Because these functional indexes help clinicians to accurately evaluate the heart status, the accurate estimation of basic ventriculometrics calls for precise segmentation of the left ventricle (LV) wall borders from cardiac images. Traditionally, the segmentation of the LV wall borders is performed manually [12,273]. However, it is a prohibitively time-consuming and labor-intensive process, being prone to intra-and inter-observer variations [288].

Segmenting the heart wall from 2D–4D cine CMRI (or CE-CMRI in Chapter 10) is under extensive studies for a long time, but still remains a challenge due to a host of difficulties [276], including large variations in the LV appearance and border shapes from one to another patient and in subsequent images of the same patient. The segmentation is affected by border discontinuities; the lack of strong edges between the epicardium and the surrounding structures, and poor image quality and noise due to patient movement, respiration motion, and artifacts from the moving blood within the ventricular cavity. Also, it is hindered by protrusions of papillary muscle structures into the cavity; partial influence of adjacent structures, such as the diaphragm, and the LV shape deformations and intensity variations at different image slices and within the same slice over the cardiac cycle, and difficulties of separating the inner border from the cavity. This is why the improvement of existing segmentation methods for efficient, robust, and accurate assessment of cardiac images remains of considerable interest.

Most successful approaches for delineating the LV wall borders have addressed these challenges by combining current and prior information about the heart, i.e., by modeling visual appearance and shape of the target objects, using, in particular, active appearance models (AAMs), active shape models (ASMs) and other models, outlined in brief in Chapter 10, Section 10.5. The shape-prior-based segmentation by the level-set guided deformable boundary (the GLS; see Section 8.4) in Reference 289 employs a linear combination of the signed training distance maps as a shape prior of the heart. Also, the LV wall borders were segmented automatically by combining the Gaussian mixtures of signals and evolving deformable boundaries, which are guided by the Dijkstra's optimal path search [153]; clustering and cardiac anatomy knowledge [192]; circular Hough transform [238]; binary classification to segment a blood pool within a predefined region-of-interest (ROI) [60]; prior knowledge of temporal myocardium deformations, which is incorporated into the level-set guidance [194], etc. The endocardium and epicardium were separately segmented in Reference 63 using discrete mathematical morphology and spatiotemporal watershed transforms.

Variational CMRI segmentation incorporates shape statistics and an edge image [54] or uses an explicit geometric deformable boundary [75], such that one coordinate of every its point depends functionally on the other coordinate, to notably decrease the computational complexity. To preserve smoothness and topological flexibility, this boundary was re-defined in Reference 14 in B-spline terms allowing for local and global regional energy terms. To evolve two fronts representing the epicardium and endocardium LV boundaries, a coupled level-set based LV segmentation in Reference 193 builds a prior from the training samples and combines both the gradient and areal data using a special coupling function. An anatomical heart atlas can be also used as a prior to constrain the image alignment and propagate labels from the atlas to the co-aligned CMRI for segmenting the ventricles.

A parametric shape model was optimized for semi-automated segmentation in Reference 290 by applying dynamic programming (DP). To delineate the myocardial borders on CMRI, a semi-automated version of the GVF-guided active contour in Reference 55 incorporates an adaptive parametric shape prior and a nonparametric background intensity model. A hybrid segmentation in Reference 176 extracted the myocardium, LV blood pool, and other adjacent structures, e.g., lungs and liver, by integrating intensity and texture descriptors and DP-based boundary detection. Bi-directional coupled parametric deformable models were introduced in Reference 276 to extract the LV wall borders using the first- and second-order visual appearance features and eventually estimate global cardiac performance indexes. In order to preserve the heart topology, a coupling factor preventing the overlap between the inner and outer borders of the LV wall was employed. A more comprehensive review of the current cardiac image segmentation techniques can be found in Reference 241.

The *wall thickness* is essential to diagnose and characterize many heart diseases, and the local *wall thickening* index, defined as changes of the wall thickness during the systole of the cardiac cycle, indicates myocardium dysfunction more accurately than the wall motion analysis [9,143,260,269]. The quantitative wall thickness measurements in CMRI are widely used in research and clinical applications to assess, e.g., the wall stress, motion, and thickening. Routinely, the wall thickness is assessed by visual inspection, being clinically preferred for practical purposes [248]. However, this process is obviously time-consuming and prone to considerable intra- and inter-observer deviations [22,111,143]. To overcome these drawbacks, local myocardial wall thickness is derived, automatically or semiautomatically, after tracing the endocardial and epicardial boundaries in all short-axis images.

The radial wall thickness and thickening estimation [220] draws a fixed number of radial lines from an approximate center of the blood pool and uses their intersections with the inner and outer borders of the heart wall. However, this intuitive method may overestimate the wall thickness if the LV cross section deviates much from a circular shape [111]. The most well-known and more accurate centerline method estimates the myocardium thickness by placing and measuring a fixed number of perpendicular chords along the computed centerline of the heart wall. Such frameworks in References 38,254 and 269 essentially required manual contouring of the LV borders. A similar measurement on a per-section basis [50] proposed in Reference 159 estimated the LV wall thickness at the end-diastolic phase only. Although the centerline method does not depend on the chosen centroid or coordinate system, like the radial method [259], inner and outer contour imperfections and image noise greatly affect its accuracy. To overcome these limitations, the myocardial thickening in CMRI was measured more reliably after establishing point-to-point correspondences between the inner and outer borders via a potential field obtained by solving a partial differential Laplace equation [247]. However, to reduce effects of segmentation errors in the wall thickness estimation, a further manual adjustment was performed by a clinical expert.

The second-order linear *Laplace PDE*:

$$\nabla^2\gamma \equiv \frac{\partial^2\gamma}{\partial x^2} + \frac{\partial^2\gamma}{\partial y^2} = 0 \tag{9.6}$$

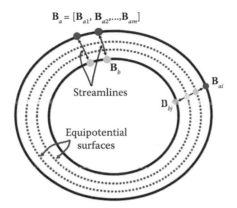

FIGURE 9.22
Point-to-point correspondences via potential field $\gamma(x, y)$ between equipotential boundaries, $\mathbf{B}_a$ and $\mathbf{B}_b$: streamlines that connect corresponding points at the boundaries are orthogonal to the boundaries and all the intermediate equipotential contours (dashed lines).

specifying a potential field $\gamma(x, y)$ between given boundaries in the (x, y)-plane, arises in various scientific and engineering applications, from electromagnetic theory to probability theory. In medical imaging applications, it has been used for colon surface flattening [130], thickness measurements [154,247], and nonrigid image alignment [163,164].

Generally, let the Laplace PDE be solved between two boundaries, such as $\mathbf{B}_a$ and $\mathbf{B}_b$ in Figure 9.22, given that all points along each boundary have the same potential, which differs for each boundary, e.g., $\gamma_a > \gamma_b = 0$. Then the obtained potential field results in intermediate equipotential contours with the potentials $\gamma(x, y) = \gamma_c$; $\gamma_a > \gamma_c > \gamma_b = 0$, e.g., the dashed lines in Figure 9.22. A streamline of the field is orthogonal to all the equipotential contours, which this line crosses, i.e., in each point the streamline is moving along the gradient of the field. The streamlines connect the boundaries and provide the desired point-to-point correspondences, such as the corresponding points $\mathbf{B}_{ai}$ and $\mathbf{B}_{bj}$ in Figure 9.22.

The generalized Gauss-Markov random field (GGMRF) of measurements $\varepsilon = (\varepsilon_\mathbf{r} : \mathbf{r} \in \mathbb{R})$, which allows for the computationally simple maximum *a posteriori* (MAP) estimates of parameters, was introduced in Reference 33. The log-likelihood of a sample ε up to a constant term is

$$\log P(\varepsilon) = -\gamma^\beta \left(\sum_{\mathbf{r} \in \mathbb{R}} a_\mathbf{r} |\varepsilon_\mathbf{r}|^\beta + \sum_{\mathbf{s} \in \mathbb{N}_\mathbf{r}} b_{(\mathbf{r}, \mathbf{s})} |\varepsilon_\mathbf{r} - \varepsilon_\mathbf{s}|^\beta \right)$$

where $1 \leq \beta \leq 2$; the factor γ is inversely proportional to the scale of the measurements ε, and the set $\mathbb{N}_\mathbf{r} \subseteq \mathbb{R}$ specifies the neighborhood of the lattice site, such as, e.g., a moving fixed-size window. The GGMRF with $\beta = 2$ is the usual Gauss-Markov, or SAR model. The closer the value β to 1, the

(b)

(a)

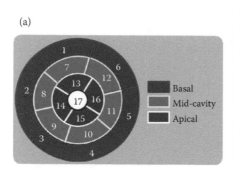

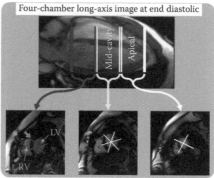

FIGURE 9.23
The myocardial 17-segment model [50]: (a) its circumferential polar plot and (b) locations of segments for the basal (left), mid-cavity (middle), and apical (right) image sections. The segment numbering starts counter-clockwise from the anatomical landmark indicated by the green arrow in the basal section.

less smooth the most probable samples. The iterative conditional modes (ICM) search for a local energy minimum for the GGMRF was introduced in Reference 25.

The *MICCAI 2009 Cardiac MR LV Segmentation Challenge*, including the data sets, scanning protocol, and evaluation criterion, is fully described in Reference 249. The *morphology-based* segmentation in Reference 190 had the highest accuracy among all the tested frameworks.

The statistical *Bland-Altman analysis* [31] assesses the degree of agreement between two clinical methods measuring (estimating) some scalar property for a number of subjects. Each pair of measurements, $(\mu_{1:i};\ \mu_{2:i})$, for the same subject i; $i = 1,\ldots,n$, is placed to the (x,y)-plane in accord with their difference, $y_i = \mu_{1:i} - \mu_{2:i}$, and average, $x_i = \frac{1}{2}(\mu_{1:i} + \mu_{2:i})$. The methods are in good agreement if their bias, i.e., the mean difference, $b = \frac{1}{n}\sum_{i=1}^{n} y_i$, is close to zero and all the points, $\{(x_i, y_i) : i = 1,\ldots,n\}$, deviate within the 95% limits around the bias, i.e., within the horizontal band between the lines $y = b \pm 1.96\sigma$ where $\sigma = \sqrt{\frac{1}{n-1}\sum_{i=1}^{n}(y_i - b)^2}$ is the standard deviation of the differences.

The *standard myocardial segments model* [50] divides the LV wall into 17 circumferential segments (Figure 9.23): six segments each at the basal and mid-cavity levels, four segments at the apical level, and one at the apex (the extreme ventricle tip).

10

Sizing Cardiac Pathologies

Modeling visual appearance on a CE-CMRI with a joint second-order MGRF offers the prospect of automatic myocardial wall assessment to identify pathological tissues in a segmented LV. The late CE-CMRI (Figure 10.1) makes it possible to estimate with high spatial resolution the transmural extent of a damaged myocardium to delineate the pathological tissue and extract useful metrics for indexing the myocardial injury. The percentage of the segmented pathological tissue with respect to the total area of the myocardial wall and the transmural extent of this tissue relative to the full LV wall thickness are two candidate metrics to quantify the myocardial viability. Section 10.5 overviews in brief some current methods to estimate the area and transmural extent of pathology.

To assist the cardiologists in diagnosing the LV dysfunction and ischemic heart disease, it is important to accurately delineate the pathological tissue area within the LV wall from the adjacent undamaged tissue and reliably measure this area (Figure 10.1), despite its identification is a challenge due to image noise, limited resolution, and imprecise boundaries. In principle, the pathological tissue can be outlined manually in order to determine its area, but such a process is time-consuming and operator-dependent. Automated or semi-automated assessment of myocardial viability can be a help in circumventing these shortcomings.

The identified LV wall pathologies are quantified by measuring the transmural extent, or *transmurality*, being a fraction of the pathological tissue, which extends across the myocardial wall (Figure 10.2). However, assessing and quantifying the LV dysfunction meets with considerable problems caused by large inter-subject and temporal variations of image intensities across the goal pathologies and their backgrounds that affect the accuracy and reliability of the segmented LV walls. Parametric shape priors often become unsuitable due to a small number of distinct cardiac landmarks, and deformable models with inadequate appearance and shape priors typically fail under excessive image noise, poor resolution, diffuse boundaries, and/or occluded shapes. Current automated sizing of a pathological area of the LV wall is also quite sensitive to imperfect myocardium borders and image noise if spatial signal dependencies between the myocardium are not adequately taken into account.

An automated framework for analyzing the CE-CMRI (Figure 10.3) overcomes in part these drawbacks by employing and learning stochastic models for both the myocardium segmentation at Step 1 and the damaged

233

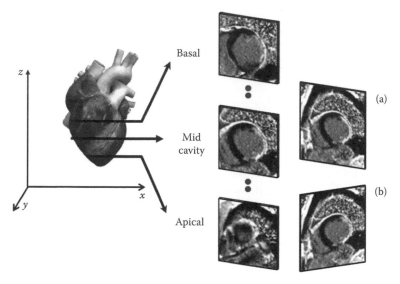

FIGURE 10.1
Basal, mid-cavity, and apical CE-CMRI cross sections and the yellow-highlighted pathological area (a) of the heart image (b).

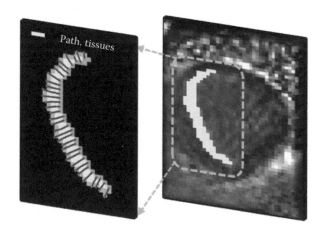

FIGURE 10.2
Transmurality of a pathological tissue in the LV wall: the CE-CMRI (right) with the yellow-highlighted pathological area and the enlarged pathology (left), its extent being shown by blue lines connecting its edges.

myocardial tissues identification and quantification at Steps 2 and 3. The accurate inner and outer LV wall borders are found by an efficient graph-cut based search for the (approximately) global energy minimum for a joint MGRF model of visual appearance and shape of the inner LV cavity. The like model was already detailed in Section 9.1. A joint MGRF model of visual

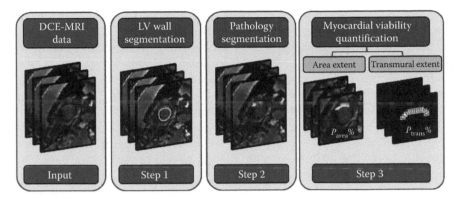

FIGURE 10.3
CE-CMRI analysis: The LV wall segmentation, pathology identification, and myocardial viability quantification by measuring the area extent and transmurality.

appearance and spatial interactions in the LV wall image is also learned to delineate the pathological tissue.

To estimate the transmural extent in a geometrically consistent way and overcome shortcomings of the more conventional radial and centerline methods, corresponding points at the inner and outer borders to measure the pathology are co-located in this framework, just as in Chapter 9, by streamlines of a potential field solving the Laplace PDE (Figure 10.4).

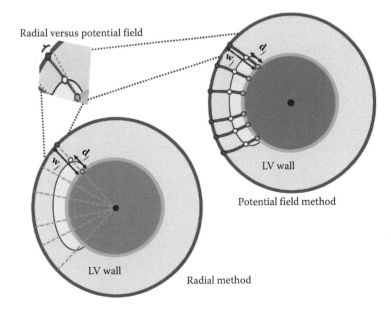

FIGURE 10.4
Deviations between the corresponding pixel pairs for radial and potential-field based transmurality estimates for a pathological LV wall tissue.

After determining segments of the pathological tissue along each stream-line, the transmural extent is estimated by the average extent of the patholog-ical tissue relative to the streamlines. Contrastingly, the radial method draws a fixed number of radial lines from the inner to the outer LV border, as illus-trated in Figure 10.4. The alternative centerline method finds a centerline between the inner and outer borders of the LV wall and draws a fixed num-ber of perpendiculars to the centerline toward each border. In all the cases the transmural extent is defined after identifying the pathological tissue along each line connecting the borders as the average pathological tissue's extent relative to these lines. However, both the radial and centerline transmurality estimates suffer from geometrically inconsistent correspondences between the inner and outer LV borders, especially, for noisy images with imperfect LV borders.

10.1 LV Wall Segmentation

Segmenting the inner cavity from the surrounding tissue is a challenge due to dynamic heart motions and image artifacts from blood circulation within the ventricular cavity. To account for these difficulties, the Bayesian MAP decision leading to a graph-cut based global energy minimization separates the inner LV cavity on a given CE-CMRI, which is modeled with a joint rotation-invariant MGRF of images and their "object–background" region maps. The model combines the first-order visual appearance descriptors (the estimated LCDGs approximating ongoing object and background sig-nal marginals) and the second-order spatial object–background homogeneity descriptors (the estimated Gibbs energy for the region map) with the learned probabilistic cavity shape prior. Then the outer LV border is segmented with a deformable boundary, which starts from the inner border and evolves as a solution of an eikonal PDE with a speed function depending on the learned shape prior and ongoing visual appearance of an outlined part of the wall.

After being co-aligned to the shape prior $P_{sp}(\mathbf{m})$, the image $\mathbf{g}$ and its region map $\mathbf{m}$ are considered a sample with the joint MGRF of Equation 9.1:

$$P(\mathbf{g}, \mathbf{m}) = P(\mathbf{g} \mid \mathbf{m}) \underbrace{P_V(\mathbf{m}) P_{sp}(\mathbf{m})}_{P(\mathbf{m})}$$

with the conditional IRF, $P(\mathbf{g} \mid \mathbf{m})$, of image signals (intensities), given the region map, and the unconditional MGRF of the evolving maps, $P(\mathbf{m})$. The map model, $P(\mathbf{m})$, contains a subject-specific spatially inhomogeneous IRF

Algorithm 14 Learning Shape Priors

---

1. Co-align a set of training CE-CMRI by rigid affine transformation maximizing their mutual information (MI).
2. Manually segment the object (inner cavity) from the aligned training set.
3. Estimate the pixel-wise empirical object–background probabilities $\{F_\mathbf{r}(\lambda) : \lambda \in \mathbb{L} = \{\mathsf{ob}, \mathsf{bg}\}; \sum_{\lambda \in \mathbb{L}} F_\mathbf{r}(\lambda) = 1; \mathbf{r} \in \mathbb{R}\}$ by counting how many times each pixel $\mathbf{r}$ is in the segmented object.

---

of region labels $P_{\mathrm{sp}}(\mathbf{m})$ as the shape prior and a second-order spatially invariant MGRF $P_\mathbf{V}(\mathbf{m})$ describing an evolving map $\mathbf{m}$.

The inner cavity shape prior $P_{\mathrm{sp}}(\mathbf{m})$ is learned from a set of co-aligned training CE-CMRI:

$$P_{\mathrm{sp}}(\mathbf{m}) = \prod_{\mathbf{r} \in \mathbb{R}} F_\mathbf{r}(m(\mathbf{r}))$$

where $F_\mathbf{r}(l)$; $l \in \mathbb{L} = \{\mathsf{ob}, \mathsf{bg}\}$, is the empirical probability that the pixel $\mathbf{r}$ belongs to the object (inner cavity) in the co-aligned training maps. The framework in Figure 10.3 employs three pre-learned shape priors, namely, for the basal, mid-ventricular, and apical levels, learned in line with Algorithm 14 (this process is illustrated in Figures 10.5 and 10.6).

To begin the inner cardiac cavity segmentation, every given CE-CMRI is aligned to a reference image, preselected from the training set (Figure 10.7). The prior pixel-wise object (ob) and background (bg) probabilities, together with the object–background signal marginals from the conditional IRF model $P(\mathbf{g} \mid \mathbf{m})$, estimated for the given CE-CMRI, are used to build an initial region map. After estimating the second-order spatial interactions in the MGRF region map model, $P_\mathbf{V}(\mathbf{m})$, from the initial map, the graph-cut based global energy minimization for the estimated joint MGRF of the CE-CMRI and region maps provides the final segmentation map.

For simplicity, the region maps are modeled here using the simple auto-binomial, or Potts MGRF with the nearest 8-neighborhood and translation/rotation-invariant potentials. The latter depend on the intra- or inter-region position of each pixel pair (i.e., whether the labels are equal or not); inter-pixel distances (1 and $\sqrt{2}$) in each pair, but not on their relative orientations. The 8-neighborhood has two types of spatially symmetric pairwise interactions: (1) the closest neighbors with the coordinate offsets $\mathbb{N}_1 = \{(\pm 1, 0), (0, \pm 1)\}$ and unit inter-pixel distance and (2) the diagonal neighbors with the offsets $\mathbf{N}_{\sqrt{2}} = \{(1, \pm 1), (-1, \pm 1)\}$ and inter-pixel distance $\sqrt{2}$. The bi-valued potentials of each type account only for the label coincidence: $\mathbf{V}_a = \{V_{a,\mathrm{eq}}; V_{a,\mathrm{ne}}\}$ where $V_{a,\mathrm{eq}} = V_a(l, l)$ and $V_{a,\mathrm{ne}} = -V_a(l, k)$

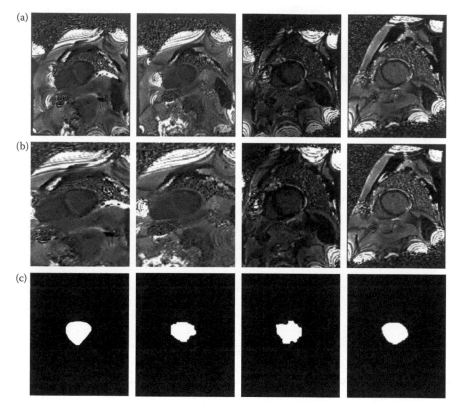

FIGURE 10.5
Learning the inner cavity shape prior at mid-ventricular level: (a) training samples, (b) MI-based affine alignment, and (c) manual segmentation.

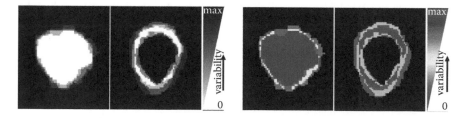

FIGURE 10.6
Gray- (left) and color-coded (right) inner cavity and LV wall shape priors.

if $l \neq k; l, k \in \mathbb{L} = \{\text{ob}, \text{bg}\}$, and $a \in \mathbf{A} = \{1, \sqrt{2}\}$. For a given training map, $\mathbf{m}$, this auto-binomial model has the approximate analytical MLE $V_{a,\text{eq}} = -V_{a,\text{ne}} = 1 - 2F_{a,\text{eq}}(\mathbf{m})$ of the potentials (Chapter 4) where $F_{a,\text{eq}}(\mathbf{m})$ is the empirical probability of the equal label pairs in all the equivalent pixel pairs

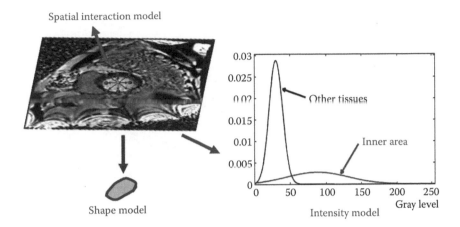

FIGURE 10.7
Aligning a joint MGRF model to the shape prior.

$\{((x,y),(x+\xi,y+\eta)):\ (x,y)\in \mathbf{R};\ (x+\xi,y+\eta)\in \mathbf{R};\ (\xi,\eta)\in \mathbf{N}_a\}$, of the training map.

The conditional LCDG models of the object (inner cavity) and background image signals are built as in Chapter 3, by assuming the two dominant modes (the cavity and its background). After the joint MGRF model of the CE-CMRI is learned, the inner cavity in a given image $\mathbf{g}$ is segmented by the Bayesian MAP decision. The goal region map with the maximum joint probability, i.e., the minimum joint energy among all region maps sampled from the model: $\mathbf{m}^* = \arg\min_{\mathbf{m}\in \mathbb{M}} E(\mathbf{m},\mathbf{g})$ where

$$E(\mathbf{m}) = -\Big(\log(P(\mathbf{g}\,|\,\mathbf{m})) + \log(P_V(\mathbf{m})) + \log(P_{sp}(\mathbf{m}))\Big)$$

is built by the efficient min-cut/max-flow optimization with positive edge weights. The corresponding two-terminal graph in Figure 10.8 contains terminal links accounting for the pixel-wise descriptors (conditional first-order LCDG appearance models of the CE-CMRI and the inner cavity shape prior), i.e., $-\log(P(g(\mathbf{r})\,|\,m(\mathbf{r})) - \log(F_{\mathbf{r}}(m(\mathbf{r})))$. The lattice-wide links between the neighbors support the potentials quantifying spatially invariant interactions between the region labels, i.e., $-\log(P_V(\mathbf{m}))$.

Segmenting the outer LV border is also a challenge due to image inhomogeneity and lack of the edges of the LV wall. To suppress these problems, the outer border of the LV wall is extracted by a robust wave propagation (Figure 10.9). A wave is emitted orthogonally from the inner border ($t = 0$) towards the external border of the LV wall. Every point on the emitted wave is classified to be the wall or the background based on the three probabilistic models, which are similar to the above inner wall models: the LV wall shape prior (Figure 10.6), the first-order LCDG model of visual appearance of the

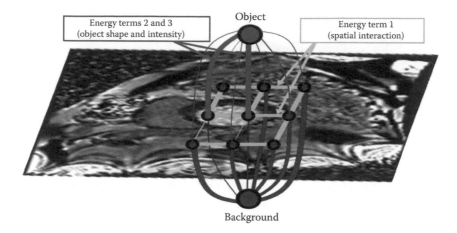

FIGURE 10.8
Two-terminal graph to be cut for segmenting the CE-CMRI: Blue and red terminal links for the pixel-wise descriptors (visual appearance and inner cavity shape prior), and orange lattice-wide links between the neighboring sites (interaction potentials). The thicker the links, the higher the affinity between the sites or terminals.

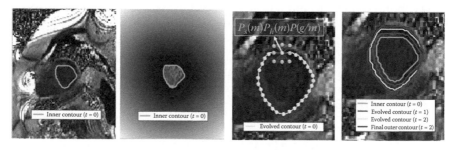

FIGURE 10.9
Segmenting the outer border: From left to right—an inner LV wall border at time $t = 0$; gray-coded normalized minimum Euclidian distances between every point in the outer area of the LV inner cavity and the LV inner border; the evolving wave at time $t = 2$ where every point is associated to the wall or background, and samples of the waves propagated from the inner LV border at different time instants; the red wave is the final segmented outer border.

LV wall, and the second-order Potts model of spatially homogeneous region label interactions. The models are learned using the same methodologies as in the inner border segmentation. Algorithm 15 to segment the outer LV wall border is based on solving the eikonal equation:

$$|\nabla t(x,y)|\Xi(x,y) = 1 \qquad (10.1)$$

where $t(x,y)$ is the time at which the wave front crosses the point (x,y) and $\Xi(x,y)$ is the known speed function. The segmentation process is illustrated

---

Algorithm 15 Segmentation of the Outer LV Wall Border

---

1. Find the inner LV wall border.

2. Find the normalized minimum Euclidian distance $d(\mathbf{r})$ between every point $\mathbf{r} = (x, y)$ in the outer area of the LV inner cavity and the inner LV border by solving Equation 10.1 with the unit speed function $\Theta(x, y) = 1$.

3. Iteratively repeat Steps 3a and 3b until no change in the position of the evolving wave.

   a. Propagate an orthogonal wave from the inner LV border by solving Equation 10.1 with the speed function $\Xi(x, y) = \exp(-\beta d(x, y))$, where the constant β controls the wave evolution ($\beta < 1$ to make the evolution smooth).

   b. Associate every point on the emitted wave with the wall or background using the Bayesian classifier based on the learned three probabilistic models.

4. Terminate and output the final wave as the segmented outer LV contour.

---

in Figure 10.9. Fast marching level sets are used to solve Equation 10.1 numerically and find the evolving wave.

10.2 Identifying the Pathological Tissue

A joint MGRF combining the first-order appearance model, $P(\mathbf{g} \mid \mathbf{m})$, and the second-order spatial homogeneity model, $P_V(\mathbf{m})$, is used also to identify (segment) a pathological LV wall tissue. Comparing to conventional signal comparisons to heuristic or user-selected thresholds, a more adequate initial segmentation threshold is found automatically by the LCDG modeling (Chapter 3) of the object and background signal marginals. This initial "object–background" map of the pathologies is refined then by learning its most likely second-order MGRF model and searching for a local minimum of the joint image-map energy with the ICM. At each step, the ICM sequentially traces the lattice and minimizes each conditional site-wise energy, given the fixed other sites, and the tracing is repeated until the total energy is not decreasing anymore.

Both the models of pathological and other (background) tissues in the LV wall are estimated just as before, using the methodologies of Chapters 3 and 4, respectively. Algorithm 16 outlines the whole process of the pathological tissue identification.

Algorithm 16 Segmenting Pathological Tissues of the Heart

---

1. Learn the LCDG models of pathological tissue and background marginals to describe visual appearance of the bounded myocardial wall at each CE-CMRI (Chapter 3).

2. Use the learned models to initially segment the pathological tissue, i.e., form its initial region map.

3. Learn the MGRF of the region maps to specify the Gibbs energy of the image and its region map.

4. Find with the ICM the final pathological tissue map corresponding to a local energy minimum.

10.3 Quantifying the Myocardial Viability

The accurately segmented pathological tissues allow for deriving two quantitative metrics: the spatial extent, or area of the pathological tissue and the transmural extent, or transmurality—which have been previously explored as potentially useful indexes of myocardial viability. The *percentage area of the pathological tissue*, $\text{Perc}_{\text{area}}(\text{Segment } i)$, is estimated, as shown in Figure 10.10, for each segment i; $i \in \{1, \ldots, 17\}$, in the 17-segment model of the myocardium wall in Figure 9.23:

$$\text{Perc}_{\text{area}}(\text{Segment } i) = \frac{\text{Area } A_i \text{ of pathological tissue in Segment } i}{\text{Area } B_i \text{ of Segment } i} \times 100\%$$

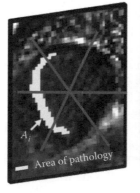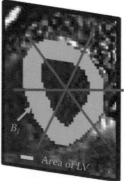

FIGURE 10.10
Estimating the percentage area, $\text{Perc}_{\text{area}}(\text{Segment } i)$ of myocardial injury; A_i and B_i denote the injury and total area of Segment i, respectively.

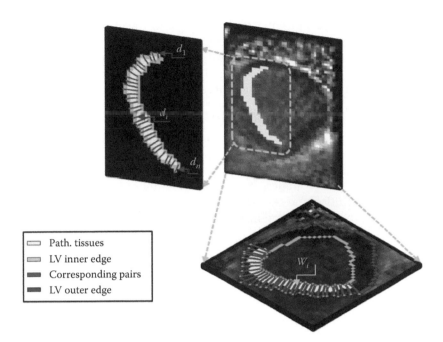

FIGURE 10.11
Estimating the transmural extent of myocardial injury: The identified pathological LV wall tissue (top right) with enlarged inter-border correspondences for the LV wall (bottom right: $W_j \equiv \text{Thickness}_j$) and the pathological tissue (top left: $d_j \equiv \text{Extent}_j$).

The *transmural extent of the pathological tissue*, $\text{Perc}_{\text{trans}}(\text{Segment } i)$, for each segment i is the average ratio between the pathology extent, Extent_j, and the wall thickness, Thickness_j; $j = 1, \ldots, n$, along the lines connecting all n pairs of the corresponding points on the borders of Segment i. These point-to-point correspondences for both the pathological tissue and the LV wall are found via the potential fields formed by solving the Laplace PDE (Figure 10.11) between the borders.

$$\text{Perc}_{\text{trans}}(\text{Segment } i) = \left(\frac{1}{n} \sum_{j=1}^{n} \frac{\text{Extent}_j}{\text{Thickness}_j} \right) \times 100\%$$

10.4 Performance Evaluation and Validation

To evaluate the framework, 14 datasets were collected from six patients by a Siemens 1.5T Espree MRI system (Siemens Medical Solutions, USA), with multichannel phased array reception coils, using late (at 15–25 min) gadolinium contrast agent enhanced (0.2 mM/kg) acquisitions (both conventional inversion time ones and phase sensitive inversion recovery). The patients had chronic heart attacks (at least 4 months before the tests) with clinically documented EF dysfunction and subsequently underwent an experimental myocardial regeneration therapy, as part of an institutionally approved trial. To ensure adequate signal-to-noise ratios, the typical spatial resolution was $2.08 \times 2.08 \times 8.0\,\text{mm}^3$. Typically, from 10 to 14 cross sections were acquired to cover the LV, and in total 168 images were examined.

To evaluate the segmentation accuracy and compare the automatically estimated infarcted tissue volumes, i.e., the total number of pathological voxels scaled by the resolution and slice thickness, to the ground truth, two experts-radiologists delineated the true inner and outer LV wall borders, as well as the pathological tissues in each image.

10.4.1 Segmentation Accuracy

The segmentation has been tested on five data sets of 2D CE-CMRI, consisting each of 11 cross sections over the LV (55 images in total). Figure 10.12 illustrates the automated LV wall segmentation in Section 10.1, and Table 10.1 compares the DSC of the segmented borders on all the 55 images to the known ground truth with the like DSC for the efficient shape prior guided level-set deformable model abbreviated GLS and described briefly in Section 8.4. Differences between the DSC for the GLS and the algorithm in Section 10.1 are statistically significant: their two-tailed p-values for the found inner and outer borders are less than or equal to 0.0001 and 0.003, respectively.

These results suggest that the framework precisely segments the LV walls on the CE-CMR images in the presence of complex shape variations. Thus, it could be suitable for segmenting other noisy and inhomogeneous anatomical structures that can be represented with the like probabilistic shape priors.

10.4.2 Transmural Extent Accuracy

Establishing the potential-field, radial, and centerline correspondences between the LV wall borders to estimate the transmural extent is evaluated on realistic elliptically symmetric synthetic phantoms with varying transmural injury extent that mimic a cross section of the heart. The infarct thickness is considered uniform to make numerical evaluations practicable, and the different thicknesses from 2 to 10 mm are taken into account to cover physiologically meaningful ranges of the pathological transmural extent: namely, small, intermediate, and large infarcts, which occupy less than 25%, 25 to 50%, and more than 50% of the wall. The wall thickness of 12 mm and an inner LV wall border from an actual patient's image

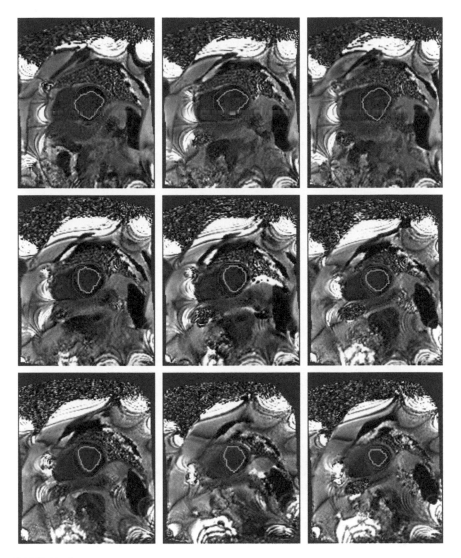

FIGURE 10.12
Inner and outer borders segmented on the CE-CMRI of one subject.

simulate a realistic heart wall size, as well as the in-plane spatial resolution of 1×1 mm^2 provides sufficient for the analysis numbers of pixels across the wall (Figure 10.13).

Figure 10.14 demonstrates how the point-to-point correspondences are established along radial lines from the center of the LV inner cavity, or along perpendiculars to the centerline, which joins midpoints of straight lines connecting the known corresponding border points, or along streamlines of the potential field between the equipotential inner and outer borders. In all the

TABLE 10.1

DSC Between the Segmentation of Section 10.1 (S10.1)
and the Ground Truth in Comparison to the GLS

DSC	Inner		Outer	
	S10.1	GLS	S10.1	GLS
Minimum	0.85	0.75	0.80	0.34
Maximum	0.99	0.93	0.96	0.91
Mean	0.94	0.83	0.92	0.81
St. dev.	0.05	0.06	0.05	0.16
p-value		<0.0001		0.003

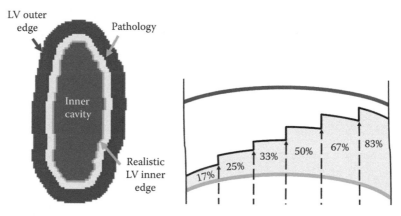

FIGURE 10.13
Simulated phantom (a) with elliptical symmetry and uniform infarct thickness, which may vary from 17% to 83% (b) to represent the small, intermediate, and large infarcts by two thicknesses per each range of the transmural extent.

cases, the total transmural extent estimate is the average of all the line-wise estimates.

Table 10.2 summarizes the estimation accuracies for the small ($\rho \leq 25\%$), intermediate ($25 < \rho \leq 50\%$, and large ($\rho > 50\%$ of the wall) actual transmural infarct sizes (Figure 10.13). The transmural extent estimates via the potential-field streamlines are much closer to the known actual sizes than their radial and centerline counterparts. Differences between the latter and former estimates are statistically significant according to the unpaired *t*-test: the two-tailed *p*-values are below 0.0001 across all the infarct ranges.

The large relative errors of the radial and centerline estimates decrease monotonously with the increasing transmural extent. Contrastingly, the potential-field estimates have much smaller relative errors decreasing fast from their largest value of 2.3% for the smallest transmural infarct and remaining then approximately flat (0.7%–0.05%) for all other pathology sizes.

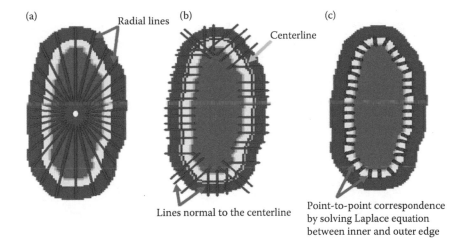

FIGURE 10.14
Radial (a), centerline (b), and potential-field (c) correspondences for estimating the transmural extent on a simulated phantom.

TABLE 10.2

Estimates of the Transmural Extent for the Radial, Centerline, and Potential-Field Correspondences on a Simulated Phantom with Different Actual Infarct Sizes

Actual Size	Estimate, mm: error, %		
mm: relative*	Potential-Field	Radial	Centerline
2: 0.17	2.0: 2.3%	2.5: 25%	2.1: 6.3%
3: 0.25	3.0: 0.5%	3.7: 24%	3.2: 6.6%
4: 0.33	4.0: 0.7%	4.9: 22%	4.3: 6.2%
6: 0.50	6.0: 0.4%	7.3: 21%	6.3: 5.1%
8: 0.66	8.0: 0.2%	9.5: 19%	8.3: 4.3%
10: 0.83	10.0: 0.05%	11.9: 19%	10.4: 4.2%

* Relative sizes w.r.t. the simulated 12-mm wall.

Such a behavior can be explained, in part, by their small absolute errors (about or less than 0.05 mm) for all the values examined, which are of importance mainly for the very small transmural infarcts. Thus the correspondence estimation via streamlines of a potential field solving the Laplace PDE outperforms the radial or centerline estimates in the full range of the infract sizes.

10.4.3 Pathology Delineation Accuracy

Typical pathology identification in comparison to the manual ground truth is shown in Figure 10.15, and Table 10.3 presents the DSC between

Original data   Ground truth pathology   Estimation

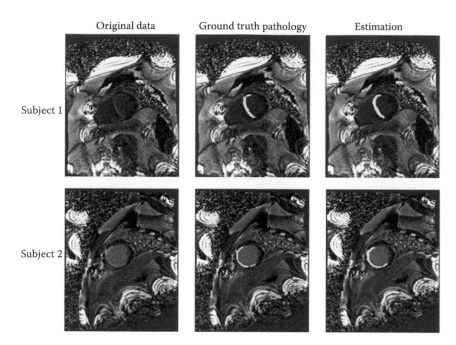

Subject 1

Subject 2

FIGURE 10.15
Automated pathology estimation w.r.t. the ground truth for two subjects.

TABLE 10.3

DSC of the Automated Pathology Estimation on the 14 Datasets (168
Images) with the Described Framework and the 2σ- or 3σ-Thresholding
w.r.t. the Ground Truth (GT) from the Two Experts: GT1 and GT2

	Framework		M01: 2σ-Threshold		M02: 3σ-Threshold	
GT	GT1	GT2	GT1	GT2	GT1	GT2
DSC mean	0.90	0.88	0.73	0.76	0.52	0.61
DSC st. dev.	0.06	0.06	0.09	0.08	0.11	0.16
p-value versus framework:			$<10^{-4}$	$<10^{-4}$	$<10^{-4}$	$<10^{-4}$

the automatically and manually segmented pathological tissue. Both the
segmentations closely agree in line with the paired t-test for each of the
two experts (p-value of 0.487). In addition, the Bland-Altman analysis
shows a good agreement between the estimated infarct volumes and their
manual ground truth from the two independent experts (i.e., almost zero
bias and most of the data points within the 95% confidence band in Figure 10.16). Both the DSC and Bland-Altman analyses confirm the robustness
and reproducibility of the described automated framework.

In addition, as evidenced by its close to the ideal unit value DSC with
the smallest standard deviation in Table 10.3, the framework outperforms in

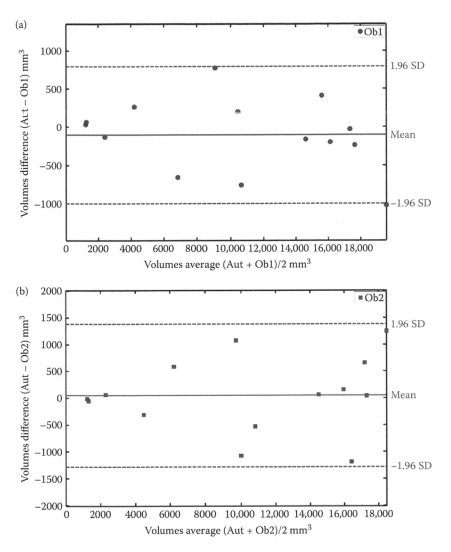

FIGURE 10.16
Bland-Altman plots for the 14 datasets: The automatically estimated (Aut) clinical infarct volume vs. the ground truth for the two experts, Ob1 and Ob2.

a statistically significant way two more conventional techniques of pathology identification by 2σ- (M01) and 3σ-thresholding (M02) (see Section 10.5, Table 10.6).

10.4.4 Clinically Meaningful Effects

The damaged tissue detection and quantification have been explored in application to indexing clinically meaningful changes. Figure 10.17

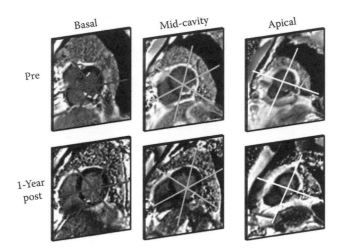

FIGURE 10.17
Changes in the injured myocardium estimated for one patient one year after the treatment.

illustrates changes of the injured myocardium, evaluated with the above framework for one typical patient over one year after the treatment. Both the extracted parameters quantifying the myocardium viability of the patient are given in Tables 10.4, and the same parameters are summarized in Table 10.5 for all the 14 datasets used in this study. Figures 10.18 and 10.19 show potentialities of both the metrics in showing treatment-related changes, being consistent with improvements in the patient status, documented by clinical indexes. Hence, the above framework is capable to detect meaningful clinical effects stemming from the treatment and physiological studies.

Because the pathology size is typically equal to or greater than the scanner's pixel size, the framework described is not tied to a specific image resolution and depends on the pathology size only implicitly, via the models learned. One might expect the higher the scanner resolution (essentially, the finer the voxel lattice), the more sophisticated inter-site interactions between the region labels have to be taken into account.

While routine clinical applications rely often on a qualitative assessment of the extent of damaged myocardial tissues, both research and testing new therapies call for efficient and accurate quantitative estimates. Heuristic intensity thresholding for such estimation are mostly inaccurate and require user interaction. The above fully automated quantification of the myocardial viability based on fast and accurate separation of pathological and normal tissues by learning LCDG and MGRF signal models facilitates a more effective CAD.

Computational practicality A MATLAB® implementation of this framework on an Intel quad-core processor (3.2 GHz each, 16 GB memory, 1 TB RAID

TABLE 10.4

Percentage Area, Perc$_{area}$, and Transmural Extent, Perc$_{trans}$, of the Pathological Tissue in the 17-segment Heart Model to Quantify the Myocardium Viability for One Patient Before (Pre) and Six Months After the Treatment (Post$_6$)

Segment	Perc$_{area}$		Perc$_{trans}$	
	Pre	Post$_6$	Pre	Post$_6$
1	0.0	0.0	0.0	0.0
2	0.0	0.0	0.0	0.0
3	2.4	2.2	2.0	1.4
4	6.4	4.3	6.2	2.9
5	0.0	0.0	0.0	0.0
6	0.0	0.0	0.0	0.0
7	0.0	2.7	0.0	0.3
8	0.0	0.0	0.0	0.0
9	2.2	0.0	0.8	0.0
10	4.6	4.7	3.8	2.7
11	27.4	12.8	20.3	10.5
12	19.1	2.6	10.1	1.3
13	5.8	0.0	2.7	0.0
14	0.9	1.2	0.2	0.03
15	9.0	2.4	9.0	2.5
16	15.9	0.0	6.9	0.0
17	0.0	0.0	0.0	0.0
Mean	4.5	2.4	3.1	1.3

TABLE 10.5

Mean Myocardium Viability over All the 14 Datasets Collected from Six Patients, S1–S6, Six Months (Post$_6$) and One Year (Post$_{12}$) After the Treatment

	Perc$_{area}$			Perc$_{trans}$		
	Pre	Post$_6$	Post$_{12}$	Pre	Post$_6$	Post$_{12}$
S1	6.5	5.2	2.0	5.3	3.6	1.3
S2	18.4	14.4	14.1	14.8	11.3	9.7
S3	4.5	2.4	–	3.1	1.3	–
S4	11.0	8.6	–	5.0	3.8	–
S5	2.1	1.1	–	0.8	0.5	–
S6	10.9	9.2	–	3.6	3.5	–

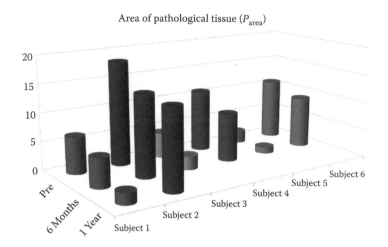

FIGURE 10.18
Mean percentage area of the pathological tissue, $Perc_{area}$, for six patients before (pre) and six months and one year after the treatment.

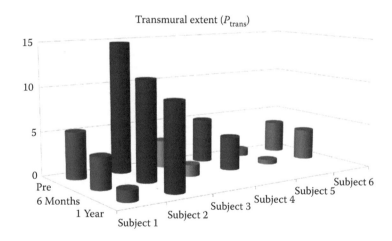

FIGURE 10.19
Mean transmural extent, P_{trans}, for six patients before (pre) and six months and one year after the treatment.

hard drive) spends approximately 3 min for identifying a pathological tissue in a CE-CMRI dataset of 12 cross sections, and less than 1 min for obtaining the two quantifying metrics for all segments of the myocardial 17-segment model. The like processing on a typical dual-core processor (2.1 GHz each, 4 GB memory) takes approximately 8 min and less than 1 min, respectively. The C/C++/C# programming environment should considerably accelerate the processing.

10.5 Bibliographic and Historical Notes

10.5.1 Appearance and Shape Priors

A multistage hybrid active appearance model (AAM) proposed in [210,211] for segmenting 2D MRI heart sections was extended then to a consistent multi-view AAM for the long- and short-axis CMRI. To improve the segmentation quality, a global shape model was then added to a set of the local 2D AAMs in order to propagate the position and size of the basal slices to the apical ones, while keeping plausible global shape characteristics. The LV segmentation was refined in [6] by fitting a 3D AAM to short-axis CMRI followed by a hierarchical 2D+time active shape model (ASM). The ASM was also combined with an AAM to segment the LV wall on short- and long-axes CMRI [314]. A reversed 3D ASM allowed for tracking better the cardiac motion and improving the shape details. A statistical ASM of the LV shape and separate models of spatial and temporal variations were used in [224]. A level-set based deformable boundary was coupled in [23] with a model of intensity marginals to segment echographic heart images.

A shape prior is often built by averaging a co-aligned training set, and for segmenting a given image the total Cartesian point-to-point distance between the current shape and the prior is minimized. Such segmentation has been successfully tested on synthetic images, functional MRI, and cardiac ultrasound images. A variational coupled level set framework in [232] combined the boundary- and region-based data into a geodesic active region (GAR) model for segmenting the LV borders in the CMRI. An anatomical module have been introduced to constrain relative positions of the endocardium and epicardium interfaces and enforce an intensity consistency over the temporal cycle. To obtain a more accurate automatic level-set based segmentation of the rat CMRI, an elliptic shape prior of the heart [244] or a dynamic prior accounting simultaneously for inter-subject variability and cardiac dynamics can be added to probabilistic areal and edge data. The LV wall can also be found by a 3D graph-based simultaneous multi-object segmentation that incorporates both the shape and context prior knowledge [277]. The same framework is applicable to, e.g., intra-retinal layers from optical coherence tomography images, or prostate and bladder 3D CT images.

Accurate assessment of myocardial viability by identifying the ischemically damaged tissue is of great clinical importance and is a standard means of diagnosing and monitoring irreversible myocardial sequelae of the ischemic heart disease, as well as guiding optimal therapies for individual patients [175]. The infarcted myocardium, after administering a gadolinium contrast agent, appears hyper-enhanced w.r.t. the normal myocardium on late (15–25 min) acquisitions [21,67,115,171,296].

Most of the automated or semi-automated myocardial viability assessment techniques use simple, heuristic intensity thresholds to detect the pathological tissue. Previous abnormality definitions set a threshold empirically at more than two [168] or three [105] standard deviations above the average intensity in a remote (presumedly healthy) myocardial region. Alternatively, an user-specified threshold was employed in [267] to distinguish between the viable and nonviable myocardium, and the full-width at half-maximum (FWHM) criterion [141] was employed in [4] to identify the pathological tissue: a seed point in the hyper-enhanced region is provided manually, and the pathological tissue includes, by definition, all the pixels with the intensities exceeding 50% of the seed intensity, which propagate from the seed point.

A study with a group of 62 patients in [217] demonstrated that infarcts segmented with a visual, user-specified threshold correlate with the manually traced ones better than their FWHM-based counterparts. The like comparisons of the FWHM and various simple thresholds in predicting segmental recovery after therapy were conducted in [20], but unlike the study in [217], there were no significant differences in accuracy for a group of 38 patients with chronic ischemic myocardial dysfunction. The classical automatic Otsu thresholding [228] of an empirical intensity marginal was extended in [287] to determine an initial infarct area, which was assessed then by connectivity filtering and region growing to reduce false positive and false negative errors. The intensity thresholding was augmented with a level-set-based regulation to exclude small noisy regions in [136], and the image intensity profile was used in [138] to initialize a watershed-based segmentation, which was refined further by analyzing connected components to fill holes and exclude small noisy regions.

However, these algorithms take almost no account of spatial dependencies (interactions) between the myocardium pixels or voxels and are too sensitive to imperfections in the myocardium borders and image noise. Table 10.6 summarizes some popular methodologies for identifying the pathological tissue on the heart CE-CMRI. The experimental results in Table 10.3 agree with the conclusions in [4] (M04 in Table 10.6) that the simple intensity-based segmentation gets worse for the cut-offs at higher proportions of the standard deviation σ.

10.5.2 Myocardial Viability Metrics

The percentage area of the pathological tissue and the transmural extent, or the transmurality, i.e., a fraction of the pathological tissue's extension across the myocardial wall [58],—have been well documented to predict patient outcomes. The seminal study [170] has established pathophysiologically meaningful ranges of the transmurality—less than 25% (a clinically small infarct) and more than 50% (a clinically large infarct). Because the transmurality is a sound predictor of clinical outcomes based on the CE-CMRI, an improved characterization and better understanding of mechanisms of the intermediate, 25%–50%, transmural extent should be of the greatest benefit.

TABLE 10.6

Methodologies (M) for Identifying Pathology (Infarct) on the CE-CMRI

Mk		N	LVS	PI	Performance
			\multicolumn{2}{Image Analysis}	
M01	[168]	26	MO	τ_2	Visually acceptable
M02	[105]	24	MO	τ_3	Visually acceptable
M03	[267]	18	MO	UT	Close to MPI
M04	[4]	13	MO	FWHM	Good BA to post-mortem data
M05	[136]	40	MO	LST	Infarct size difference 6.2 ± 6.6 ml[a]
M06	[138]	21	SA	WS+CCA	Better BA to MPI than in M2
M07	[217]	62	MO	UT vs. FWHM RG	UT is closer to MPI
M08	[20]	38	MO	FWHM vs. UT	No significant difference
M09	[287]	20	MO	HT+CCA+RG	DSC 0.83 ± 0.07 vs. 0.79 ± 0.08[b]
M10	[95]	11	DT	Fuzzy segmentation	Agreement with the expert's SA PI

Notes: N—the number of patients; τ_k—intensity threshold: mean+k×st. dev (standard deviation); BA—Bland-Altman analysis (see Section 9.4); CCA—connected component analysis; DT—deformable template; HT—intensity histogram based threshold; FWHM—full-width at half maximum threshold (50% of the maximum intensity within the infarct scar); LVS—LV wall segmentation; LST—level-set-based intensity threshold; MO—manual outline; MPI—manual PI; PI—pathology identification; RG—region growing; SA—semi-automatic segmentation; UT—user-specified threshold; WS—watershed segmentation.

[a] Between SA PI and mean MPI (3 observers).
[b] Automatic PI vs. mean MPI (2 observers).

Point-to-point correspondences between the inner and outer borders of the LV wall, as well as between the inner and outer edges of the pathological tissue (Figure 10.11) are established most accurately via the streamlines of a scalar potential field specified by the second-order linear Laplace PDE with equipotential boundary conditions [97,154,163,164]. Inaccurate correspondences lead to inconsistencies in the resulting measured transmural extent and hence affect its estimation, as illustrated in Figure 10.4. The radial and centerline estimates [270] are of much lower accuracy. The radial transmurality estimates used in [216] call for a proper selection of the central point [259]. The centerline method was introduced first for wall motion regional assessment [270] and subsequently for wall thickening analysis [203] and transmural extent estimation [264]. Unlike the radial method, the centerline depends on no centroid or a polar system of lines, but is affected by the inner and outer border imperfections and image noise.

The eikonal speed function was introduced in [3].

The Siemens 1.5T MRI system [169] was used to acquire all the CE-CMRI data sets for the above experiments.

References

1. B. Abdollahi, A. C. Civelek, X.-F. Li, J. Suri, and A. El-Baz. PET/CT nodule segmentation and diagnosis: A survey. In L. Saba and J. S. Suri, editors, *Multi Detector CT Imaging*, Chapter 30, pp. 639–651. CRC Press, Boca Raton, FL, 2014.

2. B. Abdollahi, A. Soliman, A. C. Civelek, X.-F. Li, G. Gimel'farb, and A. El-Baz. A novel 3D joint MGRF framework for precise lung segmentation. In F. Wang, D. Shen, P. Yan, and K. Suzuki, editors, *Machine Learning in Medical Imaging*, pp. 86–93. Springer, Belin, Heidelberg, 2012.

3. D. Adalsteinsson and J. Sethian. A fast level set method for propagating interfaces. *Journal of Computational Physics*, 118(2):269–277, 1995.

4. L. Amado, B. Gerber, S. Gupta, D. Rettmann, G. Szarf, R. Schock, K. Nasir, D. Kraitchman, and J. Lima. Accurate and objective infarct sizing by contrast-enhanced magnetic resonance imaging in a canine myocardial infarction model. *Journal of American College of Cardiology*, 44:2383–2389, 2004.

5. A. Amini, T. Weymouth, and R. Jain. Using dynamic programming for solving variational problems in vision. *IEEE Transactions on Pattern Analysis and Machine Intelligence*, 12:855–867, 1990.

6. A. Andreopoulos and J. K. Tsotsos. Efficient and generalizable statistical models of shape and appearance for analysis of cardiac MRI. *Medical Image Analysis*, 12(3):335–357, 2008.

7. P. Anuta. Spatial registration of multispectral and multitemporal digital imagery using Fast Fourier Transform. *IEEE Transactions on Geoscience Electronics*, 8:353–368, 1970.

8. L. Axel, A. Montillo, and D. Kim. Tagged magnetic resonance imaging of the heart: A survey. *Medical Image Analysis*, 9(4):376–393, 2005.

9. H. Azhari, S. Sideman, J. L. Weiss, E. P. Shapiro, M. L. Weisfeldt, W. L. Graves, W. J. Rogers, and R. Beyar. Three-dimensional mapping of acute ischemic regions using MRI: Wall thickening versus motion analysis. *American Journal of Physiology-Heart and Circulatory Physiology*, 259(5):H1492–H1503, 1990.

10. C. T. Badea, L. W. Hedlund, J. Cook, B. R. Berridge, and G. A. Johnson. Micro-CT imaging assessment of dobutamine-induced cardiac stress in rats. *Journal of Pharmacological and Toxicological Methods*, 63(1):24–29, 2011.

11. R. Bammer. Basic principles of diffusion-weighted imaging. *European Journal of Radiology*, 45(43):169–184, 2003.

12. E. C. Barbier, L. Johansson, L. Lind, H. Ahlstrom, and T. Bjerner. The exactness of left ventricular segmentation in cine magnetic resonance imaging and its impact on systolic function values. *Journal of Acta Radiologica*, 48(3):285–291, 2007.

13. E. L. Barbier, L. Lamalle, and M. Décorps. Methodology of brain perfusion imaging. *Journal of Magnetic Resonance Imaging*, 13(4):496–520, 2001.

14. D. Barbosa, T. Dietenbeck, J. Schaerer, J. D'hooge, D. Friboulet, and O. Bernard. B-spline explicit active surfaces: An efficient framework for real-time 3D region-based segmentation. *IEEE Transactions on Image Processing*, 21(1):241–251, 2012.

15. O. Barndorff-Nielsen. *Information and Exponential Families in Statistical Theory*. John Wiley & Sons, Chichester, UK, 1978.

16. L. E. Baum, T. Petrie, G. Soules, and N. Weiss. A maximization technique occurring in the statistical analysis of probabilistic functions of Markov chains. *Annals of Mathematical Statistics*, 41(1):164–171, 1970.

17. R. J. Baxter. *Exactly Solved Models in Statistical Mechanics*. Academic Press, London, UK, 1982.

18. G. M. Beache, F. Khalifa, G. Gimel'farb, and A. El-Baz. Fully automated framework for the analysis of myocardial first-pass perfusion MR images. *Medical Physics*, 41(10):1–18, 2014.

19. G. M. Beache, V. Wedeen, and R. Dinsmore. Magnetic resonance imaging evaluation of left ventricular dimensions and function and pericardial and myocardial disease. *Coronary Artery Disease*, 4(4):328–333, 1993.

20. A. M. Beek, O. Bondarenko, F. Afsharzada, and A. C. van Rossum. Quantification of late gadolinium enhanced CMR in viability assessment in chronic ischemic heart disease: A comparison to functional outcome. *Journal of Cardiovascular Magnetic Resonance*, 11(6):319–324, 2009.

21. A. M. Beek, H. P. Kühl, O. Bondarenko, J. W. Twisk, M. B. Hofman, W. G. van Dockum, C. A. Visser, and A. C. van Rossum. Delayed contrast-enhanced magnetic resonance imaging for the prediction of regional functional improvement after acute myocardial infarction. *Journal of American College of Cardiology*, 42(5):895–901, 2003.

22. N. Beohar, J. D. Flaherty, C. J. Davidson, M. I. Vidovich, A. Brodsky, D. C. Lee, E. Wu, E. L. Bolson, R. O. Bonow, and F. H. Sheehan. Quantitative assessment of regional left ventricular function with cardiac MRI: Three-dimensional centersurface method. *Catheterization and Cardiovascular Interventions*, 69(5):721–728, 2007.

23. O. Bernard, D. Friboulet, P. Thevenaz, and M. Unser. Variational B-spline level set: A linear filtering approach for fast deformable model evolution. *IEEE Transactions on Image Processing*, 18(6):1179–1191, 2009.

24. J. Besag. Spatial interaction and the statistical analysis of lattice systems. *Journal of the Royal Statistical Society*, B36:192–236, 1974.

25. J. Besag. On the statistical analysis of dirty pictures. *Journal of the Royal Statistical Society*, B48:259–302, 1986.

26. J. Bezdek, L. Hall, and L. Clarke. Review of MR image segmentation techniques using pattern recognition. *Physics in Medicine and Biology*, 20:1033–1048, 1993.

27. D. Le Bihan, J. F. Mangin, C. Poupon, C. A. Clark, S. Pappata, N. Molko, and H. Chabriat. Diffusion tensor imaging: Concepts and applications. *Journal of Magnetic Resonance Imaging*, 13(4):354–546, 2001.

28. S. Bisdasand, G. Konstantinou, K. Surlan-Popovic, A. Khoshneviszadeh, M. Baghi, T. J. Vogl, T. S. Koh, and M. G. Mack. Dynamic contrast-enhanced CT of head and neck tumors: comparison of first-pass and permeability perfusion measurements using two different commercially available tracer kinetics models. *Academic Radiology*, 15(12):1580–1589, 2008.

29. C. M. Bishop. *Pattern Recognition and Machine Learning*. Springer, New York, 2006.

30. A. Blake, P. Kohli, and C. Rother, editors. *Markov Random Fields for Vision and Image Processing*. The MIT Press, Cambridge, MA, 2011.

31. J. M. Bland and D. G. Altman. Statistical methods for assessing agreement between two methods of clinical measurement. *Lancet*, 327(8476):307–310, 1986.

32. C. Bouman and B. Liu. Multiple resolution segmentation of textured images. *IEEE Transactions on Pattern Analysis Machine Intelligence*, 13:99–113, 1991.

33. C. Bouman and K. Sauer. A generalized Gaussian image model for edge-preserving MAP estimation. *IEEE Transactions on Image Processing*, 2(3):296–310, 1993.

34. C. Bouman and M. Shapiro. A multiscale random field model for Bayesian image segmentation. *IEEE Transactions on Image Processing*, 3.162–177, 1994.

35. Y. Boykov and V. Kolmogorov. An experimental comparison of min-cut/max-flow algorithms for energy minimization in vision. *IEEE Transactions on Pattern Analysis and Machine Intelligence*, 26(9):1124–1137, 2004.

36. P. Brodatz. *Textures: A Photographic Album for Artists and Designers*. Dover Publications, New York, 1966.

37. L. D. Brown. *Fundamentals of Statistical Exponential Families with Applications in Statistical Decision Theory*. Lecture Notes—Monograph Series. Institute of Mathematical Statistics, Hayward, CA, USA, 1986.

38. V. G. M. Buller, R. J. van der Geest, M. D. Kool, E. E. van der Wall, A. de Roos, and J. H. C. Reiber. Assessment of regional left ventricular wall parameters from short axis magnetic resonance imaging using a three-dimensional extension to the improved centerline method. *Investigative Radiology*, 32(9):529–539, 1997.

39. S. M. Bunce, A. D. Hough, and A. P. Moore. Measurement of abdominal muscle thickness using M-mode ultrasound imaging during functional activities. *Manual Therapy*, 9:41–44, 2004.

40. R. Cabeza and A. Kingstone. *Handbook of Functional Neuroimaging of Cognition*, second edition. The MIT Press, Cambridge, MA, 2006.

41. A. Carpentier, K. R. Pugh, M. Westerveld, C. Studholme, O. Skrinjar, J. L. Thompson, D. D. Spencer, and R. T. Constable. Functional MRI of language processing: Dependence on input modality and temporal lobe epilepsy. *Epilepsia*, 42(10):1241–1254, 2001.

42. C. S. Carter, A. W. Macdonald III, L. L. Ross, and V. A. Stenger. Anterior cingulate cortex activity in impaired self-monitoring of performance in patients with schizophrenia: An event-related fMRI study. *American Journal of Psychiatry*, 158(10):1423–1428, 2001.

43. M. F. Casanova, A. El-Baz, A. Elnakib, J. Giedd, J. M. Rumsey, E. L. Williams, and A. E. Switala. Corpus Callosum shape analysis with application to dyslexia. *Translational Neuroscience*, 1(2):124–130, 2010.

44. M. F. Casanova, A. El-Baz, A. Elnakib, A. E. Switala, E. L. Williams, D. L. Williams, N. J. Minshew, and T. E. Conturo. Quantitative analysis of the shape of the corpus callosum in patients with autism and comparison individuals. *Autism*, 15(2):223–238, 2011.

45. M. F. Casanova, A. S. El-Baz, J. Giedd, J. M. Rumsey, and A. E. Switala. Increased white matter gyral depth in dyslexia: Implications for corticocortical connectivity. *Journal of Autism and Developmental Disorders*, 40(1):21–29, 2010.

46. M. F. Casanova, A. S. El-Baz, and J. S. Suri. *Imaging the Brain in Autism*. Springer, New York, 2013.

47. V. Caselles, F. Catte, T. Coll, and F. Dibos. A geometric model for active contours. *Numerische Mathematik*, 66:1–31, 1993.

48. V. Caselles, R. Kimmel, and G. Sapiro. Geodesic active contours. *International Journal of Computer Vision*, 22:61–79, 1997.

49. R. Ceppellini, M. Siniscalco, and C. A. Smith. The estimation of gene frequencies in a random-mating population. *Annals of Human Genetics*, 20(2):97–115, 1955.

50. M. D. Cerqueira, N. J. Weissman, V. Dilsizian, A. K. Jacobs, S. Kaul, W. K. Laskey, D. J. Pennell, J. A. Rumberger, T. Ryan, and M. S. Verani. Standardized myocardial segmentation and nomenclature for tomographic imaging of the heart. *Circulation*, 105(4):539–542, 2002.

51. T. Chan and L. Vese. Active contours without edges. *IEEE Transactions on Image Processing*, 10:266–277, 2001.

52. R. Chellappa. Two dimensional discrete Gaussian Markov random field models for image processing. *Pattern Recognition*, 2:79–122, 1985.

53. Q. Chen, M. Defrise, and F. Deconinck. Symmetric phase-only matched filtering of Fourier-Mellin transform for image registration and recognition. *IEEE Transactions on Pattern Analysis and Machine Intelligence*, 16:1156–1168, 1994.

54. Q. Chen, Z. M. Zhou, M. Tang, P. A. Heng, and D.-S. Xia. Shape statistics variational approach for the outer contour segmentation of left ventricle MR images. *IEEE Transactions on Information Technology in Biomedicine*, 10(3):588–597, 2006.

55. T. Chen, J. Babb, P. Kellman, L. Axel, and D. Kim. Segmentation of myocardial contours for fast strain analysis in cine displacement-encoded MRI. *IEEE Transactions on Medical Imaging*, 27(8):1084–1094, 2008.

56. L. L. Cheng, M. A. Burns, J. L. Taylor, W. He, E. F. Halpern, W. S. McDougal, and C. L. Wu. Metabolic characterization of human prostate cancer with tissue magnetic resonance spectroscopy. *Cancer Research*, 65(8):3030–3034, 2005.

57. S. G. Cho, D. H. Lee, K. Y. Lee, H. Ji, K. H. Lee, P. R. Ros, and C. H. Suh. Differentiation of chronic focal pancreatitis from pancreatic carcinoma by in vivo proton magnetic resonance spectroscopy. *Journal of Computer Assisted Tomography*, 29(2):163–169, 2005.

58. K. M. Choi, R. J. Kim, G. Gubernikoff, J. D. Vargas, M. Parker, and R. M. Judd. Transmural extent of acute myocardial infarction predicts long-term improvement in contractile function. *Circulation*, 104(10):1101–1107, 2001.

59. A. Chung and J. Noble. Statistical 3D vessel segmentation using a Rician distribution. In *Proceedings Second International Conference on Medical Image Computing and Computer-assisted Intervention (MICCAI'99)*, pp. 82–89, Cambridge, UK, Sept. 19–22, 1999.

60. C. A. Cocosco, W. J. Niessen, T. Netsch, E. P. A. Vonken, G. Lund, A. Stork, and M. A. Viergever. Automatic image-driven segmentation of the ventricles in cardiac cine MRI. *Journal of Magnetic Resonance Imaging*, 28(2):366–374, 2008.

61. D. J. Collins and A. R. Padhani. Dynamic magnetic resonance imaging of tumor perfusion. *IEEE Engineering in Medicine and Biology Magazine*, 23(5):65–83, 2004.

62. T. Cootes, C. Taylor, D. Cooper, and J. Graham. Active shape models—Their training and application. *Computer Vision and Image Understanding*, 61:38–59, 1995.

63. J. Cousty, L. Najman, M. Couprie, S. Clément-Guinaudeau, T. Goissen, and J. Garot. Segmentation of 4D cardiac MRI: Automated method based on spatio-temporal watershed cuts. *Image and Vision Computing*, 28(8):1229–1243, 2010.

64. G. Cross and A. Jain. Markov random field texture models. *IEEE Transactions on Pattern Analysis and Machine Intelligence*, 5:25–39, 1983.

65. N. Day. Estimating the components of mixture of normal distributions. *Biometrika*, 56:463–474, 1969.

66. A. Dempster, N. Laird, and D. Rubin. Maximum likelihood from incomplete data via the EM algorithm. *Journal of the Royal Statistical Society*, 39B:1–38, 1977.

67. P. Dendale, P. R. Franken, P. Block, Y. Pratikakis, and A. De Roos. Contrast enhanced and functional magnetic resonance imaging for the detection of viable myocardium after infarction. *American Heart Journal*, 135:875–880, 1998.

68. H. Derin and H. Elliott. Modeling and segmentation of noisy and textured images using Gibbs random fields. *IEEE Transactions on Pattern Analysis and Machine Intelligence*, 9(1):1919–1925, 1987.

69. L. Devroye and G. Lugosi. *Combinatorial Methods in Density Estimation*. Springer, New York, 2001.

70. M. Dewailly, M. Rémy-Jardin, A. Duhamel, J. B. Faivre, F. Pontana, V. Deken, A. M. Bakai, and J. Remy. Computer-aided detection of acute pulmonary embolism with 64-slice multi-detector row computed tomography: Impact of the scanning conditions and overall image quality in the detection of peripheral clots. *Journal of Computer Assisted Tomography*, 34(1):23–30, 2010.

71. L. R. Dice. Measures of the amount of ecologic association between species. *Ecological Society of America*, 26(3):279–302, 1945.

72. B. Dombroski, M. Nitzken, A. Elnakib, F. Khalifa, A. El-Baz, and M. F. Casanova. Cortical surface complexity in a population-based normative sample. *Translational Neuroscience*, 5(1):17–24, 2014.

73. B. A. Dombroski, A. E. Switala, A. S. El-Baz, and M. F. Casanova. Gyral window mapping of typical cortical folding using MRI. *Translational Neuroscience*, 2(2):142–147, 2011.

74. S. T. Doran, G. L. Falk, R. L. Somorjai, C. L. Lean, U. Himmelreich, J. Philips, P. Russell, B. Dolenko, A. E. Nikulin, and C. E. Mountford. Pathology of Barrett's esophagus by proton magnetic resonance spectroscopy and a statistical classification strategy. *The American Journal of Surgery*, 185(3):232–238, 2003.

75. Q. Duan, E. D. Angelini, and A. F. Laine. Real-time segmentation by active geometric functions. *Computer Methods and Programs in Biomedicine*, 98:223–230, 2010.

76. R. Duda, P. Hart, and D. Stork. *Pattern Classification*. Wiley Interscience, Hoboken, NJ, 2001.

77. A. El-Baz, G. M. Beache, G. Gimel'farb, K. Suzuki, K. Okada, A. Elnakib, A. Soliman, and B. Abdollahi. Computer-aided diagnosis systems for lung cancer: Challenges and methodologies. *International Journal of Biomedical Imaging*, 2013:1–46, 2013.

78. A. El-Baz, M. Casanova, G. Gimel'farb, M. Mott, and A. Switala. An MRI-based diagnostic framework for early diagnosis of dyslexia. *International Journal of Computer Assisted Radiology and Surgery*, 3(3–4):181–189, 2008.

79. A. El-Baz, A. Elnakib, M. F. Casanova, G. Gimel'farb, A. E. Switala, D. Jordan, and S. Rainey. Accurate automated detection of autism related Corpus Callosum abnormalities. *Journal of Medical Systems*, 35(5):929–939, 2011.

80. A. El-Baz, A. Elnakib, M. A. El-Ghar, G. Gimel'farb, R. Falk, and A. Farag. Automatic detection of 2D and 3D lung nodules in chest spiral CT scans. *International Journal of Biomedical Imaging*, 2013:1–11, 2013.

81. A. El-Baz, A. Elnakib, F. Khalifa, M. A. El-Ghar, R. Falk, and G. Gimel'farb. Precise segmentation of 3d magnetic resonance angiography. *IEEE Transactions on Biomedical Engineering*, 59(7):2019–2029, 2012.

82. A. El-Baz, A. Elnakib, F. Khalifa, M. A. El-Ghar, P. McClure, A. Soliman, and G. Gimel'farb. Precise segmentation of 3-D magnetic resonance angiography. *IEEE Transactions on Biomedical Engineering*, 59(7):2019–2029, 2012.

83. A. El-Baz, A. Farag, G. Gimel'farb, R. Falk, and M. A. El-Ghar. A novel level set-based computer-aided detection system for automatic detection of lung nodules in low dose chest computed tomography scans. *International Journal of Biomedical Imaging*, 10:221–238, 2011.

84. A. El-Baz, A. A. Farag, and G. Gimel'farb. Iterative approximation of empirical grey level distributions for precise segmentation of multi–modal images. *EURASIP Journal on Applied Signal Processing*, 13:1969–1983, 2005.

85. A. El-Baz, A. A. Farag, S. E. Yuksel, M. A. El-Ghar, T. A. Eldiasty, and M. A. Ghoneim. Application of deformable models for the detection of acute renal rejection. In J. S. Suri and A. A. Farag, editors, *Deformable Models*, volume 1, Chapter 10, pp. 293–333. Springer, New York, 2007.

86. A. El-Baz, G. Gimel'farb, R. Falk, and M. A. El-Ghar. A novel three-dimensional framework for automatic lung segmentation from low dose CT images. In A. El-Baz and J. S. Suri, editors, *Lung Imaging and Computer Aided Diagnosis*, Chapter 1, pp. 1–16. CRC Press, 2011.

87. A. El-Baz, G. Gimel'farb, R. Falk, and M. A. El-Ghar. Automatic analysis of 3D low dose CT images for early diagnosis of lung cancer. *Pattern Recognition*, 42(2):1041–1051, 2009.

88. A. El-Baz, G. Gimel'farb, R. Falk, and M. A. El-Ghar. 3D MGRF-based appearance modeling for robust segmentation of pulmonary nodules in 3D LDCT chest images. In A. El-Baz and J. S. Suri, editors, *Lung Imaging and Computer Aided Diagnosis*, Chapter 3, pp. 51–63. CRC Press, Boca Raton, FL, 2011.

89. A. El-Baz, G. Gimel'farb, R. Falk, and M. A. El-Ghar. A novel level set-based CAD system for automatic detection of lung nodules in low dose chest CT scans. In A. El-Baz and J. S. Suri, editors, *Lung Imaging and Computer Aided Diagnosis*, volume 1, Chapter 10, pp. 221–238. CRC Press, Boca Raton, FL, 2011.

90. A. El-Baz, G. Gimel'farb, R. Falk, and M. Abo El-Ghar. Automatic analysis of 3D low dose CT images for early diagnosis of lung cancer. *Pattern Recognition*, 42(6):1041–1051, 2009.

91. A. El-Baz, G. Gimelfarb, R. Falk, M. A. El-Ghar, and J. Suri. Appearance analysis for the early assessment of detected lung nodules. In A. El-Baz and J. S. Suri, editors, *Lung Imaging and Computer Aided Diagnosis*, Chapter 17, pp. 395–404. CRC Press, Boca Raton, FL, 2011.

92. A. El-Baz, M. Nitzken, G. Gimelfarb, E. Van Bogaert, R. Falk, M. A. El-Ghar, and J. Suri. Three-dimensional shape analysis using spherical harmonics for early assessment of detected lung nodules. In A. El-Baz and J. S. Suri, editors, *Lung Imaging and Computer Aided Diagnosis*, Chapter 19, pp. 421–438. CRC Press, Boca Raton, FL, 2011.

93. A. El-Baz, P. Sethu, G. Gimel'farb, F. Khalifa, A. Elnakib, R. Falk, and M. A. El-Ghar. Elastic phantoms generated by microfluidics technology: Validation of an imaged-based approach for accurate measurement of the growth rate of lung nodules. *Biotechnology Journal*, 6(2):195–203, 2011.

94. A. El-Baz, P. Sethu, G. Gimel'farb, F. Khalifa, A. Elnakib, R. Falk, M. A. El-Ghar, and J. Suri. Validation of a new imaged-based approach for the accurate estimating of the growth rate of detected lung nodules using real CT images and elastic phantoms generated by state-of-the-art microfluidics technology. In A. El-Baz

and J. S. Suri, editors, *Lung Imaging and Computer Aided Diagnosis*, volume 1, Chapter 18, pp. 405–420. CRC Press, Boca Raton, FL, 2011.

95. K. Elagouni, C. Ciofolo-Veit, and B. Mory. Automatic segmentation of pathological tissues in cardiac MRI. In *Proceedings IEEE International Symposium on Biomedical Imaging: From Nano to Macro (ISBI'2010)*, pp. 472–475, 2010.

96. A. Elnakib, G. M. Beache, G. Gimel'farb, and A. El-Baz. Intramyocardial strain estimation from cardiac cine MRI. *International Journal of Computer Assisted Radiology and Surgery*, 10(8):1299–1312, 2015.

97. A. Elnakib, G. M. Beache, G. Gimel'farb, and A. El-Baz. New automated Markov-Gibbs random field based framework for myocardial wall viability quantification on agent enhanced cardiac magnetic resonance images. *International Journal of Cardiovascular Imaging*, 28(7):1683–1698, 2012.

98. A. Elnakib, M. F. Casanova, G. Gimel'farb, and A. El-Baz. Autism diagnostics by 3D shape analysis of the Corpus Callosum. In K. Suzuki, editor, *Machine Learning in Computer-aided Diagnosis: Medical Imaging Intelligence and Analysis*, Chapter 15, pp. 315–335. IGI Global, Hershey, PA, 2012.

99. A. Elnakib, M. F. Casanova, G. Gimel'farb, A. E. Switala, and A. El-Baz. Dyslexia diagnostics by 3-D shape analysis of the corpus callosum. *IEEE Transactions on Information Technology in Biomedicine*, 16(4):700–708, 2012.

100. A. Elnakib, A. El-Baz, M. F. Casanova, G. Gimel'farb, and A. E. Switala. Image-based detection of corpus callosum variability for more accurate discrimination between dyslexic and normal brains. In *Proceedings IEEE International Symposium on Biomedical Imaging: From Nano to Macro (ISBI'2010)*, pp. 109–112, 2010.

101. A. A. Farag, A. El-Baz, and G. Gimel'farb. Precise segmentation of multimodal images. *IEEE Transactions on Image Processing*, 15(4):952–968, 2006.

102. A. A. Farag, R. Fahmi, M. F. Casanova, A. E. Abdel-Hakim, H. Abd El-Munim, and A. El-Baz. Robust neuroimaging-based classification techniques of autistic vs. typically developing brain. In J. S. Suri and A. A. Farag, editors, *Deformable Models*, Chapter 16, pp. 535–566, Springer, New York, 2007.

103. A. A. Farag, R. Mohamed, and A. El-Baz. A unified framework for MAP estimation in remote sensing image segmentation. *IEEE Transactions on Geoscience and Remote Sensing*, 43(7):1617–1634, 2005.

104. T. Fawcett. An introduction to ROC analysis. *Pattern Recognition Letters*, 27(8):861–874, 2006.

105. D. S. Fieno, R. J. Kim, E. L. Chen, J. W. Lomasney, F. J. Klocke, and R. M. Judd. Contrast-enhanced magnetic resonance imaging of myocardium at risk: Distinction between reversible and irreversible injury throughout infarct healing. *Journal of American College of Cardiology*, 36(6):1985–1991, 2000.

106. A. Firjani, F. Khalifa, A. Elnakib, G. Gimel'farb, M. A. El-Ghar, A. Elmaghraby, and A. El-Baz. A novel image-based approach for early detection of prostate cancer using DCE-MRI. In K. Suzuki, editor, *Computational Intelligence in Biomedical Imaging*, pp. 55–82. Springer, New York, 2014.

107. H. Foroosh, J. Zerubia, and M. Berthod. Extension of phase correlation to subpixel registration. *IEEE Transactions on Image Processing*, 11:188–200, 2002.

108. F. Fraioli, C. Catalano, L. Bertoletti, M. Danti, F. Fanelli, A. Napoli, M. Cavacece, and R. Passariello. Multidetector-row CT angiography of renal artery stenosis in 50 consecutive patients: Prospective interobserver comparison with DSA. *Radiologia Medica*, 111(2):459–468, 2006.

109. D. Freedman, R. Radke, T. Zhang, Y. Jeong, D. Lovelock, and G. Chen. Model-based segmentation of medical imagery by matching distributions. *IEEE Transactions on Medical Imaging*, 24:281–292, 2005.

110. K. Fukunaga and R. Hayes. The reduced Parzen classifier. *IEEE Transactions on Pattern Analysis and Machine Intelligence*, 11:423–425, 1989.

111. R. J. van der Geest, A. de Roos, E. E. van der Wall, and J. C. Reiber. Quantitative analysis of cardiovascular MR images. *International Journal of Cardiac Imaging*, 13(3):247–258, 1997.

112. D. Geman, S. Geman, C. Graffigne, and D. Pong. Boundary detection by constrained optimization. *IEEE Transactions on Pattern Analysis and Machine Intelligence*, 12(7):609–628, 1990.

113. S. Geman and D. Geman. Stochastic relaxation, Gibbs distributions, and the Bayesian restoration of images. *IEEE Transactions on Pattern Analysis and Machine Intelligence*, 6:721–741, 1984.

114. G. E. Gentle. *Computational Statistics*. Springer, New York, 2009.

115. B. L. Gerber, J. Garot, D. A. Bluemke, K. C. Wu, and J. A. Lima. Accuracy of contrast-enhanced magnetic resonance imaging in predicting improvement of regional myocardial function in patients after acute myocardial infarction. *Circulation*, 106:1083–1089, 2002.

116. G. Gimel'farb. Texture modeling with multiple pairwise pixel interactions. *IEEE Transactions on Pattern Analysis and Machine Intelligence*, 18:1110–1114, 1996.

117. G. Gimel'farb. *Image Textures and Gibbs Random Fields*. Kluwer Academic, Dordrecht, 1999.

118. G. Gimel'farb. Quantitative description of spatially homogeneous textures by characteristic grey level co-occurrences. *Australian Journal of Intelligent Information Processing Systems*, 6(1):46–53, 2000.

119. G. Gimel'farb and A. Farag. Texture analysis by accurate identification of simple Markovian models. *Cybernetics and Systems Analysis*, 41(1):37–49, 2005.

120. G. Gimel'farb and A. Zalesny. Probabilistic models of digital region maps based on Markov random fields with short- and long–range interaction. *Pattern Recognition Letters*, 14:789–797, 1993.

121. G. Gimel'farb and D. Zhou. Texture analysis by accurate identification of a generic Markov-Gibbs model. In A. Kandel, H. Bunke, and M. Last, editors, *Applied Pattern Recognition*, volume 91 of *Studies in Computational Intelligence*, pp. 221–245. Springer, Berlin, Heidelberg, 2008.

122. M. Girolami and C. He. Probability density estimation from optimally condensed data samples. *IEEE Transactions on Pattern Analysis and Machine Intelligence*, 25(10):1253–1264, 2003.

123. R. Goldenberg, R. Kimmel, E. Rivlin, and M. Rudzsky. Fast geodesic active contours. *IEEE Transactions on Image Processing*, 10(10):1467–1475, 2001.

124. N. Golyandina, A. Pepelyshev, and A. Steland. New approaches to nonparametric density estimation and selection of smoothing parameters. *Computational Statistics and Data Analysis*, 56:2206–2218, 2012.

125. A. Goshtasby and W. O'Neill. Curve fitting by a sum of Gaussians. *CVGIP: Graphical Models and Image Processing*, 56:281–288, 1999.

126. R. Grzeszczuk and D. Levin. Brownian strings: Segmenting images with stochastically deformable contours. *IEEE Transactions on Pattern Analysis and Machine Intelligence*, 19:1100–1114, 1997.

127. E. M. Haacke, R. W. Brown, M. R. Thompson, and R. Venkatesh. *Magnetic Resonance Imaging: Physical Principles and Sequence Design*. John Wiley & Sons, New York, 1999.

128. P. Hagmann, L. Jonasson, P. Maeder, J. Thiran, V. J. Wedeen, and R. Meuli. Understanding diffusion MR imaging techniques: From scalar diffusion-weighted imaging to diffusion tensor imaging and beyond. *RadioGraphics*, 26(Suppl. 1):S205–S223, 2006.

129. M. Haindl. Texture synthesis. *CWI Quarterly*, 4:305–331, 1991.

130. S. Haker, S. Angenent, A. Tannenbaum, and R. Kikinis. Nondistorting flattening maps and the 3D visualization of colon CT images. *IEEE Transactions on Medical Imaging*, 19(7):665–670, 2000.

131. J. M. Hammersley and D. C. Handscomb. *Monte Carlo Methods*. Methuen & Co Ltd, London, UK, 1964.

132. R. M. Haralick, K. Shanmugam, and I. Dinstein. Textural features for image classification. *IEEE Transactions on Systems, Man, and Cybernetics*, 3:610–621, 1973.

133. H. Hartley. Maximum likelihood estimation from incomplete data. *Biometrics*, 14:174–194, 1958.

134. M. Hassner and J. Sklansky. The use of Markov random fields as models of textures. *Computer Graphics and Image Processing*, 12:357–370, 1980.

135. W. K. Hastings. Monte Carlo sampling methods using Markov chains and their applications. *Biometrika*, 57:97–109, 1970.

136. E. Heiberg, H. Engblom, J. Engvall, E. Hedström, M. Ugander, and H. Arheden. Semi-automatic quantification of myocardial infarction from delayed contrast enhanced magnetic resonance imaging. *Scandinavian Cardiovascular J.*, 39(5):276–275, 2005.

137. K. Held, E. R. Kops, B. J. Krause, W. M. Wells III, R. Kikinis, and H.-W. Müller-Gärtner. Markov random field segmentation of brain MR images. *IEEE Transactions on Medical Imaging*, 16(6):878–886, 1997.

138. A. Hennemuth, A. Seeger, O. Friman, S. Miller, B. Klumpp, S. Oeltze, and H.-O. Peitgen. A comprehensive approach to the analysis of contrast enhanced cardiac MR images. *IEEE Transactions on Medical Imaging*, 27(11):1592–1610, 2008.

139. G. T. Herman. *Fundamentals of Computerized Tomography: Image Reconstruction from Projection*. Springer, New York, 2010.

140. N. Hidajat, M. Wolf, A. Nunnemann, P. Liersch, B. Gebauer, U. Teichgraber, R. Schroder, and R. Felix. Survey of conventional and spiral ct doses. *Radiology*, 218(2):395–401, 2001.

141. K. R. Hoffmann, D. P. Nazareth, L. Miskolczi, A. Gopal, Z. Wang, S. Rudin, and D. R. Bednarek. Vessel size measurements in angiograms: A comparison of techniques. *Medical Physics*, 29:1622–1633, 2002.

142. D. W. Holdsworth and M. M. Thornton. Micro-CT in small animal and specimen imaging. *Trends in Biotechnology*, 8(1):34–39, 2002.

143. E. R. Holman, H. W. Vliegen, R. J. van der Geest, J. H. Reiber, P. R. van Dijkman, A. van der Laarse, A. de Roos, and E. E. van der Wall. Quantitative analysis of regional left ventricular function after myocardial infarction in the pig assessed with cine magnetic resonance imaging. *Magnetic Resonance in Medicine*, 34(2):161–169, 1995.

144. A. Horská, P. B. Barker, and D. Phil. Imaging of brain tumors: MR spectroscopy and metabolic imaging. *Neuroimaging Clinics of North America*, 20(3):293–310, 2010.

145. S. Hu and E. Hoffman. Automatic lung segmentation for accurate quantization of volumetric X-ray CT images. *IEEE Transactions on Medical Imaging*, 20:490–498, 2001.

146. A. Hyvärinen, J. Karhunen, and E. Oja. *Independent Component Analysis*. Wiley-Interscience, New York.

147. J. Inglada and A. Giros. On the possibility of automatic multisensor image registration. *IEEE Transactions on Geoscience and Remote Sensing*, 42(10):2104–2120, 2004.

148. J. Jackson, D. J. Allison, and J. Meaney. Angiography: Principles, techniques, and complications. In R. C. Grainger, D. Allison, A. Adam, and A. K. Dixon, editors, *Diagnostic Radiology: A Textbook of Medical Imaging*, Chapter 6, pp. 109–128. Churchill Livingstone, New York, 2008.

149. M. A. Jacobs, P. B. Barker, P. Argani, R. Ouwerkerk, Z. M. Bhujwalla, and D. A. Bluemke. Combined dynamic contrast enhanced breast MR and proton spectroscopic imaging: A feasibility study. *Journal of Magnetic Resonance Imaging*, 21(1):23–28, 2005.

150. M. A. Jacobs, P. B. Barker, P. A. Bottomley, Z. Bhujwalla, and D. A. Bluemke. Proton magnetic resonance spectroscopy imaging of human breast cancer: A preliminary study. *Journal of Magnetic Resonance Imaging*, 19(1):68–75, 2004.

151. A. Jhamb, R. S. Dolas, P. K. Pandilwar, and S. Mohanty. Comparative efficacy of spiral computed tomography and orthopantomography in preoperative detection of relation of inferior alveolar neurovascular bundle to the impacted mandibular third molar. *Journal of Oral and Maxillofacial Surgery*, 67(1):58–66, 2009.

152. K. A. Johnson. Imaging techniques for small animal imaging models of pulmonary disease: Micro-CT. *Toxicologic Pathology*, 35(1):59–64, 2007.

153. M. Jolly. Automatic segmentation of the left ventricle in cardiac MR and CT images. *International Journal of Computer Vision*, 70(2):151–163, 2006.

154. S. E. Jones, B. R. Buchbinder, and I. Aharon. Three-dimensional mapping of cortical thickness using Laplace's equation. *Human Brain Mapping*, 11:12–32, 2000.

155. S. Joshi. *Large Deformation Diffeomorphisms and Gaussian Random Fields for Statistical Characterization of Brain Submanifolds*. PhD thesis, Washington University, St. Louis, MO, 1997.

156. I. R. Kamel, E. M. Merkle, and E. M. Merkle. *Body MR Imaging at 3 Tesla*. Cambridge University Press, New York, 2011.

157. R. Kashyap. Characterization and estimation of two dimensional ARMA models. *IEEE Transactions on Information Theory*, 2:736–745, 1984.

158. M. Kass, A. Witkin, and D. Terzopoulos. Snakes: Active contour models. *International Journal of Computer Vision*, 1:321–331, 1987.

159. N. Kawel, E. B. Turkbey, J. J. Carr, J. Eng, A. S. Gomes, W. G. Hundley, C. Johnson, S. C. Masri, M. R. Prince, R. J. van der Geest, J. A. C. Lima, and D. A. Bluemke. Normal left ventricular myocardial thickness for middle-aged and older subjects with steady-state free precession cardiac magnetic resonance: The multi-ethnic study of atherosclerosis. *Circulation Cardiovascular Imaging*, 5(4):500–508, 2012.

160. A. Kelemen, G. Szekely, and G. Gerig. Elastic model-based segmentation of 3D neuroradiological data sets. *IEEE Transactions on Medical Imaging*, 18:828–839, 1999.

161. R. Kern, K. Szabo, M. Hennerici, and S. Meairs. Characterization of carotid artery plaques using real-time compound B-mode ultrasound. *Stroke*, 35:870–875, 2004.

162. B. A. Kerr and T. V. Byzova. MicroCT: An essential tool in bone metastasis research. In L. Saba, editor, *Computed Tomography–Clinical Applications*, volume 1, Chapter 13, pp. 211–230. InTech, Rijeka, Croatia, 2012.

163. F. Khalifa, M. Abou El-Ghar, D. Abdollahi, H. D. Friebues, T. El-Diasty, and A. El-Baz. A comprehensive non-invasive framework for automated evaluation of acute renal transplant rejection using DCE-MRI. *NMR in Biomedicine*, 26(11):1460–1470, 2013.

164. F. Khalifa, G. M. Beache, M. Abou El-Ghar, T. El-Diasty, G. Gimel'farb, M. Kong, and A. El-Baz. Dynamic contrast-enhanced MRI-based early detection of acute renal transplant rejection. *IEEE Transactions on Medical Imaging*, 32(10):1910–1927, 2013.

165. F. Khalifa, G. M. Beache, G. Gimel'farb, G. A. Giridharan, and A. El-Baz. A new image-based framework for analyzing cine images. In A. El-Baz, U. R. Acharya, M. Mirmedhdi, and J. S. Suri, editors, *Handbook of Multi Modality State-of-the-Art Medical Image Segmentation and Registration Methodologies*, volume 2, Chapter 3, pp. 69–98. Springer, New York, 2011.

166. F. Khalifa, G. M. Beache, G. Gimel'farb, G. A. Giridharan, and A. El-Baz. Accurate automatic analysis of cardiac cine images. *IEEE Transactions on Biomedical Engineering*, 59(2):445–455, 2012.

167. F. Khalifa, G. M. Beache, G. Gimel'farb, J. S. Suri, and A. S. El-Baz. State-of-the-art medical image registration methodologies: A survey. In A. El-Baz, R. Acharya, M. Mirmehdi, and J. S. Suri, editors, *Multi Modality State-of-the-Art Medical Image Segmentation and Registration Methodologies*, volume 1, Chapter 9, pp. 235–280. Springer, New York, 2011.

168. R. J. Kim, D. S. Fieno, T. B. Parrish, K. Harris, E.-L. Chen, O. Simonetti, J. Bundy, J. P. Finn, F. J. Klocke, and R. M. Judd. Relationship of MRI delayed contrast enhancement to irreversible injury, infarct age and contractile function. *Circulation*, 100:1192–2002, 2009.

169. R. J. Kim, D. J. Shah, and R. M. Judd. How we perform delayed enhancement imaging. *Journal of Cardiovascular Magnetic Resonance*, 5:505–514, 2003.

170. R. J. Kim, E. Wu, A. Rafael, E.-L. Chen, M. A. Parker, O. Simonetti, F. J. Klocke, R. O. Bonow, and R. M. Judd. The use of contrast-enhanced magnetic resonance imaging to identify reversible myocardial dysfunction. *New England Journal of Medicine*, 43(20):1445–1453, 2000.

171. C. Klein, S. G. Nekolla, F. M. Bengel, M. Momose, A. Sammer, F. Haas, B. Schnackenburg, W. Delius, H. Mudra, D. Wolfram, and M. Schwaiger. Assessment of myocardial viability with contrast-enhanced magnetic resonance imaging: Comparison with positron emission tomography. *Circulation*, 105(2):162–167, 2002.

172. D.-M. Koh and D. J. Collins. Diffusion-weighted mri in the body: Applications and challenges in oncology. *American Journal of Roentgenology*, 188(6):1622–1635, 2007.

173. J. Konrad and E. Dubois. Bayesian estimation of motion vector fields. *IEEE Transactions on Pattern Analysis and Machine Intelligence*, 14(9):910–927, 1992.

174. J. G. Korporaal, C. A. van den Berg, C. R. Jeukens, G. Groenendaal, M. R. Moman, P. Luijten, M. van Vulpen, and U. A. van der Heide. Dynamic

contrast-enhanced CT for prostate cancer: Relationship between image noise, voxel size, and repeatability. *Radiology*, 256(3):976–984, 2010.

175. H. P. Kühl, A. M. Beek, A. P. van der Weerdt, M. B. Hofman, C. A. Visser, A. A. Lammertsma, N. Heussen, F. C. Visser, and A. C. van Rossum. Myocardial viability in chronic ischemic heart disease: Comparison of contrast-enhanced magnetic resonance imaging with (18)F-fluorodeoxyglucose positron emission tomography. *Journal of American College of Cardiology*, 41(8):1341–1348, 2003.

176. U. Kurkure, A. Pednekar, R. Muthupillai, S. D. Flamm, and I. A. Kakadiaris. Localization and segmentation of left ventricle in cardiac cine-MR images. *IEEE Transactions on Biomedical Engineering*, 56(5):1360–1370, 2009.

177. P. J. M. van Laarhoven. *Theoretical and Computational Aspects of Simulated Annealing*. Amsterdam Stichting Mathematisch Centrum, Amsterdam, 1988.

178. F. Lafarge, G. Gimel'farb, and X. Descombes. Geometric feature extraction by a multi-marked point process. *IEEE Transactions on Pattern Analysis and Machine Intelligence*, 32(9):1597–1609, 2010.

179. S. Lakshmanan and H. Derin. Simultaneous parameters estimation and segmentation of Gibbs random field using simulated annealing. *IEEE Transactions on Pattern Analysis and Machine Intelligence*, 11:799–813, 1989.

180. J. Lamperti. *Probability: A Survey of the Mathematical Theory*. Wiley Interscience, New York, 1996.

181. D. Langan, J. Modestino, and J. Zhang. Cluster validation for unsupervised stochastic model based image segmentation. *IEEE Transactions on Image Processing*, 7:180–195, 1998.

182. B. Lee and A. Newberg. Neuroimaging in traumatic brain imaging. *The Journal of the American Society for Experimental NeuroTherapeutics*, 2(2):372–383, 2005.

183. T.-W. Lee. *Independent Component Analysis: Theory and Applications*. Kluwer Academic, Dordrecht, 2001.

184. K. Leemput, F. Maes, D. Vandermeulen, and P. Suetens. A unifying framework for partial volume segmentation of brain MR images. *IEEE Transactions on Medical Imaging*, 22:105–119, 2003.

185. S. Li. *Markov Random Field Modeling in Image Analysis*, third edition. Springer, London, UK, 2009.

186. D. D. M. Lin, J. T. Kleinman, R. J. Wityk, R. F. Gottesman, A. E. Hillis, A.W. Lee, and P. B. Barker. Crossed cerebellar diaschisis in acute stroke detected by dynamic susceptibility contrast MR perfusion imaging. *American Journal of Neuroradiology*, 30(4):710–715, 2009.

187. X. Liu and J. L. Prince. Shortest path refinement for motion estimation from tagged MR images. *IEEE Transactions on Medical Imaging*, 29(8):1560–1572, 2010.

188. D. Lowe. Distinctive image features from scale-invariant keypoints. *International Journal of Computer Vision*, 60:91–110, 2004.

189. J. Lu, K. Li, M. Zhang, and L. Jiao. Dynamic susceptibility contrast perfusion magnetic resonance imaging in patients with symptomatic unilateral middle cerebral artery stenosis or occlusion. *Acta Radiology*, 48(3):335–340, 2007.

190. Y. Lu, P. Radau, K. Connelly, A. Dick, and G. Wright. Segmentation of left ventricle in cardiac cine MRI: An automatic image-driven method. *Functional Imaging and Modeling of the Heart*, 5528:339–347, 2009.

191. L. Lüdemann, C. Warmuth, M. Plotkin, A. Förschler, M. Gutberlet, P. Wust, and H. Amthauer. Brain tumor perfusion: Comparison of dynamic contrast enhanced magnetic resonance imaging using T1, T2, and T2* contrast, pulsed

arterial spin labeling, and H2(15)O positron emission tomography. *European Journal of Radiology*, 70(3):465–474, 2009.

192. M. Lynch, O. Ghita, and P. Whelan. Automatic segmentation of the left ventricle cavity and myocardium in MRI data. *Computers in Biology and Medicine*, 6(4):389–1407, 2006.

193. M. Lynch, O. Ghita, and P. Whelan. Left-ventricle myocardium segmentation using a coupled level set with a priori knowledge. *Computerized Medical Imaging and Graphics*, 30(4):255–262, 2006.

194. M. Lynch, O. Ghita, and P. F. Whelan. Segmentation of the left ventricle of the heart in 3-D+t MRI data using an optimized nonrigid temporal model. *IEEE Transactions on Medical Imaging*, 27(2):195–203, 2008.

195. W.-Y. Ma and B. Manjunath. EdgeFlow: A technique for boundary detection and image segmentation. *IEEE Transactions on Image Processing*, 9(8):1375–1388, 2000.

196. L. Mackelaite, R. Ouseph, A. El-Baz, and A. Gaweda. Cortical CT perfusion of the live donor kidneys as a predictor of post transplant graft function. *American Journal of Transplantation*, 12:329–329, 2012.

197. M. M. Mahon, I. J. Cox, R. Dina, W. P. Soutter, G. A. McIndoe, A. D. Williams, and N. M. de Souza. ^{1}H magnetic resonance spectroscopy of preinvasive and invasive cervical cancer: In vivo-ex vivo profiles and effect of tumor load. *Journal of Magnetic Resonance Imaging*, 19(1):256–364, 2004.

198. M. M. Mahon, A. D. Williams, W. P. Soutter, I. J. Cox, G. A. McIndoe, G. A. Coutts, R. Dina, and N. M. de Souza. ^{1}H magnetic resonance spectroscopy of invasive cervical cancer: An in vivo study with ex vivo corroboration. *NMR in Biomedicine*, 17(1):1–9, 2004.

199. J. Malik and P. Perona. Preattentive texture discrimination with early vision mechanisms. *Journal of Optical Society of America*, 7:923–932, 1990.

200. R. Malladi, J. Sethian, and B. Vemuri. Shape modeling with front propagation: A level set approach. *IEEE Transactions on Pattern Analysis and Machine Intelligence*, 17:158–175, 1995.

201. P. Mansfield. Snapshot magnetic resonance imaging (nobel lecture). *Angewandte Chemie International Edition*, 43(41):5456–5464, 2004.

202. P. McClure, F. Khalifa, A. Soliman, M. A. El-Ghar, G. Gimelfarb, A. Elmagraby, and A. El-Baz. A novel NMF guided level-set for DWI prostate segmentation. *Journal of Computer Science and Systems Biology*, 7:209–216, 2014.

203. M. J. McGillem, G. B. Mancini, S. F. DeBoe, and A. J. Buda. Modification of the centerline method for assessment of echocardiographic wall thickening and motion: A comparison with areas of risk. *Journal of American College of Cardiology*, 11(4):861–866, 1988.

204. T. McInerney and D. Terzopoulos. Deformable models in medical image analysis: A survey. *Medical Image Analysis*, 1:91–108, 1996.

205. G. J. McLachlan and T. Krishnan. *The EM Algorithm and Extensions*, second edition. John Wiley & Sons, Hoboken, NJ, 2008.

206. D. W. McRobbie, E. A. Moore, M. J. Graves, and M. R. Prince. *MRI from Picture to Proton*. Cambridge University Press, New York, 2007.

207. L. Mechtler. Neuroimaging in neuro-oncology. *Neurologic Clinics*, 27(1):171–201, 2009.

208. H. Michaely, K. Herrmann, K. Nael, N. Oesingmann, M. Reiser, and S. Schoenberg. Functional renal imaging: Nonvascular renal disease. *Abdominal Imaging*, 32(1):1–16, 2007.

209. K. A. Miles. Functional computed tomography in oncology. *European Journal of Cancer*, 38(16):2079–2084, 2002.
210. S. Mitchell, B. Lelieveldt, R. van der Geest, H. Bosch, J. Reiver, and M. Sonka. Multistage hybrid active appearance model matching: Segmentation of left and right ventricles in cardiac MR images. *IEEE Transactions on Medical Imaging*, 20(5):415–423, 2001.
211. S. C. Mitchell, J. G. Bosch, B. P. F. Lelieveldt, R. J. van der Geest, J. H. C. Reiber, and M. Sonka. 3-D active appearance models: Segmentation of cardiac MR and ultrasound images. *IEEE Transactions on Medical Imaging*, 21(9):1167–1178, 2002.
212. J. Modestino and J. Zhang. A Markov random field model-based approach to image interpretation. *IEEE Transactions on Pattern Analysis and Machine Intelligence*, 14(6):606–615, 1992.
213. J. Montagnat and H. Delingette. 4D deformable models with temporal constraints: application to 4D cardiac image segmentation. *Medical Image Analysis*, 9(1):87–100, 2005.
214. T. Moon. The Expectation-Maximization algorithm. *IEEE Signal Processing Magazine*, 11:47–60, 1996.
215. M. Mostapha, F. Khalifa, A. Alansary, A. Soliman, J. Suri, and A. El-Baz. Computer-aided diagnosis systems for acute renal transplant rejection: Challenges and methodologies. In A. El-Baz, L. Saba, and J. Suri, editors, *Abdomen and Thoracic Imaging*, pp. 1–35. Springer, New York, 2014.
216. S. Nazarian, D. A. Bluemke, A. C. Lardo, M. M. Zviman, S. P. Watkins, T. L. Dickfeld, G. R. Meininger, A. Roguin, H. Calkins, G. F. Tomaselli, R. G. Weiss, R. D. Berger, J. A. Lima, and H. R. Halperin. Magnetic resonance assessment of the substrate for inducible ventricular tachycardia in nonischemic cardiomyopathy. *Circulation*, 112:2821–2825, 2005.
217. M. Neizel, M. Katoh, E. Schade, T. Rassaf, G. A. Krombach, M. Kelm, and H. P. Kühl. Rapid and accurate determination of relative infarct size in humans using contrast-enhanced magnetic resonance imaging. *Clinical Research in Cardiolog*, 98(5):319–324, 2009.
218. F. Neues and M. Epple. X-ray microcomputer tomography for the study of biomineralized endo- and exoskeletons of animals. *Chemical Reviews*, 108(11):4734–4741, 2008.
219. K. Ngoi and J. Jia. An active contour model for colour region extraction in natural scenes. *Image and Vision Computing*, 17:955–966, 1999.
220. K. J. Nichols, A. van Tosh, Y. Wang, C. J. Palestro, and N. Reichek. Validation of gated blood-pool SPECT regional left ventricular function measurements. *Journal of Nuclear Medicine*, 50(1):53–60, 2009.
221. M. Nitzken, M. F. Casanova, F. Khalifa, G. Sokhadze, and A. El-Baz. Shape-based detection of cortex variability for more accurate discrimination between autistic and normal brains. In A. El-Baz, R. Acharya, A. Laine, and J. Suri, editors, *Handbook of Multi-Modality State-of-the-Art Medical Image Segmentation and Registration Methodologies*, volume 2, Chapter 7, pp. 161–185. Springer, New York, 2011.
222. M. J. Nitzken, M. F. Casanova, G. Gimelfarb, T. Inanc, J. M. Zurada, and A. El-Baz. Shape analysis of the human brain: A brief survey. *IEEE Journal of Biomedical and Health Informatics*, 18(4):1337–1354, 2014.
223. M. J. Nitzken, A. S. El-Baz, and G. M. Beache. Markov-Gibbs random field model for improved full-cardiac cycle strain estimation from tagged CMR. *Journal of Cardiovascular Magnetic Resonance*, 14(1):1–2, 2012.

224. S. P. O'Brien, O. Ghita, and P. F. Whelan. A novel model-based 3D+ time left ventricular segmentation technique. *IEEE Transactions on Medical Imaging*, 30(2):461–474, 2011.

225. M. E. Oest, J. C. Jones, C. Hatfield, and M. R. Prater. Micro-CT evaluation of murine fetal skeletal development yields greater morphometric precision over traditional clear-staining methods. *Birth Defects Research Part B: Developmental and Reproductive Toxicology*, 83(6):582–589, 2008.

226. S. Osher and R. Fedkiw. *Level Set Methods and Dynamic Implicit Surfaces*. Springer Verlag, New York, 2006.

227. S. Osher and J. Sethian. Fronts propagating with curvature-dependent speed: Algorithms based on Hamilton–Jacobi formulation. *Journal of Computational Physics*, 79:12–49, 1988.

228. N. Otsu. A threshold selection method from gray level histograms. *IEEE Transactions on Systems, Man and Cybernetics*, SMC-9:62–66, 1979.

229. P. Ou, D. S. Celermajer, G. Calcagni, F. Brunelle, D. Bonnet, and D. Sidi. Three-dimensional CT scanning: A new diagnostic modality in congenital heart disease. *Heart*, 93(8):908–913, 2007.

230. N. Pal and S. Pal. A review on image segmentation techniques. *Pattern Recognition*, 26(9):1277–1294, 1993.

231. A. Papoulis. *Probability, Random Variables, and Stochastic Processes*, third edition, McGraw-Hill, New York, 1991.

232. N. Paragios. A variational approach for the segmentation of the left ventricle in cardiac image analysis. *International Journal of Computer Vision*, 50(3):345–362, 2002.

233. N. Paragios. A level set approach for shape-driven segmentation and tracking of the left ventricle. *IEEE Transactions on Medical Imaging*, 22:773–776, 2003.

234. N. Paragios and R. Deriche. Geodesic active contours and level sets for the detection and tracking of moving objects. *IEEE Transactions on Pattern Analysis and Machine Intelligence*, 22:266–280, 2000.

235. N. Paragios, O. Mellina-Gottardo, and V. Armes. Gradient vector flow fast geometric active contours. *IEEE Transactions on Pattern Analysis and Machine Intelligence*, 26:402–407, 2004.

236. E. Parzen. On estimation of a probability density function and mode. *Annals of Mathematical Statistics*, 33:1065–1076, 1962.

237. E. S. Paulson and K. M. Schmainda. Comparison of dynamic susceptibility-weighted contrast-enhanced MR methods: Recommendations for measuring relative cerebral blood volume in brain tumors. *Radiology*, 249(2):601–613, 2008.

238. A. Pednekar, U. Kurkure, R. Muthupillai, S. Flamm, and I. A. Kakadiaris. Automated left ventricular segmentation in cardiac MRI. *IEEE Transactions on Biomedical Engineering*, 53(7):1425–1428, 2006.

239. X. Peng, M. Ding, C. Zhou, and Q. Ma. A practical two-step image registration method for two-dimensional images. *Information Fusion*, 5(4):283–298, 2004.

240. A. Pentland and S. Sclaroff. Closed-form solutions for physically based shape modeling and recognition. *IEEE Transactions on Pattern Analysis and Machine Intelligence*, 13:715–729, 1991.

241. C. Petitjean and J. N. Dacher. A review of segmentation methods in short axis cardiac MR images. *Medical Image Analysis*, 15(1):169–184, 2011.

242. R. Picard and I. Elfadel. Structure of aura and co-occurrence matrices for the Gibbs texture model. *Journal of Mathematical Imaging and Vision*, 2:5–25, 1992.

243. S. Pizer, G. Gerig, S. Joshi, and S. Aylward. Multiscale medial shape-based analysis of image objects. *Proceedings of IEEE*, 91:1670–1679, 2003.

244. C. Pluempitiwiriyawej, J. M. F. Moura, Y.-J. L. Wu, and C. Ho. STACS: A new active contour scheme for cardiac MR image segmentation. *IEEE Transactions on Medical Imaging*, 24(5):593–603, 2005.

245. T. Poggio and F. Girosi. Networks for approximation and learning. *Proceedings of IEEE*, 78:1481–1497, 1990.

246. R. B. Potts. Some generalized order-disorder transformations. *Mathematical Proceedings Cambridge Philosophical Society*, 48(1):106–109, 1952.

247. M. Prasad, A. Ramesh, P. Kavanagh, B. K. Tamarappoo, R. Nakazato, J. Gerlach, V. Cheng, L. E. J. Thomson, D. S. Berman, G. Germano, and P. J. Slomka. Quantification of 3D regional myocardial wall thickening from gated magnetic resonance images. *Journal of Magnetic Resonance Imaging*, 31(2):317–327, 2010.

248. S. Pujadas, G. P. Reddy, O. Weber, J. J. Lee, and C. B. Higgins. MR imaging assessment of cardiac function. *Journal of Magnetic Resonance Imaging*, 19(6):789–799, 2004.

249. P. Radau, Y. Lu, K. Connelly, G. Paul, A. J. Dick, and G. A. Wright. Evaluation framework for algorithms segmenting short axis cardiac MRI. *MIDAS Journal – Cardiac MR Left Ventricle Segmentation Challenge*, [online] http://hdl.handle.net/10380/3070: 2009.

250. B. Reddy and B. Chatterji. An FFT-based technique for translation, rotation and scale-invariant image registration. *IEEE Transactions on Image Processing*, 16:1266–1271, 1994.

251. R. Redner and H. Walker. Mixture densities, maximum likelihood and the EM algorithm. *SIAM Review*, 26:195–237, 1984.

252. T. Reed, J. Hans, and D. Buf. A review of recent texture segmentation and feature extraction techniques. *CVGIP: Image Understanding*, 57:359–372, 1993.

253. T. Reed and H. Wechsler. Segmentation of textured images and Gestalt organization using spatial-frequency representations. *IEEE Transactions on Pattern Analysis and Machine Intelligence*, 12:1–12, 1990.

254. C. Rickers, N. M. Wilke, M. Jerosch-Herold, S. A. Casey, P. Panse, N. Panse, J. Weil, A. G. Zenovich, and B. J. Maron. Utility of cardiac magnetic resonance imaging in the diagnosis of hypertrophic cardiomyopathy. *Circulation*, 112(6):855–861, 2005.

255. S. Roberts and R. Everson, editors. *Independent Component Analysis: Principles and Practice*. Cambridge University Press, Cambridge, UK, 2001.

256. S. Roth and M. J. Black. Fields of experts. *International Journal of Computer Vision*, 82(2):205–229, 2009.

257. A. Rudra, A. Chowdhury, A. Elnakib, F. Khalifa, A. Soliman, G. M. Beache, and A. El-Baz. Kidney segmentation using graph cuts and pixel connectivity. *Pattern Recognition Letters*, 34(13):1470–1475, 2013.

258. A. K. Rudra, M. Sen, A. S. Chowdhury, A. Elnakib, and A. El-Baz. 3D graph cut with new edge weights for cerebral white matter segmentation. *Pattern Recognition Letters*, 32(7):941–947, 2011.

259. F. P. van Rugge, E. E. van der Wall, S. J. Spanjersberg, A. de Roos, N. A. Matheijssen, A. H. Zwinderman, P. R. van Dijkman, J. H. Reiber, and A. V. Bruschke. Magnetic resonance imaging during dobutamine stress for detection and localization of coronary artery disease. quantitative wall motion analysis using a modification of the centerline method. *Circulation*, 90(1):127–138, 1994.

260. S. Sasayama, D. Franklin, J. Ross Jr, W. S. Kemper, and D. McKown. Dynamic changes in left ventricular wall thickness and their use in analyzing cardiac function in the conscious dog: A study based on a modified ultrasonic technique. *The American Journal of Cardiology*, 38(7):870–879, 1976.

261. C. Sato, S. Naganawa, T. Nakamura, H. Kumada, S. Miura, O. Takizawa, and T. Ishigaki. Differentiation of noncancerous tissue and cancer lesions by apparent diffusion coefficient values in transition and peripheral zones of the prostate. *Magnetic Resonance Imaging*, 21(10):258–262, 2005.

262. R. Schalkoff. *Pattern Recognition: Statistical, Structural and Neural Approaches*. John Wiley & Sons, Hoboken, NJ, 1992.

263. M. I. Schlesinger. A connection between supervised and unsupervised learning in pattern recognition. *Kibernetika*, 2:81–88, 1968.

264. J. D. Schuijf, T. A. Kaandorp, H. J. Lamb, R. J. van der Geest, E. P. Viergever, E. E. van der Wall, A. de Roos, and J. J. Bax. Quantification of myocardial infarct size and transmurality by contrast-enhanced magnetic resonance imaging in men. *American Journal of Cardiology*, 94(3):284–288, 2004.

265. D. W. Scott. *Multivariate Density Estimation: Theory, Practice, and Visualization*. John Wiley & Sons, Hoboken, NJ, 1992.

266. M. Sen, A. K. Rudra, A. S. Chowdhury, A. Elnakib, and A. El-Baz. Cerebral white matter segmentation using probabilistic graph cut algorithm. In A. S. El-Baz, U. R. Acharya, A. F. Laine, and J. Suri, editors, *Multi Modality State-of-the-Art Medical Image Segmentation and Registration Methodologies*, volume II, Chapter 2, pp. 41–55. Springer, New York, 2011.

267. R. M. Setser, D. G. Bexell, T. P. O.Donnell, A. E. Stillman, M. L. Lieber, P. Schoenhagen, and R. D. White. Quantitative assessment of myocardial scar in delayed enhancement magnetic resonance imaging. *Journal of Magnetic Resonance Imaging*, 18(4):434–441, 2003.

268. N. Shah, A. Sattar, M. Benanti, S. Hollander, and L. Cheuck. Magnetic resonance spectroscopy as an imaging tool for cancer: A review of the literature. *Journal of American Osteopathic Association*, 106(1):23–27, 2006.

269. F. H. Sheehan, E. L. Bolson, H. T. Dodge, D. G. Mathey, J. Schofer, and H. K. Woo. Advantages and applications of the centerline method for characterizing regional ventricular function. *Circulation*, 74(2):293–305, 1986.

270. F. H. Sheehan, F. L. Bolson, H. T. Dodge, D. G. Mathey, J. Schofer, and H. W. Woo. Advantages and applications of the centerline method for characterizing regional ventricular function. *Circulation*, 74(2):293–305, 1986.

271. D. Shen and C. Davatzikos. An adaptive-focus deformable model using statistical and geometric information. *IEEE Transactions on Pattern Analysis and Machine Intelligence*, 22:906–913, 2000.

272. S. Sheth and E. K. Fishman. Multi-detector row CT of the kidneys and urinary tract: Techniques and applications in the diagnosis of benign diseases. *Radiographics*, 24(2):e20 [on–line: doi:10.1148/rg.e20], 2004.

273. B. Sievers, S. Kirchberg, A. Bakan, U. Franken, and H.-J. Trappe. Impact of papillary muscles in ventricular volume and ejection fraction assessment by cardiovascular magnetic resonance. *Journal of Cardiovascular Magnetic Resonance*, 6(1):9–16, 2004.

274. B. Sitharaman, K. R. Kissell, K. B. Hartman, L. A. Tran, A. Baikalov, I. Rusakova, Y. Sun, H. A. Khant, S. J. Ludtke, W. Chiu, S. Laus, E. Tóth, L. Helm, A. E. Merbachd, and L. J. Wilson. Superparamagnetic gadonanotubes are

high-performance MRI contrast agents. *Chemical Communications*, 1(31):3915–3917, 2006.

275. H. Sliman, A. Elnakib, G. M. Beache, A. Elmaghraby, and A. El-Baz. Assessment of myocardial function from cine cardiac MRI using a novel 4D tracking approach. *Journal of Computer Science & Systems Biology*, 7:169–173, 2014.

276. H. Sliman, F. Khalifa, A. Elnakib, A. Soliman, G. M. Beache, A. Elmaghraby, G. Gimel'farb, and A. El-Baz. Myocardial borders segmentation from cine MR images using bi-directional coupled parametric deformable models. *Medical Physics*, 40(9):1–13, 2013.

277. Q. Song, J. Bai, M. K. Garvin, M. Sonka, J. M. Buatti, and X. Wu. Optimal multiple surface segmentation with shape and context priors. *IEEE Transactions on Medical Imaging*, 32(2):376–386, 2013.

278. H. Sorenson and D. Alspach. Recursive Bayesian estimation using Gaussian sums. *Automatica*, 7:465–479, 1971.

279. A. Srivastava, X. Liu, and U. Grenander. Universal analytical forms for modeling image probabilities. *IEEE Transactions on Pattern Analysis and Machine Intelligence*, 24:1200–1214, 2002.

280. W. R. Staines, W. E. McIlroy, S. J. Graham, and S. E. Black. Bilateral movement enhances ipsilesional cortical activity in acute stroke: A pilot functional MRI study. *Neurology*, 56(3):401–404, 2001.

281. P. D. Stein, A. Y. Yaekoub, F. Matta, and H. D. Sostman. Sixty-four-slice CT for diagnosis of coronary artery disease: A systematic review. *The American Journal of Medicine*, 121(8):715–725, 2008.

282. C. Studholme, D. Hill, and D. Hawkes. An overlap invariant entropy measure of 3D medical image alignment. *Pattern Recognition*, 32(10):71–86, 1999.

283. M. Styner, G. Gerig, S. Pizer, and S. Joshi. Automatic and robust computation of 3D medial models incorporating object variability. *International Journal of Computer Vision*, 55:107–122, 2002.

284. P. C. Sundgren, Q. Dong, D. Gómez-Hassan, S. K. Mukherji, P. Maly, and R. Welsh. Diffusion tensor imaging of the brain: Review of clinical applications. *Neuroradiology*, 46(5):339–250, 2004.

285. S. J. Swensen. Functional CT: Lung nodule evaluation. *RadioGraphics*, 20(1):1178–1181, 2000.

286. P. Swindle, S. McCredie, P. Russell, U. Himmelreich, M. Khadra, C. Lean, and C. Mountford. Pathologic characterization of human prostate tissue with proton MR spectroscopy. *Radiology*, 228(1):144–151, 2003.

287. Q. Tao, J. Milles, K. Zeppenfeld, H. J. Lamb, J. J. Bax, J. H. Reiber, and R. J. van der Geest. Automated segmentation of myocardial scar in late enhancement MRI using combined intensity and spatial information. *Magnetic Resonance in Medicine*, 64(2):586–597, 2010.

288. P. Thunberg, K. Emilsson, P. Rask, and A. Kahari. Estimation of ejection fraction and stroke volume using single- and biplane magnetic resonance imaging of the left cardiac ventricle. *Journal of Acta Radiologica*, 49(9):1016–1013, 2008.

289. A. Tsai, A. Yezzi, W. Wells, C. Tempany, D. Tucker, A. Fan, W. Grimson, and A. Willsky. A shape based approach to the segmentation of medical imagery using level sets. *IEEE Transactions on Medical Imaging*, 22:137–154, 2003.

290. M. Uzümcü, R. van der Geest, C. Swingen, J. Reiber, and B. Lelieveldt. Time continuous tracking and segmentation of cardiovascular magnetic resonance

images using multidimensional dynamic programming. *Investigative Radiology*, 41(1):52–62, 2006.

291. V. Vapnik. *Statistical Learning Theory*. Wiley-Interscience, New York, 1998.

292. J. J. Vaquero, S. Redondo, E. Lage, M. Abella, A. Sisniega, G. Tapias, M. L. Soto Montenegro, and M. Desco. Assessment of a new high-performance small-animal X-ray tomography. *IEEE Transactions on Nuclear Science*, 55(3):898–905, 2008.

293. P. Verro, L. N. Tanenbaum, N. Borden, N. Eshkar, and S. Sen. Clinical application of CT angiography in acute ischemic stroke. *Clinical Neurology and Neurosurgery*, 109(2):138–145, 2007.

294. P. Viola. *Alignment by Maximization of Mutual Information*. PhD thesis, MIT, Cambridge, MA, 1995.

295. P. Viola and W. M. Wells III. Alignment by maximization of mutual information. *International Journal of Computer Vision*, 24(2):137–154, 1997.

296. E. E. van der Wall and J. J. Bax. Late contrast enhancement by CMR: More than scar? *International Journal of Cardiovascular Imaging*, 24(6):609–611, 2008.

297. C. Wang, N. Komodakis, and N. Paragios. Markov random field modeling, inference & learning in computer vision & image understanding: A survey. *Computer Vision and Image Understanding*, 117(11):1610–1627, 2013.

298. L. Wang, J. Liu, and S. Li. MRF parameter estimation by MCMC method. *Pattern Recognition*, 33:1919–1925, 2000.

299. M. Wang, J. Evans, L. Hassebrook, and C. Knapp. A multistage, optimal active contour model. *IEEE Transactions on Image Processing*, 5:1586–1591, 1996.

300. A. G. Webb. *Introduction to Biomedical Imaging*. Wiley-Interscience, Hoboken–IEEE Press, Piscataway, NJ, 2003.

301. V. J. Wedeen, R. P. Wang, J. D. Schmahmann, T. Benner, W. Y. Tseng, G. Dai, D. N. Pandya, P. Hagmann, H. D'Arceuil, and A. J. de Crespigny. Diffusion spectrum magnetic resonance imaging (DSI) tractography of crossing fibers. *Neuroimage*, 41(4):1267–1277, 2008.

302. T. A. Whittingham. Medical diagnostic applications and sources. *Progress in Biophysics and Molecular Biology*, 93(1–3):84–110, 2007.

303. D. Williams and M. Shah. A fast algorithm for active contours and curvature estimation. *CVGIP: Image Understanding*, 55(1):14–26, 1992.

304. E. L. Williams, A. El-Baz, M. Nitzken, A. E. Switala, and M. F. Casanova. Spherical harmonic analysis of cortical complexity in autism and dyslexia. *Translational Neuroscience*, 3(1):36–40, 2012.

305. D. Wilson and J. Noble. An adaptive segmentation algorithm for time–of–flight MRA data. *IEEE Transactions on Medical Imaging*, 18:938–945, 1999.

306. S. R. Wilson, L. D. Greenbaum, and B. B. Goldberg. Contrast-enhanced ultrasound: What is the evidence and what are the obstacles? *American Journal of Roentgenology*, 193(1):55–60, 2009.

307. G. Winkler. *Image Analysis, Random Fields and Dynamic Monte Carlo Methods*. Springer, Berlin, Heidelberg, 1995.

308. Y. Wong, P. Yuen, and C. Tong. Segmented snake for contour detection. *Pattern Recognition*, 31:1669–1679, 1998.

309. C. Xu and J. Prince. Snakes, shapes, and gradient vector flow. *IEEE Transactions on Pattern Analysis and Machine Intelligence*, 7:359–369, 1998.

310. C. Xu and J. L. Prince. Gradient vector flow deformable models. In I. Bankman, editor, *Handbook of Medical Imaging*, pp. 493–501. Academic Press, Inc., Orlando, FL, 2000.

311. J. Yang and J. Duncan. 3D image segmentation of deformable objects with joint shape-intensity prior models using level sets. *Medical Image Analysis*, 8:285–294, 2004.

312. X. Yang and K. Murase. Tagged cardiac MR image segmentation by contrast enhancement and texture analysis. In *Proceedings 9th International Conference on Electronic Measurement & Instruments (ICEMI'2009)*, pp. 210–214, Beijing, China, Aug. 16–19, 2009.

313. S. E. Yuksel, A. El-Baz, A. A. Farag, M. A. El-Ghar, T. Eldiasty, and M. A. Ghoneim. A kidney segmentation framework for dynamic contrast enhanced magnetic resonance imaging. *Journal of Vibration and Control*, 13(9–10):1505–1516, 2007.

314. H. Zhang, A. Wahle, R. K. Johnson, T. D. Scholz, and M. Sonka. 4-D cardiac MR image analysis: Left and right ventricular morphology and function. *IEEE Transactions on Medical Imaging*, 29(2):350–364, 2010.

315. S. C. Zhu, Y. Wu, and D. Mumford. Minimax entropy principle and its application to texture modeling. *Neural Computation*, 9(8):1627–1660, 1997.

316. S. C. Zhu, Y. Wu, and D. Mumford. Filters, random fields and maximum entropy (frame): Towards a unified theory for texture modeling. *International Journal of Computer Vision*, 27(2):107–126, 1998.

317. B. Zitova and J. Flusser. Image registration methods: A survey. *Image and Vision Computing*, 21:977–1000, 2003.

Index